Langstaff

A Nineteenth-Century

Medical Life

Jacalyn Duffin offers rare insight into the life of an ordinary physician and his community during a period of revolutionary medical change. For forty years Dr James Miles Langstaff (1825–89) practised general medicine in Richmond Hill, Ontario, and kept meticulous records on every patient. Duffin investigates this average nineteenth-century doctor's reaction to the medical innovations (anaesthesia, antisepsis, germ theory, and public health) that dramatically transformed his practice. Duffin's account of Langstaff's life stands as a foil to other studies based on analysis of large groups of medical practitioners and complements the rich secondary literature on nineteenth-century medical and social history.

Langstaff's story is also a tale of Canadian social life that begins in the colonial days of sparse agricultural settlement before the Rebellions of 1837, and moves through Confederation to the era of rapid industrialization late in the nineteenth century.

A compelling, detailed picture of sickness and injury, addiction and mental illness, birth and death in a small farming community emerges.

JACALYN DUFFIN is Hannah Professor of the History of Medicine and associate dean, Faculty of Medicine, Queen's University.

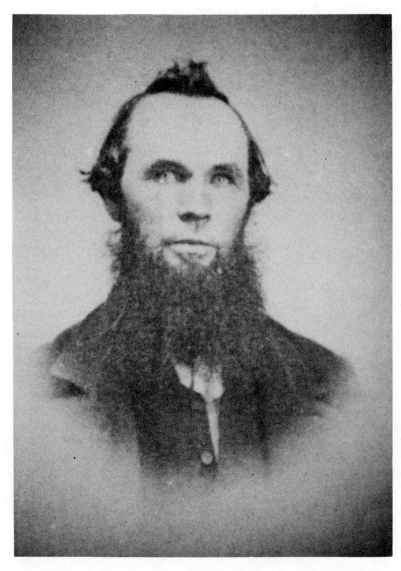

James Miles Langstaff (1825–89) circa 1865, at approximately forty years of age

Langstaff

A Nineteenth-Century Medical Life

Jacalyn Duffin

UNIVERSITY OF TORONTO PRESS

Toronto Buffalo London

© University of Toronto Press Incorporated 1993
Toronto Buffalo London
Printed in Canada

ISBN 0-8020-2908-6 (cloth)
ISBN 0-8020-7414-6 (paper)

Printed on acid-free paper

Canadian Cataloguing in Publication Data

Duffin, Jacalyn
Langstaff

Includes bibliographical references and index.
ISBN 0-8020-2908-6 (bound) ISBN 0-8020-7414-6 (pbk.)

1. Langstaff, James Miles, 1825–1889. 2. Medicine –
Ontario – Richmond Hill – History – 19th century.
3. Physicians – Ontario – Richmond Hill – Biography. I. Title.

R464.L35D8 1993   610'.92   C93-094389-9

This book has been published with the help of a grant from the Canadian
Federation for the Humanities, using funds provided by the Social Sciences
and Humanities Research Council of Canada.

For my mother
and the memory of my father

Contents

Contents

Tables, Figures, and Maps

Tables

Figures

Maps

Acknowledgments

❧

When I began with Langstaff back in 1985, I had no idea how many places he would take me, how many new friends he would bring, or how many debts he would lead me to incur. In acknowledging the people who have helped me in this work, I must start with Dr James Rolph Langstaff, his late wife, Barbara, and their family, thanking them for having carefully preserved the Langstaff records, for their permission to conduct this study, and for generous access to the daybooks. Jim's knowledge of his grandfather and the history of Richmond Hill together with his sense of humour and warm hospitality always made our meetings as pleasurable as they were productive. Langstaff's other grandchildren, especially Eileen Aiken, Helen Carroll Davis, and Phyllis Grosskurth, kindly shared their memories of the family; their continued interest was most encouraging. Other descendants of the Richmond Hill doctor answered letters and phone calls, quickly and completely, with infectious curiosity.

I have been privileged to discuss Langstaff with many other Canadians, from Halifax to Victoria; their challenging questions helped shape my own. The insights and criticisms of seminar groups at Yale University and the University of Wisconsin, Madison, were a stimulus to further work. I learned more about Langstaff and about doing history from two audiences of the Canadian College of Family Practice: the first gave their reactions to my interpretations through the dazzling medium of interactive computer technology; the second asked penetrating questions informed by their own experience with patients. Enthusiastic audiences in Buffalo and in the community of Richmond Hill, the Pennsylvania German Folklore Society, and friends of the York Central Hospital taught me that the story of Langstaff is also the exciting story of their ancestors. I hope this book addresses some of the many questions that have emerged from these diverse groups in a manner that is accessible to all.

This work would not have been possible without the willing and efficient cooperation of local historians, librarians, and archivists. I am especially indebted to Ruth Clark of the Royal College of Physicians and Surgeons of Canada; Janet Fayle, Heritage Advisor to the town of Richmond Hill; Andrew Baster, at Guy's Hospital, London, England; Laura and Alf Weaver of Thornhill; Dr Cyril Greenlands of the Greenland-Griffiths Archive; June Gibson and her colleagues at the Archives of Ontario; and the staff of the College of Physicians and Surgeons of Ontario. The editors of the *Canadian Bulletin of the History of Medicine / Bulletin canadien d'histoire de la médecine*, the *Annals of the Royal College of Physicians and Surgeons*, and *Canadian Family Physician* kindly gave me permission to use portions of the work that appeared in their journals.[1] Ross Hough of the Geography Department, Queen's University, prepared the maps.

The academic community is truly fortunate to enjoy the benefits of the Hannah Institute for the History of Medicine, which has sustained this project through a postdoctoral fellowship and the funding of my present position as a Hannah Professor. My sincere thanks belong to Dr Robert Macbeth, Dr T.P. Morley, Sheila Snelgrove, and stalwart friends at 'Hannah Central' who graciously lent support and advice.

Robert Gidney, Wendy Mitchinson, Ronald L. Numbers, Charles E. Rosenberg, and two anonymous readers for the University of Toronto Press read earlier versions of the entire manuscript; if I have done justice to their excellent recommendations, they will find my gratitude in many places throughout the revised text. I owe special recognition to scholars who willingly read chapters, answered questions, or gladly shared their expertise and their discoveries; they include Gordon Bale, Evelyn Bentley, James T.H. Connor, Jennifer J. Connor, Audrey Davis, Jody Decker, Janet Fayle, Toby Gelfand,

Mrs Wallace Graham, Bertrum H. MacDonald, Patricia Peppin, Felicity Pope, Naomi Rogers, Charles G. Roland, Stuart Ryan, John Harley Warner, Cheryl Krasnick Warsh, and Graeme Wynn. Elizabeth Severino gave spirited assistance with the research; Marian Van Bruinessen helped enormously with the tables; they both, together with Olga Kits, Dr Denis White, and Mrs Elizabeth White, were astute and surprisingly eager proofreaders, and I thank them all for their many contributions. With unfailing judgment, confidence, and good humour, Gerry Hallowell, Agnes Ambrus, and Laura Macleod at the University of Toronto Press have made the production of my first book a pleasant experience.

Robert David Wolfe participated in the study from its inception and lent his myriad talents to troubleshooting problems of every sort: technical, historical, conceptual, grammatical, and domestic. Our children, Joshua and Jessica, happily welcomed the shade of James Miles Langstaff into our home like a respected visitor and, with their tolerance and wonder, contributed to the rediscovery of his life and the writing of this book.

Kingston, Ontario
August 1992

Langstaff

*A
Nineteenth-Century
Medical Life*

Introduction

Medicine was transformed during the nineteenth century by the revolutionary principles of physical diagnosis, anaesthesia, antisepsis, germ theory, and public health. These developments and the technological changes that accompanied them led to profound alterations in concepts of disease, in diagnostic and therapeutic modalities, and in the structure and function of the profession; they laid the foundations of modern practice. A great deal of attention has been given to the discoveries and their associated protagonists or 'heroes,' the well-known men and women whose contributions fostered these changes. More recently, historians have examined the contextual origins and products of these changes as they affected large groups of physicians and the societies in which they lived; in this endeavour hospital records have been extremely useful.[1] Next to nothing is known, however, about the reaction of individual doctors to these important developments. Did they welcome the changes made by groups of their colleagues working in institutions? How did they learn about them? Did they keep up?

During forty years of this dramatic century, James Miles Langstaff (1825–89) practised in the rural community of Richmond Hill a few miles north of Toronto. He was taught by those who had seen the beginnings of anatomical diagnosis, and over the course of his career he witnessed the advent of anaesthesia, antisepsis, germ theory, and the dawn of the public health and women's movements. Langstaff had strong partisan leanings and often engaged in politics at the local level, but he was not famous, published little, and made no important discoveries. His importance lies in the precious legacy of a nearly complete set of his medical daybooks and accounts. Written in beautiful script and solidly bound, these volumes chronicle the daily practice of an ordinary doctor and represent probably the most complete, most legible, and longest-running set of nineteenth-century medical daybooks in Ontario, if not Canada. They reveal that this doctor rarely took a day off, less often left his region, and never attended a medical conference; yet he adopted the innovations of his era.

Comparatively little attention has been given to the ordinary practitioner, partly because of the nature of available sources. Physicians' diaries, biographies, and autobiographies abound;[2] some of these doctor-written accounts have been used by historians to reconstruct aspects of practice for groups and for individuals.[3] Aside from the rich immediacy of a first-person narrative, their value lies in their identification of those issues the practitioner thought to be important; however, these types of sources tend to foster hagiography because they emphasize the spectacular or the bizarre at the expense of the banal. Rarely do they comment on frequency of ordinary activities, sources of change, finances, legal difficulties, or bedside conflict either with patients or with other doctors. Medical daybooks, case books, and account books do contain such information, but sometimes in such enormous detail that their acknowledged potential has appeared to be inextricably buried under their overwhelming volume. Except for attention given by a few painstaking pioneers,[4] these daunting materials, said to be 'all too often of little value,'[5] were largely ignored until the laborious task of analysis was facilitated by recent computer technology.

Case studies, sometimes called 'microhistories,' have been made of surgical, medical, obstetrical, and financial aspects of practice, in specific locations and at precise periods of time.[6] They provide details of nineteenth-century medical life at the local level and from the perspective of the medically qualified person. But these investigations offer much more: they can enhance our understanding of the dissemination of the nineteenth-century medical innovations and allow us to test the theories put forward to explain their discovery and their impact.

I have made a computer-assisted analysis of the Langstaff daybooks and accounts in an attempt to explore and quantify all aspects of a single practitioner's activity: remuneration, professional contacts, diagnostics, therapeutics, surgery, birthing, moments of innovation, and sources of information including the doctor's library and journals. In addition, I have tried to reconstruct the perceived medical needs of Langstaff's community through identification of the usual causes of death, the prevalent diseases, accidents, and injuries affecting his patient population, and his responses to them. To situate this study, I have compared information from Langstaff's records with that in the Canada Census for the relevant decades and juxtaposed his work to other small- and large-scale studies of nineteenth-century practice. For some aspects of practice, equivalent studies have yet to be done and wider comparison cannot be made. The regrettable absence of other first-person narratives by Langstaff, such as letters or a personal diary, has prevented me from knowing (and certainly from being swayed by) the doctor's own expressly stated ideas of what was important. It has also made it difficult to uncover personal events in Langstaff's life and has doubtless caused me to miss some 'stories' altogether.[7] Partially compensating for the gap, two colourful Richmond Hill newspapers wrote copiously on village activities, often with a political slant, but the accuracy of statements made by their journalists about the town's reform-minded doctor must be viewed with some scepticism.(Further details concerning the method are given in Appendix A.)

This study is a microhistory, but it is also a medical history about an individual doctor in a dramatically changing professional world and a social history about a nineteenth-century community in an emerging country. At Langstaff's birth, Ontario was a British colony called Upper Canada with no medical school and only one hospital. Langstaff was one of the first physicians to receive formal training in Ontario, and over the course of his career, he witnessed the Rebellion of 1837, the founding of hospitals and medical schools, the restructuring of licensing bodies for medical practice, and the formation of the Canadian Medical Association within the new Dominion of Canada created at Confederation in 1867.

Langstaff's daybooks indicate precisely what his actions were, but they provide no immediate response to the perennial questions of

why or how events took place. I have attempted to answer these
questions by drawing upon the conclusions of other students of
medical, social, local, and women's history. Were Langstaff's actions
in any way related to his participation in the increasing professionalization of his discipline or to his partisan sympathies? Is there
evidence that he interacted with or was threatened by alternative
practitioners, such as homeopathists or midwives? Did he adopt new
treatments? If so, how did he come to learn about them? Was he
willing to give up outmoded forms of intervention? If women wanted
him at their deliveries, was it for the interventions of 'scientific'
medicine, for status, or because there was no other choice? Were his
motives for using or not using novelties related to political, religious,
or gender considerations? Did he appear to accept responsibility for
the prevention of illness?

This book, being a 'biography' of a practice not a person, is
organized more by subject than by chronology; changes through time
in each aspect of the doctor's work, therefore, are addressed within
each section. Chapter 1 examines Langstaff's early life, his family, his
community, and his education. Chapter 2 explores the contacts he
had with other professionals, the manner in which he worked, and
his income. Chapters 3 and 4 are devoted to how Langstaff responded
to conceptual and functional changes in medical knowledge of
diagnosis and therapeutics. Chapter 5 begins with an analysis of
rates and causes of mortality in the Richmond Hill community and
explores the nature of morbidity and the common illnesses of both
children and adults. Chapter 6 concerns special situations involving
mental illness and alcohol abuse. Chapter 7 examines the causes and
types of injuries that afflicted Langstaff's patients and how his surgical
work expanded from emergency care for wounds to include the
principles of anaesthesia and antisepsis in carefully planned elective
operations. Chapter 8 addresses Langstaff's role as a birth attendant
and his experiences with abortion, infanticide, and other situations
related to the reproductive capabilities of women. Chapter 9 uses the
framework of preventative medicine and the public health movement,
which came to Ontario in the final decade of his life, to describe
Langstaff's contacts with the law, his incursions into politics, and his
late second marriage to a much younger teacher dedicated to the
struggle for temperance and women's suffrage. The findings are
summarized at the end of each chapter and again more broadly in
the conclusion, where mention is made of unanswered questions,

both new and old, that indicate directions for future research into nineteenth-century medical life.

Finally, two qualifications must be made. First, if Langstaff had been offered the same statistically rich perspective on his work, he might not always have chosen to interpret the findings as I have done. In defence of these hypothetical discrepancies or errors, I can claim only that, as I peered at his work through the compound lenses of medical sympathy and historical cynicism, I have tried to be fair. Second, the analysis of this single practice may appear to endorse or refute certain statements made by others concerning nineteenth-century medicine, but it does not constitute proof. Only when other such documents have been examined will we begin to know whether Langstaff's practice was the exception or the rule.

CHAPTER ONE

The Making of a Doctor

On 3 October 1864 James Miles Langstaff began his day by attending Mrs Scheel during the unassisted birth of her healthy baby boy at five minutes past midnight. Within the hour, he washed and packed away his unused tools and rode home over the hard-packed country road for a few hours' sleep. He rose early to make rounds, beginning with Mrs Scheel, who did not look well and seemed to be developing the fever that would keep him coming back for another three weeks.[1]

Langstaff then went to see the other sick people in his fifteen-year-old Richmond Hill practice, most of whom had long grown accustomed to the vigorous thirty-nine-year-old doctor, with his thatch of black hair, unruly black beard, and piercing blue eyes. Some were sorry that he and his respected wife had lost so many babies, but they trusted him with their lives. He saw Mrs Badger and her children, who had been ill for three weeks with high fever, cough, and pain in the chest and stomach; the children were now better and she seemed to be improving too, but he left her some medicine. The boys at Riley's, home of the butcher's brother, had been sick with a similar ailment, possibly pleurisy, but when Langstaff looked in, he found that young Wolstan was also on the mend. Mrs Isaac Bellerby, a nursing mother, had asked him to call because of her cough; the doctor was concerned about her condition: she seemed to be losing her milk and developing a fever that just might be 'typhus setting in'; he planned to drop by again in a few days. He visited Mrs James Lymburner, as he had done practically every week since she began feeling poorly some months earlier, and he saw the painter's wife, Mrs Richardson, for the third time that week, but whatever had been her trouble seemed to have cleared up of itself.

The doctor sent William Comisky, his medical student, to town entrusted with the in-person delivery of thirty dollars' payment on the half-paid mortgage to the Reverend Henry Scadding for his properties in Toronto. In Cook's store, where Langstaff had stopped to collect a few supplies, he was accosted by McMahon, who had some minor complaint and thought he could avoid the bill for a visit by consulting the doctor in the shop.

Twice that afternoon Langstaff went to the house of his old friend Matthew Teefy to see the sick baby girl. Irish born, Teefy served as postmaster, magistrate, and village clerk out of his busy general store. He and the doctor agreed on most things political and had served together on the Grammar School Board. Langstaff had been a daily visitor in their home since late August, as Mrs Teefy, their three little girls, and young John had all suffered greatly from some strange fever that altered the mind. The sisters, 'Louie' and Clara, seemed somewhat better, but two-year-old Mary Alice was in a shocking state 'screaming almost continually and putting one hand up to [her] cheek.' He had noticed this action repeatedly and thought the child 'seem[ed] to have a pain in its jaws'; he was baffled, since the pain was unlike the symptoms of her sisters, and her behaviour unlike that of other infants with teething difficulties.[2]

On that day, Langstaff made fourteen visits in and around the village of Richmond Hill, comfortably travelling some ten or twelve miles by horse and gig as the autumn air was bracing and the roads dry. That evening he attended the regular meeting of the Vaughan township council, where, according to Matthew Teefy's careful minutes, he moved that money be set aside to provide for Sarah Livingstone, an 'aged and destitute woman,' and for the adoption of the children of F. Brown, 'if the parents' consent could be obtained.' Langstaff had been elected a councillor in the previous January and intended to stay on until some important matters were resolved. Indeed, he was already contemplating the wording and probable support for the serious motion he would make at the next meeting:

to prohibit all sale of intoxicating liquors in the township.[3]

Home the doctor went for a late supper, possibly vegetables, ham, and apple pie, certainly comprised of produce from his own farms. Then, by lamplight, he retrieved his daybook and carefully wrote a record of his day's activities, not forgetting McMahon in Cook's store. And so to bed, only to be roused again at one o'clock a.m., by a summons to attend George Hoshel, who was suffering greatly with a 'severe pain in the head.' Langstaff administered medicine right away and left some more to tide the man over until he returned later in the morning.

This day was typical of some fifteen thousand other such days in the forty-year career of James Miles Langstaff. In the two months before the next council meeting, the Teefy baby, Mrs Scheel, and the other patients he had attended on 3 October would all recover, but two other people he had not yet seen would die: Mrs Jeremy Nelson, of pneumonia late in her pregnancy, and little Daniel Barker, of diphtheria, for which the doctor partly blamed the parents, who had not sent for him as they had promised to do. There were no days without work, not even Sundays, when he was called from church; one day in November, though sick himself with an upset stomach, he managed to see four patients. In those same weeks he saved a life by reducing a man's strangulated hernia, operated on a woman's cancerous breast, corrected a child's club-foot, and helped a physician colleague in the gruesome but essential task of destroying one baby in order to spare its brother and its mother, labouring in the dreadful birth presentation of interlocking twins.[4]

Who was this Langstaff, so involved in the political, social, and emotional life of his community? What were his origins and how did he become a physician? Langstaff was a third-generation Canadian on his mother's side; his ninety-year-old father still lived nearby on the family farm, fifteen miles north of Toronto, on Yonge Street, the longest and oldest street in Upper Canada. The road, the land, and the family had always defined and secured his place in the world. Here he was born and here, at the age of sixty-four and less than three miles away, he would die.

The district extended just over thirty miles from the Lake Ontario harbour of Toronto (called York until 1834) to the southern shore of

Lake Simcoe. Deeply furrowed by tributaries of the Don and Humber rivers, the land rose slowly to a ridge covered with oaks twenty miles north of the city. A generation before the birth of James Langstaff, this territory had been densely forested with ash, maple, elm, black walnut, basswood, and white pine 'so deep that the sun's rays rarely reached the forest floor.'[5]

The first Caucasian settler to the region was Nicholas Miller (1760–1810), builder of the 'King's Mill' on the Humber River, now a restaurant in suburban Toronto. Miller's efforts to erect a log home on his Yonge Street clearing in the fall of 1793 are said to have received unexpected assistance from the troops of Governor John Graves Simcoe.[6] Other settlers soon followed. In 1794 industrious 'Pennsylvania German' people arrived under the leadership of artist and entrepreneur William Berczy, and in 1798 the Comte de Puissaye brought a handful of 'émigré' French aristocrats seeking refuge from the Revolutionary Terror. The latter group abandoned pioneer life after only two years, but the former stayed and, by the 1830s, had partially cleared the land. The farms of these tenacious settlers grew in prosperity because of their proximity to markets and government. There were still occasional stands of valuable white pine in the north; as the arable spaces became occupied, sawmills were built at frequent intervals along the many streams.[7]

The Langstaff farm was situated one lot north of the Miller homestead and had been a Crown grant to James Langstaff's maternal grandfather, Abner Miles (1752–1806).[8] Miles, who also spelled his name Mi(g)hells, may have been of German origin but was born in Massachusetts and came to York in 1794, where he ran a tavern and store that supplied the town with meat, butter, and eggs. This business eventually passed to a son-in-law, James Playter, and his brother, Ely.[9] Abner Miles acquired many properties in the vicinity and moved a mile north of his farm in 1802 to open a hotel and a potash business providing materials for soap and candles. This location was variously known as Miles' Hill and Mount Pleasant until approximately 1819, when it was renamed Richmond Hill, either to honour the visiting Duke of Richmond or to commemorate the favourite song of a local teacher, 'The Lass of Richmond Hill.' Abner Miles died suddenly in 1806 during his efforts to remove a pine stump, leaving more than 2,000 acres of land to his only son, James (1786–1840), who in turn would pass the properties on to his three older sisters, Lucy (Langstaff), Hannah (Playter), and Elizabeth (Arnold).[10]

James Miles Langstaff's mother was Abner's daughter Lucy Miles (1781–1844). Her bachelor brother, James, had taken over their father's business near Richmond Hill and, having no children of his own, became a patron of the community families, who called him 'Squire' Miles. In 1811 he founded a Sunday school, in a simple log building, with an earthen floor and split-log benches, that served as a place of worship and education. Six years later, Squire Miles brought the feisty, Scottish-born Reverend William Jenkins from his missions to the Oneida in New York State, to the growing Presbyterian flock on Yonge Street. In 1821 through the combined efforts of Miles and Jenkins, a frame church was completed at the site of the Sunday school, on land purchased from Elizabeth (Miles) Playter.[11] Presbyterianism and pedagogy were linked commitments for the Miles descendants, and this same church would become one of the doctor's charities.

James's father, John Langstaff, had come to the region on horseback from Amboy, New Jersey, sometime between 1803 and 1808. He was a fifth-generation American and one of nine children whose ancestors had left south-central England to settle in New Hampshire in the seventeenth century.[12] Legend has it that John Langstaff went back to New Jersey but returned the following year for love of Lucy Miles, who married him at the relatively late age of twenty-five. After her father's death the couple acquired the Yonge Street farm, where they raised eight children, four boys and four girls. James Miles Langstaff, the youngest, was born on 3 June 1825. Both his given names carried the stamp of family tradition: 'Miles' for his mother, uncle, grandfather, and older brother; 'James' for both maternal and paternal uncles and his paternal grandfather, who had also been James Langstaff.

John Langstaff shared his brother-in-law's interest in education and had taught in a log schoolhouse erected on the Munshaw property next to his own farm. Local schools commemorate him as the region's first teacher, but he left teaching to serve in the York militia during the War of 1812. His reasons for having chosen to fight against his native country are not clear, but many other American immigrants took part in this war; enlisting in the British militia may have helped establish patriotic credibility.[13] After the war he supplemented farming with running a store, a smithy, and factories for the manufacture of pails, shingles, and eavestroughs.

James Miles Langstaff liked to study, but the availability of schooling was a problem. In the early years education had been handled privately by willing teachers, who, like his father, were engaged by parents who deemed the exercise worthy of expense. This system had changed after the Common School Act of 1816, which guaranteed public financing[14] and, for at least some of his education, Langstaff probably attended the common school nearest his home.[15] As standards in these schools were variable, conscientious parents sometimes employed private tutors. According to one report, eight-year-old James had been sent three miles south to Thornhill to study with 'Miss Cudmore in the home of James Milbourn,' a reform-minded Quaker, and he had been taught by 'Mr Caruthers [sic], a Scots Presbyterian,' perhaps at the Sunday school founded by his uncle. His first primers were said to have been the Bible and 'other ancient books,' including the writings of the first-century Jewish historian Josephus. The eager student found he could recite all the rules of English grammar while he ploughed two turns round his father's field.[16]

On the Sabbath the family went to Richmond Hill to hear the Reverend Mr Jenkins deliver fiery sermons in which matters of religion quickly turned to politics. When one parishioner nodded off during the sermon, the preacher hurled a Bible at him, crying, 'If you'll not hear the Word of God, then feel it!'[17] Jenkins made no secret of his political sympathies and spoke openly against the Tories from his pulpit. Because young Langstaff was friendly with Jenkins's son, Ben, he was well aware of the message, even if it was not endorsed by his own father. As a former American veteran of the 1812 British militia, John Langstaff held views that were in fundamental opposition to those of his wife's liberal-leaning family and Mr Jenkins. Family legend maintains that Langstaff, Sr, always supported the Conservatives; there is abundant evidence that his older sons were lifelong supporters of the Tory party too. Only the youngest son, James, would break with Langstaff tradition to support the Reform (later Liberal) party; if glimmers of his political sympathies had not been sparked by Mr Jenkins, they were surely ignited by the 1837 Rebellion.

In Upper and Lower Canada 1837 was a year of political tension and dramatic events. For the rest of their lives people recounted the stories of that December, when discontent flared into open rebellion. After years of protest the newspaperman William Lyon Mackenzie led a revolt against the system of government and its domination by the Family Compact, a group of wealthy families who supported the status quo.[18] In preparation for an attack on Toronto, settlers, armed with pitchforks, pikes, and firearms, marched down Yonge Street to gather near Montgomery's tavern, six miles south of the Langstaff farm. Richmond Hill's Colonel Robert Moody was shot and killed outside the tavern as he rode south to warn of the rebels' plans for an attack on the garrison. Colonel David Bridgeford, also of Richmond Hill, galloped around the tavern and succeeded in reaching the garrison, only to be captured by the rebels the next day. He was saved from execution by the collapse of the Rebellion and the intervention of surveyor David Gibson, whose house, Willowdale, stood between Montgomery's tavern and the Langstaff farm.

The Rebellion could not have escaped the attentions of an alert twelve year-old; unfortunately, however, James Langstaff's own memories have not been preserved. His neighbour, play-mate, and future brother-in-law Simon Miller did leave an account of the events he witnessed at the age of eleven. Simon was a grandson of Nicholas Miller, Markham's first settler; his father, Henry, supported the rebels.[19] At breakfast early on a December morning, Simon overheard the hired hand say, 'They have been going down the road all night.'[20] It is entirely probable that James Langstaff was in class with Simon later the same day, when the booming of guns led their teacher to close the school and send the children scurrying home. Not far away ten-year-old John Wilmot Montgomery was alone with a cousin in his father's tavern when 'a cannon-ball came crashing through ... knocking down three chimneys.'[21] If Langstaff had not already met this lad, he came to know him well in medical school a few years later.

The rebels dispersed when they learned that the British troops had prepared for battle and their leaders had fled. William Lyon Mackenzie escaped cross-country through the efforts of sympathetic settlers. It was rumoured that one of the rebel leaders, Dr John Rolph, had slipped over the border even before the shooting started. Arrests, trials, and disappearances followed; more men were forcibly marched south down Yonge Street in the ensuing months than had voluntarily stridden that path in the weeks before. In April 1838 Peter Matthews and Samuel Lount, a blacksmith from north of Richmond Hill, were hanged.

Simon Miller described the scene from his home near the Langstaff farm: 'For weeks and weeks afterwards, loads of prisoners used to pass our door on the way to Toronto to stand trial on the charge of treason. Many of these had been taken by men who had actually been implicated in the uprising and took this method to divert suspicion from themselves. But the tearing of the prisoners from their families was not the worst effect of the Rebellion. The feuds it gave rise to lasted for generations.'[22]

In the following years political stability returned as changes were made to the system of government. In 1841 Upper and Lower Canada were united under one government responsible to landowning males and Upper Canada became Canada West. But the events of 1837 did divide families for many years and had devastating effects on people in Langstaff's sphere. James Milbourn, the Quaker in whose home young Langstaff had studied, was accused of being a Mackenzie supporter, stripped of his property, and exiled to Van Dieman's Land.[23] John Montgomery's father, the innkeeper, was handed a death sentence, commuted to transportation; however, he escaped and hid with his family in the United States. The Reverend William Jenkins was harassed by 'hoodlums calling themselves Loyalists,' and one of his sons fled to the United States.[24] James Langstaff's first trip away from home was a journey with Ben Jenkins to Avon Springs, New York, in the Genesee region south of Rochester.[25] The boys may have visited the exiled Jenkins brother, who had probably gone back to the Oneida territories, where his family had resided before coming to Canada. Bridgeford returned to the village, where he lived another thirty years as a prominent citizen and occasional patient of James Langstaff.

During this time, there had been more changes in James Langstaff's family. His twenty-five-year-old sister Charity succumbed to tuberculosis in October 1840. His uncle James 'Squire' Miles also died in the same year. His grandmother, Mercy Miles, died in 1843 at the remarkable age of ninety-seven. Three of his siblings were married: his oldest brother Miles (b. 1809) wed Charity Langstaff, an American first cousin; his sister Mercy (b. 1812) was now living in distant Chicago and a mother of four; and his sister Mary (b. 1810) married Wright Burkitt and moved ten miles north to Newmarket. The fourth sister, Hannah, had died in infancy long before. For four years Lucy Miles Langstaff kept house for John and their three unmarried sons, until her death on 12 December 1844.

In the autumn of his mother's death, nineteen-year-old James Langstaff left home to study medicine. It is said that the second son,

John Langstaff, Jr, made the decision to place the youngest brother with John Rolph at his school in Toronto. In Upper Canada the oldest son could usually expect to inherit the farm; since it was becoming increasingly difficult to buy land locally, education for younger sons was imperative.[26] Medicine was an attractive career for bright but landless men; however, in Canada, unlike the United States or Britain, there were few places for medical training. Montreal's McGill University, which had its beginnings in an institution founded in 1823 by graduates of Edinburgh,[27] had been the only degree-granting medical school in British North America until Toronto's University of King's College opened its Medical Department in 1843–4. At that time several other choices were available to would-be doctors, but the costs of study and the nature of the future practice itself had to be considered.

In the preceding half century, medical education had changed radically in Europe and America. The previously separate disciplines of medicine, surgery, and midwifery had been combined. A new emphasis was placed on anatomical science; the status of surgeons had improved; and practical training at the bedside became just as important for those seeking academic degrees as book-learning and lectures had always been. Association with a clinic or a hospital was essential for a successful medical school. Young Canadians who wished to become physicians went to England, France, or the United States; until the 1840s nearly all licensed doctors practising in the Toronto area were foreign-born and/or held foreign degrees.

But a degree was only one path to medical practice – not necessarily the most common. Some people with no discernible credentials practised unlicensed; others became experts in unorthodox forms of medicine such as homeopathy; an indeterminate number assisted doctors as apprentices for one or two years; still others attended privately owned, run-for-profit institutions, called proprietary schools. These institutions could not grant degrees, but they did offer respectable education that could prepare a candidate for licensing and shorten the time needed to obtain a degree abroad. Rolph's school was a proprietary school.[28]

Dr John Rolph (1793–1870) was an English-born lawyer-physician-politician who had been educated at Guy's Hospital, London, and at Cambridge, England. In the 1820s he founded a medical school in St Thomas, Upper Canada, but this tiny institution survived just two years and graduated only one student. Nothing daunted and by this

time embroiled in politics, Rolph continued to teach medicine from
his home in Toronto until the 1837 Rebellion. Although he was linked
to Mackenzie, his role in the uprising has come under scrutiny and
his allegiance to the rebel cause has been questioned. When it was
clear the uprising was doomed, one of Rolph's medical students,
Henry Hover Wright, helped the doctor escape by waiting with a
saddled horse in the winter dark on the night the Rebellion died.[29]

Rolph continued teaching during the five years of his exile in
Rochester, New York. H.H. Wright and James H. Richardson both
followed him there. The latter described his experience living in the
attic of Rolph's own small home and dissecting cadavers preserved
in whisky barrels that had been shipped secretly across Lake Ontario
by the seemingly ever-faithful Wright.[30] When amnesty was granted
in 1843, Rolph returned to Toronto, where he practised and taught
from a house on Lot Street (now Queen Street West). He remained in
the public eye as a politician and as an eloquent speaker on matters
of temperance and biology. Richardson followed his teacher once
again; but he was 'run down by incessant study' and had developed
sciatica, which obliged him to use crutches for several months.[31] With
two other students he carried out more anatomical dissections in a
back room adjoining the stable, where 'the four legged occupants of
the very adjacent stalls ... could be distinctly heard heartily enjoying
their ... material aliment.'[32]

Rolph attempted to give his students thorough training in anatomy,
the science that had become the new cornerstone of medical knowledge. He also taught surgery and provided clinical experience by
taking his students on house calls and rounds at the Toronto General
Hospital. The observation of patients and operations, though highly
desirable, was not easily available and sometimes became quite controversial because of public disapproval and bitter rivalry between
physician-educators.[33] Richardson later fell out with his teacher for
political and academic reasons, but he described Rolph as 'dignified,'
'quiet,' 'precise,' a 'charming and persuasive orator,' with 'absolute
self-control,' 'profoundly versed in all branches of medical and surgical science ... I must do him justice to say that it would have been
impossible to find anyone more competent to teach, more indefatiga-
ble in teaching and more considerate and pleasant in his general
intercourse than he.'[34]

On 10 September 1844 James Miles Langstaff travelled the fifteen
miles down Yonge Street to begin his medical career. Years later

he commemorated the anniversary of this important day with a note
in his medical daybook, 'This day 35 years [ago] went to study at
Dr John Rolph's, Queen St Toronto. Drove out with Dr Morrison:
took my first dinner at Rolph's.'[35] Dr Thomas D. Morrison was yet
another of the legendary physician-rebels of 1837, who had been
arrested for treason that December and jailed until June 1838.[36] If not
heroes, these men were certainly impressive from the socio-political
perspective of Langstaff's youth. He was joined by a few other students, including Edward Bull, George Coulter, William T. Aikins,
and John Wilmot Montgomery, who had returned at amnesty from
his father's exile and was chosen by the class to be demonstrator in
anatomy.

Despite the personal upheaval his mother's death may have caused,
Langstaff excelled in his studies and, at the end of his first year, was
awarded a book prize for his achievement on a public examination in
anatomy. Further displaying his reverence for his medical début, he
wrote on the inside cover of his new book: 'The examination was on
9th Sept. 1845 lacking one day of being a year from the day I went to
Dr Rolph's.'[37]

Rolph had incorporated his school as the Toronto School of Medicine (1843); he charged his students fees and board but could not
grant medical degrees. Since 1795 there had been various acts pertaining to the licensing of medical practice in Upper Canada. There
was also the examining Medical Board, which from its inception had
conferred combined licences in the three domains of medicine, surgery, and midwifery. Often, however, the Medical Board members
were linked to the persons and values of the Family Compact. This
was perceived to be one reason why licence to practise was automatically granted to those holding an MD degree (or its equivalent)
from British institutions, but colonial authorities were obliged to respect the privileges of British credentials and were somewhat mis-
trustful of Americans. An examination was necessary for all others
with or without degrees from the United States or elsewhere.[38] From
the mid-1840s, when they first appeared, graduates of Toronto's King's
College Medical Department were said to pass the examination more
easily than others.

Rolph thought the practices of the Medical Board were discrimina-
tory; given his political orientation, it is entirely probable that the
system did somehow disadvantage his pupils. In a text prepared for
a Toronto School of Medicine annual announcement, he claimed, 'the

medical professors of the University principally compose the acting members of the Medical Board appointed by the Government and have almost exclusively conducted the examinations for licence and decided upon the merits not only of their own pupils but also of those of the Toronto Medical School [*sic*], thus giving to the former an important if not an improper advantage in the acquirement of professional licence, as is a matter of notoriety and complaint throughout the country generally.'[39] This problem persisted for the students of Rolph's school throughout the entire period of Langstaff's education.

Rolph encouraged his students to go elsewhere to complete their training. Study at other schools may have helped with the licensing problem, but it was increasingly popular for medical students in all western countries to spend time at other institutions. After two years with Rolph, Richardson had taken several courses at the new King's College; similarly, Langstaff and Edward Bull enrolled in the King's course in materia medica while they were still with Rolph.[40] Some students went to Europe. James H. Richardson left for Guy's Hospital in London, England, in October 1844, one month after Langstaff's arrival at Rolph's school. Richardson managed to secure a passage at a reduced rate: he worked on deck, took his meals and bunked with the second mate, and happily remembered being as 'active as a monkey in the rigging.' In London he was disappointed to discover that Rolph, notorious for his involvement in the 1837 Rebellion, was not fondly remembered by his alma mater. When Bransby Cooper, nephew of the illustrious Sir Astley Cooper, with whom Rolph had studied, read the young Canadian's letter of introduction, he cried, 'Rolph! He ought to have been hung long ago!' Then he stalked off. Richardson later said, 'this fairly staggered me ... of course, I could but turn and slink away'; other students soon recognized 'I was in dead earnest' and had a good knowledge of anatomy and surgery, but 'Cooper took no notice of me for a long time, only asking me about some persons he knew in Toronto.'[41] Richardson spent part of 1846 in Paris[42] and returned to Canada in 1847, having passed the examinations of the Royal College of Surgeons of England. Possibly annoyed about his rude reception at Guy's or somehow swayed against his old teacher, he associated with Rolph's foes, completed a medical degree at the university, and became the anatomy professor in the rival school.

While Richardson was in Paris, Rolph sent James Langstaff to Guy's Hospital. Nothing is known of Langstaff's voyage, nor is there any evidence to suggest that he was supplied with an introductory letter of potentially dubious value.[43] The hospital does have a record of Langstaff's registration in two sessions, 1846–7 and 1847–8, indicating that he was placed with the third-year students upon arrival and left with part of his fee unpaid.[44]

Guy's Hospital, founded in 1726 through the partly philanthropic vision of the publisher, Thomas Guy, had been considered one of England's best institutions for medical training for some time. When Langstaff enrolled, the hospital's director, Benjamin Harrison, was completing the last two years of his twenty-three-year tenure. Following his retirement, economic conditions would result in a relative decline, the closing of wards, and a period of stagnation for the medical school. During Langstaff's sojourn, however, there was no more exciting hospital in London. Changes had just been made to the education program as of 26 March 1846 to bring the training in line with contemporary trends. Students were to be charged fees up to £40 a year depending on their level and were to hold clerkships (junior internships) so that they would learn 'not only by exposition but by practice and experience.'[45]

In this academic milieu, emphasis was placed on anatomical pathology and physical diagnosis, both having increased in medical significance since R.T.H. Laennec's 1816 invention of the stethoscope. Rolph's teacher, Sir Astley Cooper, had maintained an interest in Guy's until his death in 1841. At his own request and in keeping with the new scientific preoccupations, Cooper's body had been dissected by his colleague John Hilton in the presence of the physician Richard Bright and Cooper's nephews, the surgeons Edward Cock and Charles Aston Key.[46] A succession of Sir Astley's relatives held important positions at Guy's and were among Langstaff's surgical instructors, including Key, Cock, and Bransby Cooper, who had so terrorized James Richardson. Hilton taught Langstaff anatomy.

Medicine at Guy's Hospital had been equally illustrious. Thomas Hodgkin had transferred to nearby St Thomas Hospital in 1842. Richard Bright, for whom the hospital had created Britain's first special ward for the investigation of kidney disorders, had retired in the year of Langstaff's arrival, but Thomas Addison continued to work there, gathering material for his study of adrenal gland insufficiency (later called 'Addison's disease'). Hodgkin and Bright had already published their classic descriptions of the diseases that now bear their names; these masterpieces of medical observation were a matter of recent pride at Guy's.

TABLE 1.1
Lectures heard by Langstaff at Guy's Hospital, 1846–8

Professor	Topic	Date (if given)
W.W. Gull	Physiology	2 Oct. 1846 – 19 March [1847?]
Carpenter	Nervous system	
T. Addison	Disease of the heart	15 March [1847?]
Chevers	Arteries	
John Hilton	Nervous system	Oct. 1847 – 13 March 1848
	Ossification	Oct. 1847 – 13 March 1848
	Veins	Oct. 1847 – 13 March 1848
Stephens	Piles	
Bransby Cooper	Piles	

TABLE 1.2
Operations observed by Langstaff at Guy's Hospital, 1848

Date		Patient, age (years)	Operation	Surgeon
9	Feb.	Female, 40	Umbilical hernia	Key
19	Feb.	Adult male	Hydrocoele	Hilton
22/3?	Feb.	Boy, 4	Stone (chloroform)	Cock
23	Feb.	Female, 21	Perianal abscess	Cock, Barlow
?	Feb.	Adult male	Knee (chloroform)	Hilton
?	Feb.	Adult male	Knee	Cock
1	March	Adult male	Leg amputation	Cooper
1	March	?	Fatty tumour	Cock
8	March	Boy, 4	Stone (uric acid)	Key
8	March	Female	Mastectomy	Key
14	March	Female, 40	Bleeding piles	Cooper
15	March	Male, 35	Cystic tumour	Cooper
15	March	Female, 30	Fatty tumour	Cooper
12	April	?	Antrum polyp	Cooper
13	April	Female, 21	Repeat perianal abscess	Cock, Barlow

One document compensates for the absence of other records pertaining to Langstaff's London experience: a small leather-bound book containing his handwritten notes on the lectures given by seven of Guy's physicians and surgeons and his observations concerning thirty-five medical cases and thirteen operations (see Tables 1.1, 1.2, 1.3).[47] From this notebook Langstaff's medical education can be reconstructed and his teachers identified as some of the medical luminaries of his age.

TABLE 1.3
Medical cases attended by Langstaff at Guy's Hospital, 1848

Date	Patient, age	Diagnosis	Physician
19 Jan.	?	?	Addison
?	Thin female, 45	Paralysis, arm	Hilton
?	Child, 3 and 4 months	Paralysis, foot	Hilton
?	Female, 16	Fever	
?	Martha, 23	Catamenia increased	
?	Catherine Ryan	Rheumatism	
?	Prostitute, 20	Inflammatory rheumatism	
?	Charity, 21	Chlorosis, aortic bruit	Addison
?	Elizabeth Keller	Amenorrhea, mitral disease	
?	Naom male, 16	Injury	
23 Feb	Dorcas, 35	Eczema	
?	Mary, 35	Eczema	
?	Male, 35	Steatomous tumour	
?	Child, 11	Burned arm	Key, Syme
?	Male, 14	Concussion	Key, Withrow
?	Male, 40	?	
1 Mar	Dorcas, 22	Abscess arm, bruit	Key, Tiny, 'myself'
?	Mary Jackson	Scirrhous breast cancer	Key
?	Jane	Weak digestion	
2–3 Feb	Dorcas	Swollen knee	
?	Mary, 35	Cough	

Langstaff followed Addison's clinics and lectures and faithfully attended the physiology teaching of William Withey Gull. He was a clinical clerk for Golding Bird,[48] said to be the first in the hospital to use the flexible stethoscope. Bird also had a special interest in diseases of children and the relationship between physiology and electricity. Langstaff learned Bright's method for demonstrating the presence of protein in urine by heating a sample in a spoon held over a candle. He probably encountered the well-liked Benjamin Guy Babington, who had invented the laryngoscope, an instrument for examining the throat, in 1829.[49] Although no record has been kept of Langstaff's midwifery experience, he may have witnessed blood transfusion experiments in cases of severe maternal haemorrhage or at least heard of the earlier transfusion attempts of the Guy's physiologist, James Blundell (1791–1878).[50]

Hilton's anatomy lectures were designed to emphasize the function of bodily organs as much as their structure, and thereby linked the more traditional subject of anatomy to the newer realm of experimental physiology. Langstaff related Hilton's lectures to his earlier medical experience in Toronto, annotating his notes on 'ossification' with a reminder that 'the same [condition] existed in the Indian at Rolph's '44–45.'[51] He learned confidence in the power of medical intervention, but he also learned the value of patience from a fortuitous opportunity to observe the therapeutic caution of Edinburgh's famous James Syme. Now known for several operative procedures and as the teacher of the surgeon Joseph Lister, who later promoted antisepsis, Syme consulted at Guy's while on a visit to London following the 1847 death of his rival Robert Liston. Impressed with Syme's management of a burn on the arm of Key's eleven-year-old patient, Langstaff wrote, 'a week ago, it was said by some high authority that the arm could not be saved, [but] now [it is] a great measure healed.'[52] This lesson was entirely in keeping with Syme's influential reputation as a conservative surgeon.[53]

The most exciting medical development while Langstaff studied in Britain was the advent of general anaesthesia. This decidedly American achievement, which had been some years in the making, swept the world following a public demonstration of the effects of ether at the Massachusetts General Hospital on 16 October 1846 – precisely two weeks after Langstaff began his studies at Guy's. British publications on surgical anaesthesia appeared the following month. News of the technique spread rapidly: ether was first used in Canada in early 1847.[54]

In late 1847 another anaesthetic, chloroform, was introduced by James Young Simpson of Scotland; it also was adopted quickly. Although Syme is said to have been one of the first in Europe to use ether, sources at Guy's Hospital maintain that chloroform was first used there in 'early 1848' by Charles Aston Key.[55] The exact date is not known, but Langstaff may have been present, since he appears to have been on a surgical rotation in early 1848 and to have attended several procedures done by Key.

On at least two occasions at Guy's, Langstaff did witness the use of chloroform. On 22 (or 23) February he watched Mr Cock operate 'for stone' on a four-year-old boy. 'The chloriform [sic] acted beautifully,' he wrote. The same day, he saw Hilton perform an operation on a man's knee, during which the anaesthetic 'acted with tolerable success.' On these two occasions only did he specifically mention anaesthesia, although he observed several other surgical procedures in the ensuing weeks.

During the long break between April and October 1847, Langstaff

may have visited medical France, as his colleague Richardson had
done the previous year. No proof for this conjecture can be found,
but mid-nineteenth century Paris was a popular destination for British and American students and Langstaff is known to have understood French.[56] According to family tradition, he curtailed his studies
in London and did not take a qualifying examination, because he fell
seriously ill and there was concern for his life.[57] Sickness among
hospital-based students of medicine was common: while at Guy's,
Richardson had contracted erysipelas, a severe skin infection, and
had been treated with purging and mercury by Dr Gull, who also
shaved the student's head and ordered him to drink Roussillon wine
when he went to Paris.[58] The admission records contain no indication
that Langstaff was ever treated as a patient at Guy's Hospital; despite his illness, he is said to have been awarded an 'Honorary Certificate of Distinction,' the existence of which cannot be confirmed.

Langstaff returned to Canada sometime in 1848; however, his activities for an entire year cannot be traced, a difficulty that lends
credence to the stories of ill health. In April 1849 he sat the licensing
examination of the Upper Canada Medical Board. Despite his lack of
written credentials and the Board's possible bias against Rolph's students, he passed on his first attempt.[59] Gestation in a British hospital
may have had a laudatory effect on the young man's performance or
on the examiners' receptivity to him.

Langstaff's personal experiences at Guy's may not have been sufficiently inspiring for younger students to wish to follow him; in 1849,
possibly hoping to find a more receptive atmosphere, Rolph sent
William T. Aikins to Jefferson College in Philadelphia for two years
of study with Samuel Gross and Robley Dunglison. The licensing
problems of Rolph's students finally improved in 1851, when he succeeded in 'alter[ing]' the 'construction of the Medical Board, long the
subject of public animadversion,' by having himself and former pupils placed on it.[60] Back from Philadelphia and now a member of the
board, Aikins claimed that the newcomers' examination questions
shamed the old members into revealing their ignorance on many
aspects of anatomy and therapeutics and made them reluctant to
present their own pupils. He reported to Rolph after one such meeting, 'many were the curses heaped upon you.'[61] In 1853 the University of King's College Medical Department was closed, partly through
the political influence of John Rolph.

Upon his return to Richmond Hill young Doctor Langstaff encountered two grieving siblings. His sister Mary Burkitt had been widowed while pregnant with her fourth child in August 1847; her forty-year-old husband, Wright, had died of an illness contracted as he 'engaged in the service of mercy' attending to Irish immigrants with cholera in a makeshift hospital set up in an old Newmarket brewery.[62] Langstaff's sister-in-law Charity had died in childbirth, leaving his oldest brother, Miles, to raise their four children, including the newborn James. This namesake nephew was always special to the doctor, who supported him financially into adult life.

Langstaff's second brother, John, Jr, had built and was operating a sawmill on a tributary of the Don River and would eventually take over the family farm. The younger sons, Lewis and James, were each given large parcels of land, but Miles, the oldest, was virtually cut off from their father's lifetime generosity and eventually out of his will.[63] The reasons for the harsh treatment of the widowed firstborn son are not clear. Perhaps John, Sr, felt that Miles was already financially secure, with two hundred acres of his own.[64] Miles may also have inherited some of his 'Squire' uncle's estate at his mother's death. But one other consideration probably served to distance the oldest son from the youngest son if not the rest of his family: Miles had become a distiller.[65] Old John Langstaff was known to take a nip from time to time, as the storekeeper Matthew Teefy could readily testify, but the temperance-minded young doctor would scarcely have approved of his brother's presiding over the daily production of fifty gallons of liquid evil.[66]

❧

James Langstaff emerged from his upbringing and education as a doctor imbued with the new ideas of anatomical and physiological science, and as a disciple of John Rolph, committed to reform in matters of politics, education, social welfare, and drink. His own experience with sickness, together with the loss of his mother, his two sisters, a close sister-in-law, and several infant relatives, gave him firsthand knowledge of disease as it ravaged his community. In his career, medicine, science, politics, and empathy would always be intertwined, just as they were in the autumn of 1864.

CHAPTER TWO

The Professional and Social World of a Nineteenth-Century Doctor

In the settling lines of darkness o'er the sky
The storm-clouds hung with ominous suspense;
The air was solemn, sombre, dull and dense,
As though some power oppress'd it from on high;
Swift lightning flashes suddenly did fly,
Illuminating the vaults of Heaven immense
And ere the thought could overtake the sense
Vanished with cleavage swift in vacancy.
After a length of silence there did rise
The thrilling trumpeting of thunders vast,
As through the universe with awful blast,
The power of God went echoing down the skies;
And as I saw and heard the blazonry of heaven
My soul found that sweet peace for which it long had striven.

'Storm Rest' – E.G.G.

Newspaper clipping pasted in Langstaff's account book, 1885

In May 1849, one month after receiving his licence, Langstaff set up a medical practice in Unionville, a village five miles east of his home.

That slow summer he made seventy visits in four months, to a score of different people, giving out advice and medicines, attending deliveries, and pulling teeth. He saw no patients at all from 23 August to 8 September 1849, when he moved back to Richmond Hill and purchased the practice of Dr John Reid, including house, lot, horse, and buggy, for the considerable sum of £500 and an extra '£30 for the good will.'[1]

John Reid had emigrated from Ireland in 1841, but by 1849 he may have decided to concentrate on nearby Thornhill, where his son, Dr John N. Reid, would take over in 1853, or he may have moved temporarily to Philadelphia, where Matthew Teefy seems to have pursued him with an outstanding bill from the general store.[2] With the Richmond Hill property came a bound notebook containing medical student lecture notes, a list of debtors to the practice, and Reid's signed oath of abstention from all alcoholic beverages. Langstaff began his own account-keeping in the same ledger, sketched the plans for his house, and listed his acquisitions: a cow, a cutter, a watch, and a violin. In a separate book, the first of many, the young doctor began keeping day-by-day records of his own medical activity.

Langstaff did not practise in isolation; even in the 1850s there were colleagues within easy reach. The British-trained Dr John Duncomb had located in Richmond Hill two years previously. Langstaff seems never to have sought Duncomb's opinion as a consultant, but he did refer to him thirteen times over the next twenty years, usually as patients' former (and presumably less competent) doctor. The cool relations between the two physicians may have stemmed from their competition for the same market or the fact that they stood on opposite sides of the political spectrum.[3] Duncomb seems to have had difficulties with patients as well as colleagues, as he was the subject of both a satirical broadside implying that he overcharged the poor and an outraged letter that demanded an apology for his tasteless diatribe against a colleague. These, together with the aggrieved doctor's response that his assailant would have no apology because he was a 'dirty, impudent fellow,' were carefully placed in the town scrapbook by Matthew Teefy. The postmaster seems to have been no fan of Duncomb and, like James Langstaff, tended to side with Reform.[4]

John Reid, Jr, and possibly his father were three miles south in Thornhill, where W.S. Durie, a graduate of Edinburgh, also resided, but Reid, Sr, was the only other physician Langstaff mentioned in his first year of practice. Cornelius Philbrick and Orlando Winstanley, both British-trained physicians, lived at Yorkville, between Thornhill and Toronto; American-trained J.J. Hunter worked ten miles north in Newmarket; while a short distance east, in Stouffville, were located James Freel, trained in Ireland and the United States, and A.C. Lloyd, both of whom seemed to maintain a loose association with Rolph. Many other doctors with whom Langstaff occasionally had contact lived in Toronto, including James H. Richardson, S.J. Stratford, and Joseph Workman, who was superintendent of the Provincial Lunatic Asylum, which opened a new building in 1853.

In the early years of Langstaff's practice more Canadian-trained doctors began to occupy places in the interstices: H.H. Wright had family and property in neighbouring Markham township; Edward Bull settled a few miles west in Weston; Walter Geikie, another of Rolph's students, moved north of Richmond Hill to Aurora; and more doctors moved to Newmarket, Bradford, and Barrie. Gradually, the ratio of physicians to population increased and the character of the profession changed from foreign-trained to predominantly Ontario-trained, with a few McGill graduates.[5] In other words, when Langstaff began, a doctor lived within five to ten miles in any direction; later the distances between doctors became shorter and sometimes there were several doctors in a single small town available and competing for ready consultation.

For brief periods Langstaff went into formal partnership with younger colleagues (Appendix B1). The first such agreement was made in May 1852 with Dr J.V. Parker (or Parkin), about whom almost no information can be found; however, the arrangement lasted less than a year. Increasingly busy, Langstaff practised alone for twenty-five years, until the 1880s, when he was in declining health and seems to have tried to engage an associate at all times. Two of the later associates were nephews, Elliott and Garibaldi, the sons of John Langstaff, Jr; another was the doctor's brother-in-law Jerry Palmer. As if the situation constituted a makeshift internship, these young partners stayed for precise periods of time, either one or two complete years, immediately following their graduation. Langstaff paid a salary for their assistance: Elliott, for example, received $450 per annum in 1880. Langstaff advanced sums for books, travel, and clothes against the annual salary and let the young doctor calculate what was owing at the end of his service in December 1881.[6] In his agreement with

Palmer a 'coon skin coat' was part of the written bargain.[7]

Langstaff also had contact with medical students. The calendar of the Toronto School of Medicine listed him as a professor in 1850–1, but it is not clear when, where, or what he taught, and his name was absent the next year.[8] The title may simply have recognized his willingness to receive students in Richmond Hill, which he did at several times and in every decade of his career beginning in 1852 (Appendix B1). Student apprenticeships seem to have been common in Canada and the United States, although the extent of the practice has not been documented and there are few indications of the exact requirements, if any.[9] A single account suggests that Langstaff may have given lessons in anatomical dissection.[10] The last two student assistants were his own sons, only one of whom completed medical training. Students usually accompanied the doctor on his rounds, but they were also sent alone on uncomplicated visits; patients were billed for their services. In Langstaff's rare absences his students sometimes managed alone, but their daybook entries indicate that they relied on 'back-up' from seasoned practitioners and that visits were few, perhaps because patients knew the doctor was away and did not want to bother with or be subjected to his young replacement. Langstaff provided temporary financial support for at least two of his preceptor students, but he expected to be repaid.[11] When F.R. Armstrong, one of the young doctors, had failed to settle his debt nearly a decade after it had been incurred, Langstaff recorded a trip to his home in Markham Village 'to dun him.'[12] More than two years later Armstrong arranged a settlement in which Langstaff took over his farm.[13]

Canadian medicine had been fairly pluralistic before Langstaff entered practice, but during his career there was a trend towards increasing homogeneity. A general reorganization of the Ontario profession took place in the 1860s. First, homeopathic and eclectic practice were legalized in 1859 and 1861 respectively; thus two more examination boards, in addition to the one that had licensed Langstaff, were created. Second, the General Council of Medical Education and Registration was formed in 1865. Finally, the three separate examining boards merged when the College of Physicians and Surgeons of Ontario was created in 1869 with powers to license, regulate, examine, and discipline members of the combined profession, including alternative practitioners. Local and national professional associations were created for the purposes of setting tariffs and discussing issues of professional and medical importance. In 1867, shortly after the Confederation of Canada, the Canadian Medical Association was formed and new regional medical associations joined those already in existence.[14]

Sparse entries in the daybooks suggest that Langstaff had little to do with professional legislation, medical associations, or controversy over the legislative changes. On 5 June 1866 he was duly registered with the new council, probably through a grandfather clause that did not require examination for established practitioners; he twice went to Toronto 'to vote for Aikins' in Medical Council elections; and he contributed to the costs of publishing medical fees.[15] Presumably as a service for a medical association, he prepared a list of physicians practising in York County as of 4 November 1867.[16] Given the great changes taking place in the structure of the medical world around Langstaff, his relative silence on these issues seems significant, possibly indicative of indifference or complacency, as if he were confident that practitioners like himself would prevail and were therefore willing to leave these matters of medical bureaucracy to his Toronto colleagues involved in academe.

There is little evidence that Langstaff had much contact with unorthodox practitioners. Twice he mentioned 'Granny Hall,' whom he told one family to 'keep away' from their sick child and whose ministrations he blamed for a delay in care that led to a child's death.[17] The word 'quack' also appeared only twice;[18] homeopathists and other specific sectarians, were not recorded at all. Dr Dellenbaugh, possibly an alternative practitioner who billed himself as 'the old and original German Physician of Buffalo,' was named as having been present during a minor surgical procedure, but he was not consulted.[19] Dentists appeared fairly often after 1860, since Langstaff assisted them by giving anaesthetic, but a veterinarian was mentioned only once. Women attendants from the patient's family were present, not only in obstetrical cases but throughout the entire practice; however, a 'nurse,' in the sense of a trained medical assistant rather than a nanny or wet nurse, did not appear until after 1880 (Appendix B2).[20] The doctor tolerated women assistants, although occasionally he thought they infringed inappropriately and inaccurately on his prerogative to make the diagnosis (see chapter 8).

Langstaff's contact with other members of his profession seems to have been strictly social or clinical. Periodically, he dropped in on old friends working at the hospital to observe their operative procedures. He took tea with John Rolph on at least two occasions, once only a few months before his old teacher's death.[21] Langstaff also attended several of the Toronto School of Medicine's glittering banquets in the late 1870s.[22] The doctors at dinner usually opened their self-congratulatory festivities by welcoming dignitaries such as Premier Oliver Mowat and representatives of the rival schools and by reading regrets from the governor general, the prime minister, the opposition leader, or the physician-politician Charles Tupper, before tucking into a 'recherché [but dry] bill of fare' that ended with an eclectic medley of songs: 'La Marseillaise,' 'The Vicar of Bray,' and 'My Name It Is Dr Quack.'[23] A cryptic entry in the daybooks, written six months after one of these dinners, suggests that Langstaff had found a financial solution to the embarrassing fact that he did not have an 'MD' diploma, although he had always written the letters after his name: he paid his old friend W.T. Aikins, now head of the Toronto School of Medicine, the sum of twenty dollars 'for degree.'[24]

Langstaff's main contact with colleagues came through clinical consultation. In forty years of practice he consulted more than 750 times, with over 150 different colleagues (Appendix B3). Arrangements would be made, either by messenger or, after 1870, by telegraph, for two or more doctors to gather at the patient's bedside. In the early years Langstaff asked for advice from more experienced doctors; in the later years he became the sought-after, experienced doctor. Most consultations took place within his region, but occasionally he went further: to Kleinburg, Toronto, Barrie, Bradford, Whitby, Collingwood, and once, more than two hundred miles to Wallaceburg, where the local doctor may simply have taken advantage of Langstaff's having made a custodial visit to his properties there. Sometimes the patients he saw in distant places were relatives of the Richmond Hill families he had tended for years.

Many factors appear to have influenced consulting practice, including the perceived need for help on the part of either the patient or the physician, the availability of other doctors, and indeed the weather and the passability of the roads.[25] From an average of one consultation every two or three months in the 1850s, there was a steady rise in frequency to an average of approximately two consultations every month in the early 1860s – the increase was partly due to the practice, common in that decade, of inviting two or more colleagues to consult at the same time on a single patient, instead of only one. The consultation rate declined slightly from 1865 to 1874 and then rose again to approximately twice a month from 1875 until Langstaff's death in 1889 (Table 2.1). The peak came in 1878, when he made forty-one consultations over a twelve-month period; on a single day in December of that year, he met Dr Rupert of Maple no fewer than eight times at the bedside of a man dying of fever and abdominal pain. Each visit was duly recorded as a consultation.[26]

The daybooks tend to confirm the impressions, gained elsewhere, that the profession was crowded and possibly somewhat confused in the mid–1860s.[27] A 'tenacity index' can be constructed of the probability of physicians' remaining in the vicinity of Richmond Hill by grouping Langstaff's named colleagues into five-year cohorts based on their first appearance in the daybooks and examining how many were still present fifteen years later. There was a steady influx of new doctors over the four decades, but those doctors whose names first appeared in the 1860s were far more likely to leave the region than those who came before or after (Table 2.1).

The consultation was a forum and a proving ground for new ideas; there is evidence of friendly debate. Langstaff kept track of those occasions when his dissenting judgment had been borne out by therapeutic success or failure, the opinion of eminent colleagues, or the final proof of autopsy.[28] In the context of consultation he disputed the merits of the heart drug digitalis and argued over whether or not a limb could be saved from amputation by antiseptic dressings. He consulted with some doctors vastly more often than with others, and his preferred consultants were not always those that lived closest. In decreasing order, the doctors he consulted most often included his brother Lewis Langstaff, John N. Reid, Rolph Lloyd, and Walter Geikie, all former students of John Rolph.

At least ten per cent of the consultations involved rivalry, if not frank hostility. Financial competition was a factor, especially if one doctor was thought to be poaching on another's turf. A patient told Langstaff of being 'forbidden' by John Hostetter to consult with him as she lived on one of Hostetter's properties and 'had no right.'[29] Another, who also preferred Langstaff, confided his fears that Hostetter would 'overcharge' him for having discontinued.[30] Less crass reasons for hostility depended on perceived infractions of medical decorum or deficiencies in knowledge, fully demonstrated in an ugly incident with Hostetter at a birth (see chapter 8).

John Hostetter was the physician Langstaff disagreed with most often. He thought little of the man's clinical judgment and found his

TABLE 2.1
Frequency of consultations, arrival of new doctors, and 'tenacity index' in Langstaff's records, 1849–89

Year	1849–55	1856–60	1861–5	1866–70	1871–5	1876–80	1881–5	1886–9
Average number of consultations a year	7.4	10.2	22	18.6	24.8	31.4	22	23.4
Number of new doctors in 5-year period	25	14	22	25*	17	18	23	11
Tenacity index (%)**	20	50	4.5	12*	12	33		

* Fourteen of these twenty-five doctors were named only once on the list of York County doctors that Langstaff wrote on 4 November 1867 (Account book 1867 inside back cover). If they are excluded, the corrected tenacity index for this group is 27.2 per cent.

** Tenacity index is defined as the percentage of doctors in a five-year cohort of new doctors still present (i.e., mentioned in Langstaff's daybooks) in the period fifteen years later. For example, 50 per cent of the doctors who were first mentioned in the years 1856–60 were still being mentioned on or after 31 December 1870. For the period 1876–80, ten years only could be analysed.

Source: Based on analysis of over 750 consultations and the names of over 150 doctors who were mentioned as consultants, or for other reasons, in Langstaff's daybooks

therapies too aggressive, but some of his intolerance may have been political, since the English-trained Hostetter stood on the conservative side of Ontario politics and had even offered himself for election (albeit unsuccessfully).[31] It may also have been because Hostetter was the first newcomer to challenge Langstaff's financial coexistence with Duncomb in the domain of Richmond Hill; furthermore, his talents were recommended over Langstaff's by the vacationing Dr Duncomb. This published announcement caught the eye of Matthew Teefy, who sarcastically wrote, 'Dr Duncomb! recommending his talented friend Dr Hostetter!!' on his own issue of the *York Herald*.[32] Seven years into Hostetter's sojourn the animosity seemed to subside slightly following their shared experience of a sobering case of tetanus – neither doctor had been able to alleviate the patient's horrifying symptoms.[33] Possibly they simply grew accustomed to each other; yet, after twelve years of strife, Hostetter finally left the village. His successors seem to have had better relations with Langstaff.

John N. Reid of Thornhill, the son of the doctor from whom Langstaff had purchased his practice, was one with whom disagreement was almost as common as collegiality. According to Langstaff's records, their frequent disputes centred most often on Reid's inept diagnoses and on whether or not alcohol should be used as medication. Like his abstemious father, Reid was, if possible, an even more staunch proponent of temperance than was his colleague three miles north; however, he did sometimes prescribe brandy as a stimulant. The two doctors seem to have been trying to outdo each other, alternating in their advocacy or rejection of alcohol, almost as if one's recommendation automatically implied the other's interdiction. Disappointingly, Langstaff never mentioned Reid's charismatic servant, 'Holy Ann Preston,' supposedly endowed with healing powers; however, Matthew Teefy, who shared her Irish roots, carefully placed her obituary complete with a photograph into the back of his book on the duties of magistrates.[34]

Langstaff also had an antagonistic relationship with Thomas Eckhardt of Unionville, with whom he disagreed over financial, medical, and even personal issues. In the case of a young woman who was a relative of Eckhardt, Langstaff was offended by his colleague's arrogance and annoyed by the frightened family's inability to decide which doctor was in charge. The patient had refused Eckhardt's attentions, although 'her sister [was] trying hard to persuade her.' It seems Eckhardt had been promising a cure; Langstaff wrote, 'I said, "if he says he can cure her, let him prescribe when he comes tonight."'[35] In another case, Eckhardt refused to accept Langstaff's diagnosis of fluid in the chest, and made a wager that 'he would leave it to any respectable doctor in Toronto and if he was wrong he would pay all costs.' Duly summoned from Toronto, H.H. Wright decided that there *was* fluid in the chest and came to his conclusion, wrote the triumphant Langstaff, 'without knowing our opinions.'[36] So common were consultation disputes that Langstaff's relief is apparent in the note he made after a consultation with Dr E.B. Knill: 'disagreed but did not quarrel.'[37]

Perhaps the highest compliment physicians could pay one another was to ask for help with illness in their own families. Langstaff was deemed worthy of this honour by several fellow practitioners. In addition to the last illness of his brother Lewis, he was summoned to sickness in the homes of F.R. Armstrong, Isaac Bowman, William Comisky, Walter B. Geikie, Rolph C. Lloyd, John D. McConnell, Edward Playter, John Reid, Oliver Rupert, and T.C. Scholfield. The ravages of alcohol were evident in at least three of Langstaff's colleagues, two of whom died. After the suspicious death of F.R. Armstrong, who had been the former student unable to repay his debt, Langstaff wrote that he 'had been drinking hard' and was found with a 'bottle of laudanum in his pocket.'[38] Possibly as a reflection of the bias of late nineteenth-century historians, the names of those doctors who, according to Langstaff, were given to drink are now the most difficult to find in local histories.

Leaving problems of alcohol aside, any illness among physicians was a matter of some delicacy, since public knowledge of the doctor's infirmity usually meant an immediate loss of income. Dr John N. Reid published a denial of gossip that he had cancer of the tongue, claiming that he had been suffering from a cut that would not heal. He later announced his return to full activity; however, another rumour circulated that he would not attend to night calls, and he had to have 'a number of notices printed to deny' the allegation.[39] The reassurances take on a peculiar significance, since the beleaguered doctor died only a few weeks later; the local press cryptically said he had been 'called by the most dreaded of all diseases,' but a medical source bluntly named his ailment as 'malignancy of the tongue.'[40] Langstaff seems not to have tended Reid in his last illness.

Sudden death visited medical people on rare occasions. When the testy Dr Thomas Eckhardt collapsed lifeless in the home of a patient, the papers reported that 'a far more powerful and mysterious messenger had called him.'[41] Notwithstanding the animosity that may have existed between them, Langstaff carried Eckhardt's casket to the grave, as he did those of Reid and Armstrong.

Medical books and journals were an important source of information. Langstaff's library has been dispersed, but his accounts show that he owned at least a few medical books on specific topics, including orthopaedics and breast cancer, and he subscribed to Quebec and Ontario medical journals published during his career as well as to some American publications (Appendix c). These publications, like his contact with other medical people, kept him current with the many innovations of his era; however, for the vast majority of his time Langstaff worked and travelled alone and his closest associates were the people of his community.

Langstaff's practice began slowly; during the first five years he made an average of only 3.5 visits daily, but this number increased within the first ten years to a relatively steady average of just under ten visits (Table 2.2). Once established, he published regular office

TABLE 2.2
Langstaff's medical activity

	1850s	1860s	1870s	1880s
Average no. visits/year	1,453	3,423	3,491	2,739
Average no. visits/day	3.9	9.4	9.3	7.7
Average no. days off/year	37.6	0	0.33	8.5
Calls at night (% of visits)	5.2	5.9	3.5	4.6
House calls (% of visits)	> 57	77.5	77	77.1

Source: Langstaff's daybooks: all visits May 1849 to June 1854; Jan. to Dec. 1861; Feb. 1872 to Feb. 1875, 1 Jan. 1880 to 31 Dec. 1882

hours, usually following the mid-day meal; however, he always saw the majority of patients in their own homes. Night calls came two or three times every week; there is no indication that he ever waited until daylight to respond. Although he often went out at night, he seems to have preferred to return home rather than stay over. Perhaps returning made it easier for the next messenger to find him.

The geographic boundaries of Langstaff's daily practice remained relatively constant, with a radius of approximately five miles in all directions. He seems to have tried to coordinate visits to people in the same region, but attempts at efficiency were not always convenient; he could be called to go from one extremity of his practice to another in a single day. The nearby railroad was completed in 1853 and Langstaff used it to make occasional forays, usually at the request of another physician, to cases twenty or more miles away, in Collingwood, Bradford, and Barrie (Map 1). Rare journeys even further afield were taken for social or financial reasons. With age the doctor seems to have become increasingly preoccupied with the number of miles he travelled on a busy work day. It is not known if he actually went greater distances in later life or simply recorded distances more often. Thus, after the age of fifty, he noted having ridden '75 miles in 16 hours from 10 am to 2 am' and, on a different day, 38 miles before midnight, followed by another 24 miles in answer to a four o'clock a.m. telegram; and at the age of fifty-nine, he went 110 miles by horse to see a patient without stopping for sleep.[42]

Messengers, often family members, were sent to fetch the doctor for urgent problems. In less dramatic situations, neighbours or shopkeepers were asked to pass word that a certain family would appreciate a visit from the doctor when he was 'out their way.' In the early 1870s Langstaff began receiving messages by telegraph. The telephone was not mentioned until 1889, the final year of his practice, although the first Ontario exchange had been established a decade before.

Illness was a social occasion. For very sick patients, the doctor was only one invited guest among a group of concerned attendants who kept vigil at the bedside. Referred to in the daybooks as an anonymous 'they,' these people washed, fed, and changed the clothing of their ill relative and administered medications. Sometimes, especially in the later period, they sought specific recommendations; often, however, they had already established a treatment program and turned to the doctor simply for advice or minor adjustments to their routine.[43] Social aspects of sickroom gatherings are described in more detail in other documents from the period. For example, Ely Playter recorded his visit to another man's sick daughter and wrote passages on the illness of his own 'little Franklin'; the doctors' visits were mentioned but given no more emphasis than those of the 'women [who] all come here in the evening to see the sick child.' When Playter's boy died, many visitors assembled and two men laid out the corpse.[44]

Another diarist, thirteen-year-old Sophia MacNab, described her mother's illness, the sickroom, and the doctor's visits in 1846. Fear of 'dear Mamma's' impending fate dominated the child's narrative of the constant watch maintained by sisters and aunts as they carefully presided over the invalid's diet and medication and made meticulous observations concerning her alarming fits of coughing, weakness, and fainting. The visits of Dr Hamilton and Dr King were extended sometimes into the following day with little effect on the bedside routine, except for the calming influence of their platitudinous remarks about the lack of danger. When her two preferred physicians were not available, 'Dear Mamma' refused to see 'Dr Craigie and ORiely [sic],' and although she was surrounded by family, no doctor was present at her death.[45]

Langstaff was accustomed to the presence of relatives and friends and relied on them to fill his orders. It seems the greater the anxiety, the larger the crowd. A young woman, 'moaning with every breath,' was attended by 'her relations standing round and think[ing] her dangerous.'[46] The doctor observed a man's 'friends are all staying' because he took to his 'bed expecting his death and has drunk a cup of nature wine.'[47] Langstaff worried that too many well-wishers could

Langstaff: A Medical Life

Map 1 The regional extent of Langstaff's practice and his land holdings in the vicinity of Richmond Hill. Yonge Street runs north from Toronto through Richmond Hill and forms the boundary between Vaughan and Markham and between King and Whitchurch townships.

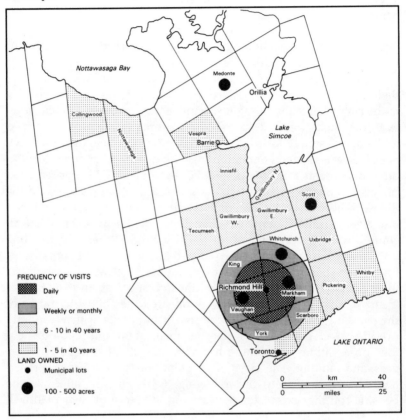

Map 2   The distribution of Langstaff's properties in southern Ontario

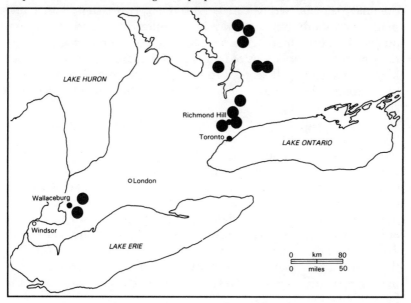

hamper convalescence: after his visit to a woman with severe abdominal pain, he wrote, 'all her brothers, two sisters, father and
mother are there, but they stay in the outer room and she is kept
quiet.'[48] In most situations he seems to have welcomed the ministrations and the observations of family attendants: at the end of a boy's
long illness, Langstaff seemed to regret that there had been 'no one
in the room when he died' either to comfort the patient or to relate
clinical information.[49]

Those without relatives sought care from their employers and
friends, who could be generous or indifferent. Female domestic servants fared better than male workers. On a visit to a hired man,
Langstaff discovered 'his two attendants asleep on the floor.'[50] Another labourer was even less fortunate: 'no one will wait on him,' the
doctor wrote, and since it was 'a fine day,' he decided to 'send him to
the hospital.'[51] This was a frightening proposition, used rarely and
only as a last resort, especially in the 1850s, since the hospital in
Toronto was thought to be filthy and the attendants unkind.[52] In fact,
there were fewer than a dozen hospitals in the entire province during most of Langstaff's practice; in his forty years of record-keeping
he mentioned hospitals only eight times.[53]

Some of the doctor's activity was seasonal, as he was always busier
in late spring than at any other time of the year. This variation was
due as much to the improved passability of the roads in May over
the early spring snow and mud as it was to cycles of epidemic disease, especially diphtheria, which tended to peak in the spring. For
transportation he relied on his horse, sometimes harnessed to a gig
or a sleigh. By the end of his practice his stables accommodated
sixteen horses, with such evocative names as 'Messenger,' 'Whirl-
wind,' 'Lightning,' and 'Charley Horse.' The doctor took an interest
in their breeding and care: only once did he record having lamed a
mare, and among his papers he kept a diagram that explained how
to examine a horse.[54]

The weather figured prominently in the daybooks, with thermometer readings ranging from 96 degrees Fahrenheit above zero to 40
degrees below; on a morning he called 'the coldest day,' Langstaff
found bottles frozen inside his office.[55] Storms hampered his rounds,
but people did venture out in the driving wind, even when it was
'too cold for teams,' and he saw 'plenty of frozen faces.'[56] He wrote
with awe how a 'very great snowstorm' in February 1868, 'blowing
direct from the East ... fill[ed] Yonge Street clear across from the top

of one fence post to the top of the other.' A day short of one year later (Langstaff seemed impressed with the coincidence) all the roads were again closed by another storm, which 'came down from the north' dropping 'small snowballs too heavy to drift.'[57] Frequently caught in squalls, he recorded long dismal trips 'home through incessant rain.'[58] Some of these descriptions are vivid, if terse: 'Robinson rode back with me; [the roads] drifted ... had to get out and tramp ahead of Rose [the] little brood mare.'[59]

The doctor experienced the same kind of accidents that generated part of his business. One February he upset both his horse and cutter; when he 'got free,' he left the cutter behind and continued bareback.[60] After a spring rain he was 'stuck in lane with [his] gig and horse down and the wheel sinking.'[61] The wheels and other parts of his gig were wont to break. When an axle split just before Christmas in an 'excessively cold wind,' he 'rode home on [a] buffalo skin on horseback.'[62] One January morning, after two nights without sleep and sixty miles of travel, Langstaff's gig tire broke and he had to walk back one mile through the snow to find two bolts to put it together.[63] On the odd night when he could not reach home, he would quietly let himself into an open house; according to his grandson, local people grew accustomed to the morning discovery of Dr Langstaff sleeping by the hearth. These experiences were shared by most members of the profession who worked in rural areas. The description of another doctor's journeys emphasized the constant danger in solitary travel by horse and the battle with the painful cold of the Canadian elements, especially when 'a frosty wind blowing against his face, shrivelling the skin and making his eyes water,' made him 'inclined to curse the hour when he had decided to become a physician.'[64]

The town apparently took a sympathetic interest in the travails of a medical life. The paper published a report concerning an unidentified physician who 'tied his horse beside a board fence,' unaware of the beehives behind it. The 'horse howled like a "condensed earthquake"' and was doused in water by the doctor, who came 'too close to the enraged little insects and received a stirring welcome ... on a smooth spot on his head.'[65] The anonymity of the victim is dispelled by Langstaff's daybook: above an entry concerning a patient, in tiny script, he wrote the single word 'Bees.'[66]

Langstaff seems to have enjoyed the opportunities provided by his work to discover the scenery around him. He went to 'one quarter mile from the highest part of King [township],' where the view north was breath-taking, allowing one to 'see over Lloydtown, Chomberg [sic], Bond Head, Bradford, and Lake Simcoe.'[67] A month later he described the hills and valleys seen on another trip past Oak Ridges to Scott township: 'a little over thirty miles. Started at 8 1/2 pm, the weather not very cold but got stinging cold during the night, horses white. Stopped at Ballantrae ... took along crackers & cheese ... & took off our boots and warmed our feet ... then north to opposite Mount Albert ... thence East ... to where a well-travelled road turns into Scott ... The cream mare "Curley" took all the turns coming back of herself.'[68]

Going in and out of the district homes entailed a certain amount of social interaction. Occasionally the doctor stayed to tea or a meal; as this type of hospitality was recompensed with a discount from the bill, he noted 'horse and myself fed' or, hinting at an even warmer reception, '[I] dined and horse fed.'[69] Since the young doctor would have been considered a suitable future husband for the community daughters, there may have been ulterior motives behind the invitations. He too may have been looking for a spouse. After a trip to Toronto, where he had dined with several people including Victoria University's Professor Rowell, he noted that 'Miss Rowell [was] there.'[70]

During Langstaff's fifth year in practice he was summoned to the home of Henry Miller to attend Andrew, younger brother of his old friend Simon. The boy was suffering from his second bout of rheumatic fever. The doctor made many visits throughout Andrew's illness and convalescence and commented on the presence of 'Miss Miller.'[71] Langstaff had probably known Simon's sister for many years, but as the now nineteen-year-old Mary Ann nursed her brother, the twenty-nine-year-old doctor may have been led to a reappreciation of her qualities. They were married six months later, in September 1854 – a union of two established families; their offspring, descended from the region's two earliest pioneers, Abner Miles and Nicholas Miller, would be fourth-generation Canadians.

Unfortunately, the daybooks for the months surrounding Langstaff's marriage have been lost and it is not known how his practice might have changed. The accounts and other records show that he added a second storey to his house and began buying more land, possibly as an investment or as a means of diversifying his income and providing for his future family. Certain changes in decorum may have accompanied the domestic alterations: Teefy sold Langstaff a spittoon.[72]

Less than two years into their marriage and a few weeks before their own first child was to be born, Langstaff and his Mary Ann became the guardians of eight-year-old Susannah and ten-year-old Henry Burkitt, orphaned children of his sister Mary, who had succumbed to lingering illness, or grief, in February 1852.[73] The five-year period of Mary Burkitt's widowhood seems to have been particularly difficult: a baby girl had not survived infancy; another boy, who seems to have had a chronic illness, died just nine months after his mother. Her tombstone was inscribed, 'She longed for death to ease her suffering.'[74] Mary Burkitt had named her 'affectionate brother Lewis [Langstaff]' as guardian of Susannah and Henry, but four years later Lewis decided to go to medical school; since he was married and about to become a father himself, he turned to the younger but more established brother, James. Care of the orphaned children, administration of the Burkitt estate, and dealing with Henry's ongoing troubles would consume many hours of the doctor's time over the next thirty years.

The young Langstaff couple may have had a ready-made family with the adopted niece and nephew, but they were to experience much sadness over Mary Ann's eleven births. Their first baby, Lucy, was born eighteen months after their marriage, but she died nine months later. The second child, a blond, blue-eyed boy named Wickliffe, died at the age of two in January 1863; another baby girl died six months later at the age of one; and several other babies died within days or weeks of birth. In October 1863, after five of their own children had died, the Langstaffs adopted the robust two-and-a-half year-old boy Ernest, who was said to resemble Wickliffe. It was not until 1866, twelve years after their marriage and the birth of their sixth child, that they had the first of their three natural children who would grow to adult life: two girls, Mary Lillian (Lily) and Louisa Eleanor (Nelly), and a son, Rolph Lewis, named for Langstaff's teacher and his medical brother. The doctor attended Mary Ann in all but one of her deliveries, leaving careful descriptions, but wrote about the death of only one child (see also chapter 8). The natural parents of their son Ernest are not known, although it seems the doctor would have been given ample opportunity through his work to learn of children in need of adoption.

Holidays were rare in Langstaff's practice. In his first full year in practice, there were 121 days without work, but four years later, only four; he worked almost every day, including Sundays, Christmas, and New Year's Day. After the first five years there was usually less than one free day a year. In the entire period from February 1872 to February 1875, he took only one day off, but it was likely given to unrecorded care for a sick relative. After twenty-five years in practice the doctor went on his first vacation: a two-week train journey with his family to the 1876 United States Centennial celebration in Philadelphia. Typically, Langstaff did not record his own impressions of the 1876 American Centennial but equally typically, his loquacious brother did. From his own voyage to Philadelphia and beyond, John Langstaff, Jr, regaled the home town with detailed letters, replete with political jokes, smugly contrasting life south of the border with the delights of Richmond Hill: 'If Ontario were farmed in the same slovenly way [as is Eastern Virginia],' he railed, in 'ten years our whole country would be brought to starvation.' He advised 'settlement of a few Canadian farmers on the land' and claimed that in just a few years the results 'would astonish the [American] nation.'[75] The 1876 Centennial seems to have had a profound effect on Canadians in the nine-year-old Dominion;[76] at the same time the medical press commented favourably on the parallel International Medical Congress, with much talk of Lister and Pasteur, held at the College of Physicians in Philadelphia.[77] The Centennial trip seems to have caused Langstaff to reflect on the benefits of regular vacations; thereafter, he went 'north' for a one- to three-week holiday in the summer or early fall of alternate years.[78] A student or another physician always served as locum tenens and continued to use the daybooks.

Less spectacular recreational activities were far more common. While the doctor's 'stopping' for tea or a meal with various colleagues and patients seems to have been common, there is no information on how he reciprocated, although he did write about social events outside his home. The church, temperance societies, and the Mechanics Institute provided entertainments in the form of speeches, plays, debates, and musical soirées. The doctor's presence occasioned comment in the local newspapers, as did the gifts he gave at wedding and anniversary parties. In the fall Langstaff usually went to the county fair at Markham; sometimes he travelled by train to bigger exhibitions in Toronto, Guelph, or Hamilton, where he was once in a crowd of 20,000, said to have caused the floor at the gate to sink two feet, while rain and pickpockets put a damper on festivities.[79]

The proximity of Toronto had a great impact on Langstaff's medical, financial, and social life. He made the round trip of thirty miles into the city more than 300 times – approximately once every two or three months. In the busy years from 1862 to 1864, however, he was in Toronto only four times. A third of the 300 visits were for business reasons, especially real estate affairs; another quarter were for legal matters; and a significant minority were for an eclectic variety of cultural events, including the visit of the Prince of Wales, a performance of Handel's *Messiah*, a show by P.T. Barnum's circus, medical dinners, and 'to hear Kennedy sing.'[80]

Langstaff seems to have been religious in a social sense: he went to church regularly, subscribed to Presbyterian publications, supported the Upper Canada Bible Society, and contributed to the minister's salary and to building projects of all local denominations. Perhaps the pantheistic sentiment of the poetic epigraph to this chapter resonated with those feelings he may have experienced in his numerous solitary rambles across York county.

Religious devotion notwithstanding, the townspeople viewed their doctor and his colleagues as 'men of science.' Indeed, the increasingly scientific trappings of medical practice have been cited as both reason and pretext for the rising status and enhanced control physicians would have over their own profession; these trappings have been variously seen either as a guise adopted by a monopoly-seeking profession or as laurels thrust upon practitioners by an increasingly satisfied public.[81]

Langstaff's opinion on the science of medicine cannot be determined, but he was not adverse to innovation. It is tempting to speculate on what he may have thought of the new theory of evolution, which made its popular début with Darwin's *Origin of Species* in 1859. His agricultural interests, especially in horse and poultry breeding, gave him the necessary conceptual tools to understand the idea of natural selection, but there are no specific references to Darwin, nor does he appear to have owned any of the publications of the early evolutionists. He did, however, attend a lecture given by the American liberal clergyman Henry Ward Beecher, who had accepted the theory of evolution, claiming it was compatible with religious belief because it demonstrated the organizational design of the Creator. Beecher's views were controversial and his credibility had been undermined by a scandal involving a parishioner's wife. Whether or not Langstaff agreed on the subject of Darwinian evolution is unknown, but the significance of his possibly sarcastic rendition of Beecher's title, widely advertised as 'Evolution and Revolution,' invites contemplation: Langstaff wrote, 'evolution and Involution.'[82]

🌰

It is generally accepted that the average Ontario doctor did not earn a large salary until the second half of the twentieth century. A reader of Langstaff's day-to-day financial notes frequently encounters entries such as 'nothing on hand,' but these comments create a false impression. Despite the common lack of ready cash, Langstaff became a wealthy man within a few years, and his prosperity was only partly related to medicine.

A complete study of nineteenth-century medical earnings has yet to be made. In 1946 George Rosen published a useful collection of nineteenth-century medical tariffs; however, the frequency with which the average doctor was reimbursed fully is, for the most part, unknown.[83] The fees published by Langstaff's colleagues were fairly constant throughout the period under study and resemble those applied in his practice (Table 2.3).[84] Detailed analysis has been given to the income of the nineteenth-century Canadian practitioner Dr Harmaunus Smith, who billed no more than $750 for his medical services in any year.[85] Recent surveys of American and French doctors at specific times and in certain localities have suggested a wide range in earnings despite generous fees.[86] In his examination of Canadian general practice of the half-century following Langstaff's career, S.E.D. Shortt stated that most doctors enjoyed a 'comfortable but not affluent income' and that true wealth came from other earnings.[87] Langstaff may not have been typical of his own era, since he earned far more than did Harmaunus Smith, but his finances seem to correspond to the non-medical earning pattern described by Shortt.

Langstaff kept a chronological record of his daily income and expenditures in the back of his medical daybooks. At intervals this information, together with the services rendered to various patients as noted in the front of the daybook, would be copied into a separate ledger or account book, arranged roughly in alphabetical order by family. There is evidence that the intervals were long and errors occurred. Since the doctor was often absent, he usually authorized someone else at the house to receive payment on his behalf: his students, the son of Ben Jenkins, his own sons, and his wife. A receipt

TABLE 2.3
Tariffs for medical services in nineteenth-century Ontario ($)

	1855*	1875**
Visits within 1 mile	1.00	1.00
At night		2.00
Each subsequent visit	.50	
First extra mile	1.00	1.00 (2.00 at night)
Each subsequent mile < 10	.50	.50 (.75 at night)
Over 10 miles (per mile)	.40	
Unusual detention (per hour)		.50 (.75 at night)
Consultation (excl. mileage)	.75	1–2.00
Midwifery cases	5.00	5.00
Complicated		10.00
Fracture, dislocation (excl. mileage)	5.00	5–30.00
Major operations (excl. mileage)	20.00	20–50.00
Minor operations	4.00	5–10.00
Cupping	1.00	.50–2.00
Administration of anaesthetic		2–4.00
Advice, bleeding, vaccination, tooth-drawing, opening abscess	.50	.50–2.00

  * Converted from £/s/p, at £1 = $4; W.B. Geikie for the Simcoe Medical Association, *Globe*, 5 Feb. 1855
** 'North Ontario Medical Association,' *Canada Lancet* 7 (1874-5): 220–1

was provided, but Langstaff sometimes forgot to mark the settlement in his book. Finally, further clouding this issue, he used more than one account book at a time; thus, the records overlap considerably and contain debts as much as twenty years old.

Reconstruction of Langstaff's annual income can be only approximate at best; however, the variety of sources he has left allow for cross-checking and lend some strength to the estimates. Throughout the period under consideration, the average labourer's wage was one dollar a day – in the later decades $1.50, if the work was particularly heavy.[88] These were the wages Langstaff paid his own hired men. Female servants earned less cash, although they did have board.[89] With a six-day work week, the average yearly income of a labourer could be $300; however, much of the work in the community was seasonal and many people took home far less. In contrast, the doctor's annual fees could be ten times this amount. He usually received payments equivalent to half his billings. From an initially low medical income of about $500 in 1851, Langstaff seems to have enjoyed a steady increase in each decade: $2,000 in 1861, $2,500 in 1871, $3,000 in 1880.[90] These are only approximate figures, but they are much higher than the $1,200 a year claimed by one medical writer to be the typical wage of Ontario's poverty-stricken doctors in 1875.[91]

Four account books and a list of estate debts have been subjected to detailed analysis (Table 2.4). These items are well placed at the beginning, middle, and end of the practice and contain a few lists of all known debtors as of a specific date. Comparison of two pairs of consecutive years shows there was great variation in income from year to year (Table 2.5). Several hundred families owed Langstaff money during his active practice. His own father and brothers were expected to pay, but other doctors and clergymen were exempt. Payments taken in a given year were sometimes applied to debts many years old. An examination of accounts standing more than five years and still owing in 1879 shows that fewer than twenty per cent received any payment over a two-year period. After the doctor's death, his executors listed only 153 families with outstanding debts; others may have settled quickly once they learned of the doctor's illness, or the executors may have considered them either unable or unwilling to pay. In the 1850s Langstaff charged interest on accounts unpaid after four years, but for sixteen per cent of these he accepted payment in the form of food, produce, lumber, animals, and labour. In the 1870s the interest charges disappeared, and only two per cent of debts were settled with goods rather than money.

Matthew Teefy's account books are strikingly similar to his doctor's and show that Langstaff's indebted patients were the patrons of the general store. Running accounts in Teefy's records tend to be just as large as if not larger than the doctor's and invite speculation on what the average person's overall debt to all other merchants and professionals may have been. Teefy also adopted the practice of dissolving debts in exchange for labour and goods: Langstaff's father managed to pay off some of his bill for whisky and sundries with a side of beef and by 'teaming.' From modest amounts in the early years, Langstaff's bill seems to have been allowed to grow much larger than those of other patrons, including physicians, perhaps because Teefy was similarly indebted to him. The doctor and the postmaster seem periodically to have conducted a simultaneous consultation of their records and cancelled their debts to each other.[92]

Since Langstaff continued to enter payments in the 1869–70 ledger for six more years, a few statements about size of debt, size of payment, and proportion of non-payment can be made (Table 2.6). Fewer

TABLE 2.4
Account book debts and proportion paid to Langstaff

	1851*	1857–8*	1869–70	1879	1889
No. of debts	115	411	846	492	153
Total debt	$684.00	$3,156.50	$10,397.82 ($5,198.91/yr)	$5,356.80	$2,490.00
No. (%) of debts paid (full or part)	65 (56.5)	82 (20) (in 1 yr)	462 (54.6) (up to 6 yrs)	123 (25) (over 2 yrs)	na
Amount paid	$402.35	$1,011	$4,816.75 ($2,408.38/yr)	$1,183.54	na

* Conversion 1£ = $4; na = not available

Sources: Account book, 1847: only 115 of the 283 families seen in 1851 were named in this account. Account book, 1852: list made at the end of 1857, probably in order to convert debts to the new dollar system. Account book, 1869–70: including all debts incurred in the two years. Account book, 1879: 'Debts as of January 1879,' summaries at end of each alphabetical section. Account book, 1889: list of debtors to Langstaff's practice, probably assembled by executors

TABLE 2.5
Day-to-day income recorded in back of daybooks

	1869	1870	1879	1880
Medical	$568	$2,042.65	$2,675.90	$3,432.88
Rent	$69.75	$146.75	$853	$571.70
Other	$460	$567.40	$824.61	$870.15
Burkitt estate	$583	$792		
Total	$1,680.75	$3,548.80	$4,353.51	$4,874.73

Source: Daily entries in the back of Langstaff's daybooks

than half the debts were paid in full; reimbursement could take ten years or longer. People were more likely to pay something on very large debts and totally neglect small ones. Similarly, Langstaff seems to have been more inclined to give discounts on settlement of larger debts. It would be interesting to relate the relative wealth of patients to their payments on debts, as was done by Roland and Rubeshewsky in their study of Dr Harmaunus Smith.

The record indicates that some medical work took place in Cook's

TABLE 2.6
Relationship of size of 846 debts to payment and discounts*

Bill	No payment (%)	Partial (%)	In full (%)	Discounted (%)
> $50	23.2	35.1	41.7	13
> $6	59	3	38	2.4
> $2	56.7	6.7	36.6	0
< $2	61.7	3.7	34.6	4.3
All bills	45.4		37.7	

* A 'discount' is an account considered by the doctor to have been 'paid in full,' although the amount given was less than the bill; it is not a partial payment.

Source: Account book, 1869–70, containing payments up to 1876: average bill, $12.29 (median, $5.50); average amount paid, $5.69 (median $0.50)

store or the local hotel, where the doctor may have been consulted by a patient trying to avoid the cost of a house call. If Langstaff could recall the time and place, these fortuitous consultations were also added to the patient's account. Sometimes there was heated disagreement over what was owed. When large accounts were not paid, the doctor sued his patients or their estate; these cases were dealt with, several at a time, by the regular visits of the Division Court. Specific details are scant.[93]

Although Langstaff expected remuneration, he seems to have been a little absent-minded about collection. In fact, his ability to take care of his finances is remarkable, given the many indications that he gave far less than his complete attention to the business. He misplaced large amounts of cash, as did some of his helpers; once he rewarded 'little John Dixon' with twenty-five cents for returning the twenty dollars he had dropped in the newspaper office.[94] The distracted nonchalance exuded by the well-heeled doctor may have amazed the poorer townsfolk, especially when they read Langstaff's embarrassingly vague front-page advertisement offering a reward for return of the unregistered deed to one of his many properties, 'lost or left at some private home some months ago.'[95]

In his first year of practice the doctor failed to note the names of more than ten per cent of his patients. Most of the unidentified people were unsupported women and their children. Lack of a name made it impossible to collect the fee. In later years Langstaff usually recorded names, but he always had some trouble remembering addresses, vital information when it came to distinguishing one 'Smith' from another. In the second year (1851), he may have resolved to collect his debts promptly: a code of lines and slashes in the daybooks (*not* the account books) indicates that over fifty per cent of patients paid their bills at the time of the visits. This figure declined rapidly over the next few years to fewer than ten per cent. By the 1870s more than ninety-nine per cent of patients simply had the amount owed added to their accounts. In the 1880s Langstaff's adopted son, Ernest, took a great interest in the family finances and, in exasperation with his father, wrote a procedure in the cover of an account book: 'I. addresses; II. accounts not collectable by J.L; III. November render accounts; IV. December – send blank notes to those who have not paid or shown cause; V. January – send notice that unless paid or responded to action will be taken; VI. Enter in court – send bailiff.'[96]

There were other sources of medically related income: drugs, consultations, coroners' business, and spas or special clinics. Langstaff obtained his medicines from a pharmacist, with whom he maintained long-running accounts. He appears to have mixed the remedies for each patient and sold them at little more than cost. Consultations often resulted in large fees, usually guaranteed or paid by the physician who had asked for help.[97] Other income came from doing autopsies or giving evidence in coroners' cases (see chapter 9).

Spas or small institutions devoted to water cures were popular in mid-nineteenth-century Ontario. Langstaff's brother, the enterprising John, Jr, made his own personal contribution to this industry in 1884, when he discovered 'a very valuable Spring of Mineral Water on his farm at Thornhill.'[98] Analysis by Thomas Heys of the Toronto School of Medicine confirmed the curative properties of the 'very pleasant' water. Thereafter, the 'beautiful grove' was offered for national holidays and the local festivities of all religious denominations and political persuasions. The water itself could be purchased for fifteen cents a gallon; visitors could find accommodation at 'reasonable rates' in the quickly created 'Hawthorn Mineral Springs Residence.' The bracing 'country air,' patrons were reminded, was free. Of John's three sons who eventually became physicians, two were intimately associated with this venture. Hawthorn Springs was developed just as interest in Ontario spas began to decline – a process J.T.H. Connor attributed to the emergence of the modern hospital and the triumph of the germ theory over the miasma and epidemic constitutions of old theories that had been rooted in analysis of atmospheric conditions.[99] James Langstaff appears to have kept a distance from his brother's claims for the mineral water, but there is insufficient evidence to say whether or not he was sceptical. He occasionally consulted for the doctors working at Hawthorn Springs, but he took no part in the business; by this time he seems to have accepted the idea that diseases came from micro-organisms, not from airs and waters (see chapter 9).

The source of Langstaff's great prosperity was not medicine; it was land (Appendix D, Maps 1 and 2).[100] From the earliest days, he acquired lots in the village of Richmond Hill, but shortly after his marriage he began purchasing out-of-town properties, whenever he had some extra cash. He first invested in real estate in 1856, at a time when Lambton and Kent counties were being opened to settlement. This extreme southwestern part of the province, more than two hundred miles from Langstaff's home, had been developed very slowly because of its marshy land. The whole Langstaff family seems to have been involved. In 1856 John Langstaff, Sr, bought five hundred acres in Kent and many lots in the town of Wallaceburg; Dr James Langstaff bought three hundred acres in Lambton. The latter investment promised some return from the planned digging of drainage ditches, but it reaped far more as the result of a serendipitous discovery one year later: Canada's first oil well. Great speculation followed the founding of the towns of Oil Springs and Petrolia.[101] Langstaff's oldest brother, Miles (the distiller), temporarily moved to nearby Wallaceburg and advertised no less than 60,000 acres for sale.[102] James Langstaff continued to hold one hundred acres near the oil wells; however, he sold the remainder in 1865, when he inherited his father's five hundred acres and town properties.[103] This land was the only distant part of the province with which Langstaff developed any familiarity; his six trips there as visiting landlord provided him with the chance to discover the miracle of train travel.[104]

Also in 1856 Langstaff bought his first Toronto property, from the Reverend Dr Henry Scadding, Anglican minister, historian of Toronto, and founder of the York Pioneers. This was a piece of land at the corner of Esther (now Augusta) Street and Queen Street West, just a few blocks from the original site of John Rolph's school. When development was complete, the lot comprised three stores on Queen Street and six houses on the back streets. Langstaff agreed to a price of

$5,400 and the Reverend Doctor gave him a fifteen-year mortgage at six per cent interest. Payments were made in a somewhat irregular fashion, either hand-delivered by family members or students or sent in letters registered by Postmaster Teefy as 'containing money or supposed to contain money.'[105] With the final receipt, Langstaff had a personal note from Scadding, 'Am sorry for my own sake that you are paying off.'[106] From 1875 at the latest, Langstaff received rents of up to ninety dollars each month. Furthermore, when the city widened Esther Street, he was compensated for the expropriation with $3,000. These sums were vastly higher than his medical earnings; moreover, the doctor's land-owning had only just begun.

One year after he bought the Scadding property Langstaff purchased another Queen Street lot, slightly west of the first, for a price of $3,500, managed on another six per cent mortgage.[107] In 1875, with both mortgages paid and upheaval over the widened street ongoing, the doctor had four new rental houses built on the quiet alley at the back of the second lot. Although he did not sell any of his Toronto properties, they increased in appraised value more than threefold during the thirty years he owned them. At the time of his death these lots comprised well over half his personal wealth.[108]

Langstaff also owned many town properties in Richmond Hill and in Wallaceburg. He had rental houses constructed and was the landlord to the local Temperance Hall and Mechanics Institute. Certain tenants were chosen to collect the rents in their vicinity, in exchange for a reduction in their own. Periodically the doctor sold town lots to raise cash, and he seems to have engaged in a stiff competition to sell land for a village park. In October 1872 a sale of twenty-nine town lots in Wallaceburg, a few with water frontage, brought nearly $1,250; three years later an auction of some of the forty lots offered in Richmond Hill brought between $50 and $150 per lot.[109] The doctor kept running advertisements in the papers to ensure occupancy of his rental properties and further sales.

When Langstaff inherited land in Chatham from his father, he immediately sold some of his Lambton acreage and put the money into a farm near his home, on the second concession of Vaughan. This was purchased from the bursar of University College in Toronto, also on a mortgage. He completed payment in six years and added smaller parcels to the land. A tenant managed the farm, but Langstaff participated in decisions about crops and livestock and took a portion of the harvest. According to the 1871 census, he owned 1,054 acres, the most land in his district, three times as much as the next most-endowed landowner, and no less than fifteen per cent of all the land held in his census district. He also acknowledged ownership of eighteen town or village lots, sixteen dwelling houses, six barns or stables, five carriages or sleighs, five wagons or sleds, six ploughs or cultivators, two reapers or mowers, one horse rake, ten swine, eight horses, three colts, three cows, and two sheep, and he claimed an annual produce of a hundred pounds of butter, fifty pounds of wool, and twenty-five yards of cloth or flannel.[110] Unfortunately, the 1881 census data have not been preserved in equivalent detail; it is not known if his agricultural wealth waxed or waned.

Langstaff seems to have become interested in agriculture partly for financial reasons, but also as a hobby. He occasionally helped tenants and hired hands with haying and threshing, and he devoted much time to his horses, pigs, cows, poultry, and various crops. He seems to have had a passion for chickens: he kept a detailed record of his varieties and the products of their cross-breeding, and named his 'Fowls' for their characteristics or after the people from whom he had acquired them. But his success with poultry did not match his enthusiasm: several clutches of eggs failed to hatch, some broods died as chicks, and adult birds died too. One evening he walked out into his yard and found 'Silver Grey and Tovell dead ... lying together having fought,' but, he added hopefully, 'Silver Grey [had] treaded the three Toronto hens in morning.'[111]

Apples were another favourite. Langstaff kept a recipe for grafting wax on the inside cover of a medical account book (just below Ernest's instructions for debt collection), and in 1867 he began an orchard. He 'did not quite fill the holes & planted deep [but] a warm rain set in at night & a very cold wind for the next two days.' A week later he replaced those trees that 'had not taken well.'[112] Tantalizing lists of nostalgic varieties and their properties are scattered throughout his professional papers. A tree he called 'Ernest's Apple' (probably for his adopted son) bore a 'yellow white fall apple in the middle of September'; the 'Yellow Transparent' bore 'very early in July.' He repeated a saying that 'The Alexander [was] "good for nothing but to look at"'; however, the doctor had high praise for the 'Seek-no-further': 'good table, good cooker, good bearer, hardy tree.' At the age of sixty he planted 500 apple trees in a single day, and in 1889, while suffering from his last illness, he carefully grafted nine new species into his beloved orchard and mapped their locations. Perhaps he conducted a friendly rivalry with the town druggist, acclaimed for his giant apples.[113]

The doctor's investments extended to industry. Sawmills were a major part of the early Ontario economy; in the late 1840s Langstaff's brother John built a mill powered by water from a dammed tributary of the Don River.[114] A cryptic note in the 1851 census suggests it was capable of a modest production.[115] The doctor had been involved in the construction of the millpond dam and spillway and the acquisition of saws, and may briefly have owned the property while John paid rent.[116] In the late 1860s James Langstaff began buying timber stands in Muskoka townships and sent crews to clear part of the bush, for fifty cents a cord. Some of his loggers were people who owed money for medical services; while they were away, Langstaff provided for their families.[117] The lumber from these lots was milled in Bracebridge or Gravenhurst. Later Langstaff received several offers to buy the remaining pine trees from his Muskoka woods, but he appears to have refused all of them, until the early 1880s.

In the mid-1870s, with his many construction projects in Toronto and at the Vaughan farm, Langstaff had often bought planks from a local miller and member of parliament, Amos Wright. The two men had done a colourful business settling medical debts with lumber and vice versa.[118] Perhaps the doctor reasoned that owning a sawmill would be a way of reducing the costs of his housing developments. Thus, in 1875 he acquired the sawmill originally built by his brother, together with an adjoining planing mill and a door-and-sash factory. The transaction seems to have taken place less than one month after he had received the $3,000 for the street widening in Toronto. Improvements were made almost immediately; a cross-cut saw and other new machinery were shipped by rail.[119]

Few accounts remain from Langstaff's mill; what proportion of his income was derived from its product is unknown. Some benefits may not have appeared in cash, as he likely used some lumber in his own buildings or traded it against other debts. A single statement gives some measure of capacity: in the two months of January and February 1879 his employee milled 24,098 feet of lumber and was paid one dollar for every 1,000 feet.[120] The doctor rented the door-and-sash factory for twenty dollars a month, until he sold it in 1879.[121]

Still needing 'grist' for his sawmill, Langstaff began to acquire wood lots closer to home; once logged, these lots would eventually become farms. Thus, he acquired acreage in Markham and Whitchurch townships and Simcoe, Ontario, and Victoria counties. His delighted anticipation on seeing one of his new properties is evident: 'rolling *heavily* timbered would make great sugar bush.'[122] He accepted property to settle medical debts, sometimes assuming outstanding mortgages. In 1881 he made his largest purchase: nearly 2,000 acres in Victoria county, bought for the low price of $323. Some of this land would be logged. By the time of his death and discounting the town and village lots, Langstaff owned or had been the owner of 4,000 different acres of Ontario real estate. In fact, property made up over eighty per cent of his personal fortune, valued by his executors at close to $60,000 in 1889 (Table 2.7).[123]

Langstaff appears to have conformed to Michael Bliss's description of late-nineteenth-century Canadians, who only gradually became accustomed to depositing money in banks, because 'real property was the asset everyone had or wanted to have.'[124] Bank notes and cheques, including some rejected for not sufficient funds, are mentioned in his records from the 1850s, but the doctor appears to have used banks only when his debtors and creditors required he do so. More often, he carried out his property finances through the Freehold Building Society, one of the many savings and loans societies.[125] Throughout the 1860s and 1870s he arranged for several private loans, ranging from $300 to $1,300, which were applied to his mortgages, repaid, and promptly reborrowed. Among those from whom he borrowed was the wealthy landowner John Lauder, who became a financier of public as well as private enterprise: the school board's long overdue debts to Lauder were explained in placating letters penned by Matthew Teefy in his capacity as village clerk.[126]

In 1880 the doctor took an unprecedented step and purchased '30 shares in the new loan company in Toronto.'[127] Perhaps he felt compelled to diversify his finances so heavily weighted in real estate; more likely, he was encouraged by his son Ernest and tempted by relatively low prices following the financial scare in the summer of 1879.[128] According to Bliss, these companies were run in 'imperfect markets' by 'knowledgeable insiders' who were connected by 'myriad webs' comprised of social and financial filaments.[129] Within a year Langstaff had become a director on the board of the Ontario Industrial Loan and Investment Company (OILIC). Over the next eight years he made no fewer than sixty-eight trips to Toronto for meetings to deliberate on the plans for a $95,000 'arcade,' the construction of a 'music hall,' and the sale of real estate. How many of the projects

TABLE 2.7
General description of property in Langstaff's Estate File
(amounts in dollars)

Household goods and furniture	854
Farming implements	226
Stock in trades	270
Horses	760
Book debts and promissory notes	2,490
Bank shares and other stock	6,320
Cash on hand	90
Farm produce	620
Subtotal	11,630
Real estate	
Toronto (bought of Scadding)	20,526
Toronto (bought of Houghton)	12,980
Richmond Hill	4,750
Other	9,333
Subtotal	47,589
Total	59,219

Source: Archives of Ontario, Estate Files, GS1-1015, no. 7529,
Cabinet 2, microfilm 478, Dr James Langstaff

were realized is not known. This enterprise seems to have operated on a modest scale or in relative secret, since its dealings and annual shareholders' meetings do not appear to have been published in the newspapers. Langstaff became involved just before the boom year of 1883 and, from that time on, enjoyed dividends from $100 to $221 every six months. He put roughly two-thirds of his profits back into the company. At the time of his death he held over $6,000 in paid-up stock.[130]

With the passage of time Langstaff appears to have become somewhat bored or annoyed with the business of high finance. He was impatient with wrangling over lawyers' fees and noted how two directors had had a 'set to' over company dealings. Twice in the spring of 1885, he made the long trip to town only to discover that the meetings were 'just over'; dismay is evident in his comment that the directors 'could not have sat one half hour.' In 1887 he grumbled about attending an OILIC meeting 'on important business,' and on his return 'it rained hard all the way out.' He kept up his Toronto travels for OILIC for two more years, until shortly before his death. But it is abundantly clear where his priorities lay: in 1888 he wrote, 'I was on my way to Toronto ... when I met a man coming full gallop in a gig. I returned with him tho' subpoenaed to a crown case & notified to attend [a] meeting of oi[LIC] directors.'[131] The doctor's choice caused him to miss his engagements, but it did allow him to attend the birth of a healthy baby girl. Whatever the sources of his personal wealth, when it came to personal identity, Langstaff was first and last a physician.

James Langstaff joined the medical profession of the mid-nineteenth century Ontario as a 'regular' practitioner without a medical degree, but he readily passed his licensing examination and continued to fulfil the necessary criteria for ongoing status. He seems to have been little concerned with medical politics; however, he maintained steady contact with colleagues, students, and partners in the form of bedside consultations roughly once every two to six weeks. Although Langstaff was not isolated, he usually worked alone and conducted his medical activity in patients' homes in the village or the countryside within a five- to ten-mile radius of his own home, through all weathers, and with rare opportunities for rest. Married to Mary Ann Miller, a third-generation Canadian like himself, he became a father, began investing in land, and took part in the social, intellectual, and cultural diversions of his community in a manner that befit an Ontario gentleman and a Protestant man of science. Only partially through his medical practice, he became moderately wealthy and invested profitably in land and stock. The next chapter explores how Langstaff brought the diagnostic medical science of his era to the bedside.

CHAPTER THREE

Medical Knowledge in Diagnosis:

Physical Signs at the Bedside

Whenever Langstaff visited sick people, he tried to find an organic diagnosis for their ailments. Commonplace as this statement may appear, he was among a generation of physicians for whom 'physical' diagnosis was an increasingly important part of disease recognition or the process of conceiving of, naming, and classifying patterns of illness. In the eighteenth century, diseases were recognized usually by symptoms, the subjective aspects of illness, as obvious to the patients as they were to their doctors. The change in diagnostic emphasis took place at the beginning of the nineteenth century and resulted from a variety of social, political, and intellectual factors; it brought with it new techniques, such as percussion (or tapping on the chest) and use of the stethoscope and other instruments, to allow detection of structural abnormalities inside the body before the patient's death, sometimes even before the patient felt sick. This development, sometimes cited as the advent of a doctor's ability 'correctly' or 'accurately' to determine what was wrong with the patient, has been called the advent of 'modernity' and 'scientific' medicine; however, as John Harley Warner has said, 'Medicine did not simply become more scientific during the nineteenth century; what was considered science, and what was not, changed.'[1]

After the advent of physical diagnosis, symptoms remained essential for 'sickness' to exist and to point to the diagnosis, but detection of internal organic alterations was emphasized; some disease names were changed and new ones invented. For example, in the late eighteenth century, diseases identified by their symptoms might have been 'dyspnoea' (difficult breathing) or 'consumption' (wasting), but after the change to organic-based diagnosis, these same conditions would be recognized only as symptoms or characteristics of diseases such as 'pleural effusion' (fluid in the chest), emphysema (loss of lung tissue), bronchitis (inflammation of the airways), or 'tuberculosis' (the existence of organic tubercles throughout the body).

Knowledge of anatomy, both normal and pathological, was increasingly important for the well-informed physician. In the last decade of Langstaff's career a theory that germs could cause disease came to be accepted. The diseases proven to have been caused by germs had always been fairly easily recognized by their symptoms; physical signs and laboratory facilities for the detection of germs were not available until much later. The advent of germ theory, therefore, had little impact on Langstaff's diagnostic practice, although it did impinge on his therapeutics.

Langstaff's teacher John Rolph was a proponent of anatomy, but how much of his 1840s teaching was devoted to physical diagnosis is not known. For example, it is not known when he first began to use the stethoscope, only that he was aware of it by 1837.[2] If James Langstaff had not been instructed in the new 'anatomo-clinical' medicine before, he was certainly exposed to it at Guy's Hospital. He had done dissections in his study of normal anatomy and witnessed autopsies for post-mortem diagnosis to learn about the changes wrought by disease. As a practitioner he brought an understanding of pathology to the bedside and, for both diagnostic and medico-legal reasons, conducted autopsies on some patients who died while in his care.

To determine what was wrong with his patients, Langstaff first took a detailed history, sometimes noting tendencies that ran in the patient's family or peculiarities of the patient's own physiology that made him or her 'disposed' or 'subject' to certain conditions. This interest reflected the ancient theory of 'temperaments,' a word that had considerable use even in Langstaff's day, but which is absent in his record. Sometimes the diagnosis could be made on the basis of the patient's history alone; further examination was an exercise in confirmation of this initial impression.

Communication could be difficult. He wrote of an older woman, '[she] cannot express herself but manages to make herself understood'; of a similarly afflicted man, 'cannot speak, but knows me.'[3] When the patient was unable to talk, the doctor consulted family members and, in the case of a child, noted if the parents could understand when he himself could not.[4] Level of consciousness was graded in a cursory manner: 'coma,' 'stupor,' 'responsive to pain,' and 'drowsy but rousable' were categories used frequently. He noticed if a somnolent person gave appropriate answers and once observed that a patient had 'an idiotic look but slowly puts out tongue when asked: – only sign of intelligence.'[5]

Before touching his patients Langstaff watched them closely, sometimes while he was taking the history. Aspects of their appearance and behaviour helped to indicate the diagnosis and were also important measures of the degree of illness and its possible outcome (prognosis). He noted wasting, pallor, blueness, staring, and 'the death rattle,' all of which were ominous signs. None was as sinister or as meaningful as the 'hypocratic' [sic] or 'sunken,' 'cadaverous countenance,' which is the special appearance, recognized since antiquity, of the face of a person about to die. Unusual actions, such as 'picking' or 'clawing' at the skin and bedclothes, or shaking tremors, such as 'subsultus tendinum,' indicated brain dysfunction and signified a poor prognosis. When one boy claimed he could not 'see straight,' Langstaff watched him eat and concluded in agreement, since he 'put spoon under plate instead of in.'[6] Some patients, especially children, were found to 'look wild' or 'horrible'; Langstaff wrote that one little girl, who had swallowed a piece of glass, 'stared at every face in the room as I have seen in fatal cases before'; she then 'clinched [sic] the edge of [her] cradle & died.'[7]

Some behavioural signs heralded improvement, as when wasted patients ate 'greedily' or sick children laughed, played with their toys, or helped their parents, and these were duly noted. Incongruities or conflicting signs were unusual and of special interest: Langstaff said of one man with a puzzling ailment, 'feel of his pulse and you would think he was dying, look at his face and his eyes [and you] would say he is going to live.'[8] Despite the hope inspired by the contradictory signs, this patient died.

Langstaff carefully described the appearance of rashes or unusual 'spots,' such as the 'darkish spot of congestion in the cheek [of a child] indicating debility or dissolution.'[9] The colour, texture, and progression of a rash was also noted, especially if it did not conform to recognizable patterns, as in the case of one man: 'body [was] deep scarlet. Arms *spotted* like measles but brighter ... [next day] arms *now* uniformly red.' Tongues that were coated, furred, blistered, and 'strawberry' were given daily inspection. He noted the deviation of the tongue to one side after a stroke. Aware that physical changes could eliminate inhibitions and conscious that his record might be read someday, the doctor was scrupulous about preserving his patients' dignity. For example, he wrote of a woman, 'had a stroke right arm & right face; tongue protruded (at my request) to the left.'[10] For more sensitive information pertaining to genitalia or suspected venereal disease, he resorted to Latin.[11]

The doctor referred to his earlier records as part of his continuing learning. In 1853 he described without naming a skin eruption suggestive of erythema nodosum: 'circular blotches on front of limb [leg] the size of a sixpence to 3 in. in diameter of a blueish red colour, the borders abrupt & elevated above the surrounding skin, just as in erysipelas but presenting rounded papulae ...'[12] The top of the next page is annotated with the words 'erythema nodosum,' apparently added after the page was written, as if he had later discovered the name of the clinical entity and then searched back in his record until he found the original entry to give it its appropriate label.[13] Later still, when he became quite familiar with erythema nodosum, he used it as a touchstone to describe variant clinical appearances. For example, he said that the spots on the thigh of one patient resembled 'erythema nodosum but several vesications form on the top & a core has come out of one.'[14] This is another manifestation of the doctor's continuing education and the importance of his daybook in the process.

Langstaff uncovered significant changes in the eyes of the patient, especially the pupils, in which he observed smallness, dilatation, inequality, irregular outlines, failure to react to light, and spasmodic contractions 'even while looking at the same object.'[15] He also recorded instances of intolerance to light.[16] Instruments to aid inspection were sparse. The loupe or magnifying glass does not appear in the record; the 'ophthalmoscope,' which was expensive and difficult to use, was mentioned only once, in reference to another doctor's consultation in 1886.[17] Specific attempts to measure defects in motor function and visual or auditory acuity were sparse and crude: patients with paralysis were 'palsied' either 'completely' or 'partly'; those with hearing difficulties of any sort were uniformly 'deaf.' Langstaff's only recorded attempt to assess day-to-day changes in vision took place in 1869–70, when he followed a patient's ability to count fingers or read the clock at varying distances ranging from two feet to across the room.[18] No reference was ever made to an eye chart.

The most commonly cited measure of well-being was the pulse, carefully timed with his watch, unless, as happened once, it had 'run down.'[19] The quality of the pulse was also significant and many varieties were described: strong, weak, natural, small, splashing, unequal, quick, hard, silky, faltering, falling, water hammer, 'with a backstroke,' and absent. If the 'pulseless' patient continued to breathe, Langstaff recognized 'death beginning at the heart.'[20] He once observed the opposite situation in a death attributed to 'hyperpyrexia,' recording that 'the pulse continued to beat some time after [the patient] ceased to breath[e].'[21] In the later years, he recorded the time lapsed between cessation of the palpable pulse and cessation of respiration.[22] Sometimes he could not feel the pulse for more mundane reasons, as was the case for a patient who had been well 'oiled with hen's fat' by his attentive family.[23]

The hot or cold feeling of the skin was important in cases of fever, but prior to Langstaff's use of the thermometer, the course of a fever was directly related to the rise or fall of both pulse and respiration: the more rapid the heartbeat or breathing the more dangerous the fever. Thus, he spoke of 'high' fever even before he used a thermometer. The pulse, which could be counted, appeared to be a more reliable and more sensitive indicator of the course of a fever, because it seemed to reveal subtle differences that could not be detected by the subjective feeling of the skin.

Respiratory rate was measured approximately half as frequently as the pulse. The quality and pattern of respiration was also important. Langstaff used palpation to determine the texture and shape of organs in the abdomen. He knew the significance of a bulging or depressed fontanelle in a baby with fever or dehydration.[24] He commonly percussed or tapped the chest to determine areas of 'dullness' in the lungs which represented the consolidation or collections of fluid, denoting pneumonia or pleurisy. The location of these findings also conveyed meaning: any indication of cavity or congestion in the apex or upper parts of the lung was a sign of tuberculosis.

The sciences of anatomy and physiology were never far from Langstaff's consciousness. He sought organic explanations for functional disturbances; if he was unable to find them, he pondered the significance of the apparent paradox. Thus, when he saw a patient in whom he suspected pericardial effusion or fluid around the heart, he observed her rapid breathing and the small pulse and reasoned that her 'blood cannot get through the heart.'[25] When he saw a young woman whose 'lung [was] clearing up' after pneumonia, he asked himself, 'why the quick respiration?'[26] Metabolic acidosis may have accounted for the increasingly rapid breathing despite an increasingly healthy lung, but it had yet to be described. It is significant, however, that Langstaff's concern to find a physiological explanation for his patient's condition brought the incongruity of her physical signs to his attention.

From the earliest days, Langstaff used the monaural stethoscope, or 'tube' as he called it, and sometimes he made special visits for the purposes of lengthy 'examination of the chest,' presumably to rule out phthisis (his word for tuberculosis). This was a slowly acquired skill and he made frequent use of the terminology invented by René T.H. Laennec (1781–1826) to designate the normal and abnormal sounds of the heart and lungs: first and second heart sounds and splitting of the latter; 'friction,' 'crunching,' 'sawing,' 'creaking,' 'grating,' 'rubbing,' and 'to and fro' noises suggestive of pericarditis, or as he once said, 'fibrin in pericardium'; 'bruits,' 'murmurs,' and 'whiffs,' which he attributed to physiological alterations including anaemia or to dysfunction of specific valves; 'natural respiration' and 'bronchial,' 'puerile,' 'whistling,' and 'wheezing' breath sounds, related to conditions of the airways; and 'egophony,' 'bronchophony,' 'pectoriloquy,' and altered 'fremitus,' indicative of disorders in the lung tissue itself.

A stethoscopic chest examination was a serious matter in the age of tuberculosis. It was probably with some trepidation that Matthew Teefy consulted Langstaff for a cough and a pain in his side in January 1854. The young doctor must have spent a long time listening to the postmaster's chest, for he wrote a fairly detailed description of a 'slight pleuritic [friction] rub on the left' and a 'distinct but soft' murmur of the heart; he was able to reassure his patient that the trouble was pleurisy and not serious. Indeed, two days later Teefy was convalescent. The young doctor's accurate prediction and his evident facility with medical technology may have helped confirmed the patient's allegiance for the next thirty-five years.[27]

Langstaff purchased a 'flexible stethoscope' on 25 May 1865, although he had probably seen Golding Bird use one at Guy's Hospital long before.[28] The next day he attended one of the town's prominent mill owners, in whom he detected 'pleuritic friction sounds synchronous with systole' – suggestive of inflammation around the lung and heart.[29] With experience the doctor dispensed with recording details about the sounds he could hear through his stethoscope and wrote only what he construed the underlying anatomical change to be. Thus, nearly ten years after his careful examination of Teefy's chest, he was invited to examine the lungs of the postmaster's oldest daughter, Clara. He would have taken a history, inspected with his eyes and his hands, and used his stethoscope, but the record indicates only an anatomical finding. 'Right apex phthisical' was all he wrote, an indication that he suspected tuberculosis in the right upper lung of the thirteen-year-old girl.[30]

As with other aspects of examination, Langstaff contemplated auscultatory incongruities, such as the 'bruit ... like a soft hum' heard in the heart of a woman patient that did 'not correspond to either side of the heart'; he thought it was caused 'perhaps [by] the venous blood entering the auricles.'[31] Similarly, he saw a male patient in whom 'fremitus was *increased* though pleurisy [was] present.'[32] He was confident of his technique in auscultation and openly disagreed with colleagues about interpretation of the sounds, as on the day he 'examined the lung and urine' of a man and 'found both healthy in the presence & in opposition to [Dr] Reid.'[33]

Langstaff's only known contribution to the medical literature was an observation concerning the physical diagnosis of pneumonia – a brief letter to the editor of the *Canada Lancet* about the complete consolidation of a little girl's lung.[34] He admitted that he used to think 'dulness [sic] over one side would indicate effusion,' but after seeing a similar case four years previously, he came to realize that the combination of dullness, bronchial breath sounds, louder transmitted voice, and rapid clearing indicated not fluid in the chest but inflammation and congestion of the lung tissue itself. The letter seems to have been intended as a guide for other doctors seeking to determine the precise state of the organs of the chest.

Inspection of body fluids and excreta was a major part of the process of physical diagnosis. From early in his practice Langstaff noted the quantity and appearance of urine, especially the colour and the presence of blood. He tested urine for albumin (protein) by applying heat, as Bright had first demonstrated at Guy's Hospital in 1827.[35] Again, he seems to have been sure of his skill: he wrote that he found nothing wrong with the urine of a young woman patient, although a nurse had boiled it and found it 'thick with albumen.'[36] In the three cases of diabetes, however, the diagnosis seems to have been based on generalized wasting and copious urine rather than on a demonstration of sugar in the urine.[37] In 1861 Langstaff once distinguished albumin from 'lithates,' but it seems unlikely he used a microscope for the purpose.[38] He also used a 'urinometer' to measure specific gravity and compared changes in this parameter over time, especially when he suspected a renal origin for dropsy (swelling).[39] It appears that, unlike some colleagues, Langstaff did take the time to perform these measurements on home visits during the 1860s.[40]

Microscopy did not enter medical practice until the 1830s, although the microscope had been invented centuries before. In Canada several clinicians are known to have promoted the instrument prior to 1860, including James Bovell of Toronto and Andrew Holmes of Montreal. The Faculty of Medicine at Toronto's Trinity College promised to provide 'microscopical demonstrations' during the 1855–6 academic year, and four years later a course in anatomical microscopy was offered in Quebec City.[41] Articles on microscopy and the topics it inspired, such as cell theory, had begun to appear by the late 1860s in the Canadian journals Langstaff received.[42] The instrument became useful, especially in laboratories for pathology and forensic medicine, but whether or not it was a common item for a country doctor to apply to his practice is unknown. Amateur applications were popular in the United States and in Canada; even in Langstaff's community the educated public displayed an interest in microscopy: Dr Geikie spoke at the the Mechanics Institute on 'Cell Life through the Microscope,' and the local press carried articles on the 'Wonders of Microscopy.'[43]

Langstaff purchased a microscope in November 1879. Exactly how he employed this forty-dollar instrument is not clear. The estate inventory listed the microscope as part of his office equipment,[44] and certain clinical descriptions suggest that it may have been used in physical diagnosis, especially urinalysis. For example, he declared a patient's urine to be 'very purulent.'[45] Nevertheless – possibly hinting at a more amateur application – the purchase account was entered in the hand of the doctor's adolescent son, who recorded the simultaneous acquisition of a two-dollar telescope.

Langstaff also examined sputum, noting colour, texture, and, on rare occasions, whether it floated or sank in water.[46] The presence of blood was an indicator of pneumonia, but there is nothing to suggest that he ever used a microscope to examine sputum for red or white blood cells. A man expectorated 'about a pint in twelve hours' of 'dark grumous [i.e., clotted] mucopurulent [sputum], floating in watery liquid & thicker purulent mucous at bottom. They thought there was a little blood but not certain.'[47] Once only, Langstaff commented on the tenacious quality of expectorated sputum, recording that it 'sticks where it strikes, the size of a cent piece'; on another occasion, he wrote that a little child, who did eventually recover, lay gasping with 'ropes of mucus hanging down to the floor.'[48]

The doctor viewed constipation as a dangerous state, requiring intervention with 'physic,' enemata, magnesium salts, or more violent preparations intended to prevent auto-intoxication with the poisonous effects of uneliminated bodily waste. He inspected the stools of patients with abdominal pain and knew the significance of blood, pus, and 'black tar-like motions,' or 'melaena.'[49] He also was alert to unusual appearances, as in the case of a child with diarrhoea who had 'transparent slimy gelly constantly running from him.' He used the term 'rice water stools' in the context of cholera.[50]

Since bleeding was a major part of Langstaff's therapeutic armamentarium, he was given ample opportunity to observe changes in the blood and relate them to the clinical situation. When a thick creamy layer, visible to the naked eye, formed at the interface between the red blood and its straw-coloured fluid, Langstaff said the blood was 'buffed and cupped.' This appearance in blood left standing, now attributed to an increase in white cells and proteins, was used by Langstaff as a reliable sign of internal inflammation; he viewed a decrease in the buffy layer as a sign of improvement. If the blood was 'dark' or 'black,' a change he recognized as caused by too little oxygen, he concluded that the patient's lungs were failing. He seemed to impute the same meaning to 'thick' blood that flowed slowly. Once at the end of a venesection for a man with pneumonia, he noted that the 'very dark [blood] ran a little lighter near the last,' suggesting the treatment had brought some benefit even before it was complete. Despite the favourable sign, this man died.[51]

The one diagnostic instrument Langstaff learned to use often was the thermometer. Although the instrument had been invented centuries before, clinicians did not generally adopt it until the 1880s. Early thermometers were fragile, especially the twelve-inch model, and posed difficulties for itinerant physicians. The change in attitude has been attributed to the meticulous 1868 monograph of Karl Wunderlich (1815–77),[52] but others consider that the work of Edouard Séguin (1812–80) had a greater impact on North American medicine than did that of Wunderlich.[53] Articles on medical thermometry appeared in the Canadian medical literature even before 1868, but with greater frequency in the late 1870s.[54]

From at least 1856 Langstaff had used either newspaper reports or his own thermometer readings to measure atmospheric temperature, especially on very cold days. He did not, however, record a clinical reading until May 1878, while consulting with a younger colleague on a comatose child with a pulse of 140 and a temperature of 103.5 degrees.[55] The timing of Langstaff's use of clinical thermometry tends to endorse the theory of Séguin's influence. Langstaff may even have read the review of Séguin's treatise, which had appeared in one of the journals he received during the previous year.[56] Two and a half years later, his accounts show he purchased a 'clinical thermometer' through Postmaster Teefy.[57] The daybooks suggest that despite this acquistion he did not use his new instrument very often. In fact, two years passed before he mentioned it a second time, seemingly while attending alone; then another eighteen months went by before the third reference, which was written by his physician nephew, who worked with him.[58] By November 1884, however, and until the end of his practice, Langstaff recorded clinical temperatures at least once a month. It is possible that he actually used the instrument earlier and more frequently than the daybooks indicate, especially if he recorded only abnormal or significant normal temperatures.

The growing use of instruments in medical practice may have been influenced by insurance companies and their required physical examinations, as Audrey Davis has shown.[59] The vast majority of the persons Langstaff attended looked and felt sick; the insurance company physical offered virtually the only situation in which he examined healthy people. These examinations appear to have begun in December 1868, and from then on they took place several times a year, often in clusters of three or four. What constituted such an examination is not recorded, but the doctor was faithfully paid three or four dollars for each, usually a few weeks later; seven different companies were named in his record.[60] He often examined several family members in a day: Matthew and Betsy Teefy were examined for life insurance a month after their twenty-three-year-old son; on one exceptional day, possibly following the visit of a convincing sales-man, Langstaff examined twenty-one people, including eight couples, and charged a bargain rate of one dollar each.[61] A single 'certificate' for what may have been a physical examination for employment in the 'Civil Service' appears in his record; and there was one 'certifi-cate for sickness,' perhaps a document required by a school or an employer.[62]

Just as Langstaff occasionally examined healthy people, so he was occasionally summoned to examine the dead. If an organic diagnosis had not been made before the patient died or there had been any suspicion of foul play, an autopsy would be performed. From March 1852 until October 1888 Langstaff made approximately one post-mortem examination each year; this figure rose to a peak of three per year in the 1860s and declined slowly to the last decade, during which he performed only five such examinations. Of the thirty-seven autopsies identified, seven concerned children. Most of the post-mortem examinations were intended to satisfy a medical need for explanation, but roughly one-quarter were done for legal reasons (see chapter 9). Langstaff does not appear to have used a microscope in this context; his report usually consisted of a brief description of the findings visible to the naked eye. For example, he wrote, '[I] went and opened abdomen, all cancerous.'[63] Sometimes he confined his inspection to the body part that had offered symptoms, such as the head of a fifteen-year-old boy who had been 'shouting' and 'clawing, know[ing] a person one minute & next does not.'[64]

Not all autopsy descriptions were so cryptic. A boy whose rheu-matic heart murmurs Langstaff had followed for four years died a 'very easy' death: 'on taking him from the rocking chair to the bed, he just lay down and was gone.' The 300-word description of the cardiac abnormalities shows that, for this attending physician, the post-mortem inspection was the final interpretation of the strange heart sounds he had studied for months on end. It included mention of the 'small bodies less than the size of a pin head [sic] placed quite close to each other forming a fine crest ... along the free margins of the mitral and semi-lunar valves.'[65] These lesions appear to be the same ones Laennec recognized as valvular 'vegetations,' an abnor-mality that was not interpreted until this century.[66]

In his elegant study of hospital therapeutics, John Harley Warner noted that, during the nineteenth century, there was a change in the adjective used to describe aspects of patients who were not sick, from 'natural' to 'normal.' He related this shift to increasing quantification of physiological disturbances.[67] It is interesting to note that Langstaff, an individual, made the change Warner documented as having been made by large groups and institutions. In all periods studied, Langstaff frequently wrote the word 'natural' to describe healthy appearances. The word 'abnormal' appeared quite early, though rarely, and was applied exclusively to heart sounds.[68] Langstaff did not write the word 'normal' until June 1882, when he described a patient's chest after rupture of an abscess.[69] The word next appeared three years later in a passage pertaining to body temperature written by the aforementioned physician nephew.[70] Langstaff himself used the word to describe a temperature some four months after that.[71] From then on, 'normal' appeared occasionally, usually in the context of temperature measurement. 'Natural' seems to have pertained to a range of different conditions, but 'normal,' which refers to a precise norm, possibly even a numerical indicator such as temperature, seems to have accommodated less variation, thereby tending to narrow and facilitate the definition of health. Whatever may be the epistemological and psychological significance of this tiny shift in nomenclature, its appearance in the language of this physician suggests a causal link to the increasing use of instruments in medical practice.

Always fond of evocative images, Langstaff was most eloquent in his description of physical signs. The heart could be 'tumultuous' and 'boisterous,' or a murmur 'like strong milking into a frothy pail of milk'; and a rattle in the chest was 'louder than I've ever heard, like pouring potatoes down boards into a sellar [sic].'[72] A man who had ridden to Scarborough in a winter wind of the southwest had a 'face mottled like cheese.' An inflamed mouth 'looked as if seared with [a] hot iron.' A convalescent patient sat by the 'hot stove' with a 'singular expression of [his] countenance.' Another, who 'ate 24 oysters' on the previous night, had 'very offensive' breath that could be 'smell[ed] across the room.' An old man, treated aggressively by another doctor, had been 'purged and puked severely'; a one-and-a-half-year-old child, similarly mismanaged for some time, was like 'a skeleton ... crying, the picture of distress.'[73] In a few words, Langstaff conveyed a vivid impression of the scenes that confronted him: the 'perfect quiet' in the room of a seriously ill child; the stretching figure of a woman in her 'death struggle' from some sudden and unexplained cause; his pleasant surprise the moment he arrived to visit a young girl who, for months, had lain 'on the lounge' and found her up, playing 'on the melodeon, her brother working the pedals.'[74]

A medically qualified person cannot read these documents without attempting to 'diagnose' Langstaff's complete descriptions, even if such a diagnosis was not established until long after the doctor's death. The vivid accuracy of his clinical narrative, often more than sufficient to allow for a modern diagnosis, proclaims Langstaff's excellent powers of observation. This is not to suggest he deserves priority for the physical signs described later by others: he did not publish his descriptions; more important (and possibly also a reason for not publishing), he usually failed to connect them to the underlying condition. Nevertheless, his clinical observations, at least four of which had been made without the prior sensitization of gaze that follows a classic description, serve to situate this country doctor in the intellectual centre of his medical milieu. Several examples are cited.

An elderly woman who 'sometimes stop[ped] breathing as if dead for a minute' clearly demonstrated Cheyne-Stokes respiration, a periodic irregular breathing pattern suggestive of a problem with neurological control; Langstaff did not use the word 'periodic,' but he may have read or heard of this sign, which had been published during his training.[75] For an unconscious man who lay dying on Christmas Day 1886, Langstaff wrote that his family had given up, yet he was 'blowing breath whole length of bed. A well man could not blow harder.'[76] This seems to be Kussmaul's breathing, indicative of diabetic ketoacidosis, which had been described in the German literature just twelve years before. A woman with pain and vomiting was found to have an enlarged liver and a palpable gall-bladder and may have demonstrated Courvoisier's sign of pancreatic cancer, thirty-six years before its publication.[77] Several patients in the Langstaff daybooks had illnesses suggestive of appendicitis, but a man who was 'tender in one spot' in the right lower abdomen had the unmistakable sign of acute appendicitis – pain at the precise spot known as McBurney's point – described twenty-eight years later, in the year of Langstaff's death.[78] A fifteen-year-old youth who was six feet two inches tall and had dropsy of the abdomen and another young man described as a 'strippling with heart disease' both seem to have suffered the developmental condition that would come to be called Marfan's syndrome,

after the doctor who first wrote about it two decades later.[79] Thrice
Langstaff described numbness and partial palsy involving the limbs
of people who had suffered influenza, which most likely represented
the infectious polyradiculoneuritis described by G. Guillain, J.A. Barré,
and A. Strohl in 1916.[80] Finally, the 'small lumps on tendons of wrists
and about joints of fingers' of a boy with rheumatic heart disease are
without doubt examples of Osler's nodes, observed by Langstaff when
William Osler was still a boy of ten living at the Bond Head rectory a
few miles away.[81]

❦

Langstaff's diagnostic practice reflected the preoccupation of the academic physicians of his era, with its emphasis on internal organic
explanation for sickness. He relied on a careful patient-history and
physical examination and tried to integrate his knowledge of anatomy
and physiology with the clinical situation. From the outset of his
career he made precise observations about the patient's condition
and changing behaviour, measured pulse and respiration, and used
percussion and auscultation; however, the record also shows that he
made at least one change in vocabulary and learned to use new
instruments, especially the thermometer and urinometer. Innovation
in his diagnostic practice was owing to the influence of younger
colleagues, the medical literature, and social factors such as the examinations of apparently healthy people required by life insurance
companies.

CHAPTER FOUR

Medical Knowledge in Therapy:

Old Stand-bys, Innovations, and Intangibles

The history of medical therapeutics was long ignored by medical historians, partly because much of the therapy given by doctors in the previous century was considered to be worthless or even harmful in the present. Only recently have scholars sought to understand the social and medical reasons why dangerous drugs and practices were commonly used and to document the extent of their use.[1] An image of the caring, patient pioneer-doctor, who had little to offer but his presence, has been dispelled by studies of prescribing practice that show nineteenth-century doctors tended to use large numbers of different medications, sometimes several drugs at a time.[2] John Harley Warner has demonstrated that use of remedies with very strong side effects slowly declined over the course of the century. There may have been a variety of reasons for the change in prescribing practice, including increasing therapeutic scepticism as a manifestation of so-called scientific medicine and competition from unorthodox practitioners who used milder forms of treatment.[3] In the second half of the century several new agents with specific physiological actions were introduced. The Langstaff daybooks afford an opportunity to examine if and how an individual practitioner, who rarely left home, responded to the trends of his era with respect to both giving up the old remedies and adopting the new. The record shows that he did accept some of the changes embraced by large groups of his contemporaries.

Langstaff prescribed medications to nearly every patient he saw. This is not to suggest that the less tangible manifestations of his care, such as psychological support, were unimportant; they were important, but they operated in conjunction with numerous material therapies. Langstaff's prescriptions of drugs increased over the four decades of practice from 59 to 72.1 per cent of all visits (Table 4.1). He rarely gave medication to surgical and obstetrical cases; if they are excluded, the proportion of patients receiving drugs is much higher. Most often he simply wrote 'Med.' to indicate a drug had been left, but sometimes he supplied the names and dosages of the medications given (Appendix E). Unfortunately, however, only qualified conclusions can be drawn about the frequency of drug use, as he became decreasingly diligent about recording details of his prescriptions. He named the remedies in one-quarter of his early cases and in only one-tenth of the later.[4] Thus, in reconstructing Langstaff's pharmacopoeia, we can identify only the most commonly *mentioned* drugs, which may not have been the most commonly used drugs in each decade (Table 4.2). It is possible that Langstaff was more careful to record use of highly active drugs as opposed to less toxic remedies, which sometimes appear simply with nondescript indicators such as 'bottle,' 'pills,' or 'laxative.' If so, the list of frequently mentioned drugs may indeed contain a measure of the relative use of strong remedies one to another, but there is little evidence to endorse or refute such an assumption.

Langstaff obtained his drugs from pharmacists in Toronto, with whom he appears to have kept running accounts. The few surviving bills reveal that he stocked up on his medicines at infrequent intervals and sometimes sent his students to collect the orders.[5] The doctor probably made the final preparation of pills and liquid mixtures himself from his supplies. Occasionally, he wrote that he had wished to use a certain drug but had none left.

In the 1850s, quinine was the most commonly recorded drug in the first five years of Langstaff's practice, in keeping with the prevalence of malaria or ague in his region. Prescriptions peaked in the late summer and fall, reflecting the activity of ague-bearing mosquitoes, but patients suffered recurrent fever even in late winter. Ironically, Langstaff once gave quinine, which was later shown to cause bleed-

TABLE 4.1
Visits, prescriptions, and identification of medications in Langstaff's practice

	1850s	1860s	1870s	1880s
Total number of visits	7,265	3,423	10,472	5,477
Visits with a prescription	4,288	2,150	7,125	3,951
Percentage of all visits	59	62.8	68	72.1
Prescriptions identified	1,839	475	687	356
Percentage of all prescriptions	42.9	22.1	9.6	9

Source: All entries in Langstaff's daybooks for 1849–54, 1861, 1872–5, 1880–2

TABLE 4.2
Ten therapies most frequently mentioned by Langstaff in each decade (descending order)

1850s	1860s	1870s	1880s
1 Quinine	Opium	Cupping	Cupping
2 Opium	Tartar emetic	Opium	Opium
3 Venesection	Cupping	Milk	Tartar emetic
4 Tartar emetic	Quinine	Tartar emetic	Chloroform
5 Calomel	Blister-plasters	Alcohol	'Stop' order
6 Blister-plasters	Calomel	Bromide	Bromide/Ergot
7 Ipecac	Venesection	'Stop' order	Aconite
8 Cupping	'Stop' order	Venesection	Chloral hydrate
9 Iron	Ipecac	Chloral hydrate	Enema
10 Jalap	Alcohol	Chloroform	Milk

Source: All entries in Langstaff's daybooks for 1849–54, 1861, 1872–5, 1880–2

ing problems, to a patient with bruising.[6] From the 1870s the drug appears not to have been used for fever, but as a strengthening tonic, almost always in conjunction with iron.

Langstaff used opium, a narcotic extracted from the poppy, for pain relief, sedation, control of diarrhoea, and suppression of cough. It appears to have been the most commonly recorded drug in the later part of his practice. He knew that its side-effects included constipation, stomach upset, drowsiness, contracted pupils, stupor, and slow breathing. When patients were in great pain, Langstaff 'left plenty of opium.' He tolerated coma in 'narcotized' patients, especially if he thought they were dying.[7] Opium's analgesic power was welcomed by patients such as the woman who had accidentally burned her face and 'beseeched not to be left without her [opium] pills.'[8] The doctor's confidence in this drug remained constant throughout his practice: in 1886 he criticized himself for stopping it too soon in a woman suffering post-partum complications.[9]

Laudanum, another narcotic like opium, also appeared in the record, but less often. In at least half the cases of laudanum use, the drug seems to have been administered by the patient before the doctor arrived. Although addiction to this readily available remedy was recognized, there is nothing to confirm or deny Langstaff's awareness of the problem. He did, however, treat a child for an accidental overdose of laudanum; the outcome is unknown.[10] Occasionally, he prescribed it for pain, perhaps to avoid increased costs, if the patient already had some on hand. Once he claimed it cured hiccups that had lasted three days.[11]

The most commonly recorded drugs in the 1850s include jalap, calomel, and tartar emetic (antimony potassium tartrate), all strong remedies with violent side-effects. Medical historians have sometimes mocked these drastic therapies, but they may actually have had some benefit even if they were not always comfortable for the patient.[12] Charles E. Rosenberg has argued convincingly that physicians derived a prestige and authority from their knowledge of these drugs and their ability to manipulate the side-effects.[13] The long-recognized danger of overdose notwithstanding, and in keeping with Warner's observation that the use of drastic remedies declined in nineteenth-century American hospitals, a survey of the Canadian medical literature for the 1860s and 1870s seems to suggest an increasing number of publications on 'poisoning' by these previously well-established medications.

Calomel (mercurous chloride), a cathartic, was used for severe fevers, such as acute rheumatism and hepatitis, especially when accompanied by constipation.[14] Its side-effects included increased salivation, 'sore gums,' and characteristic odour of the breath, which Langstaff called 'mercurial fetor,' but unless it was severe, the toxicity did not cause him to stop the treatment. He was especially critical of overdose or inappropriate use of mercurials by some of his colleagues;[15] however, in the absence of their records, we should not conclude that other doctors were never given similar opportunities to criticize him. Perhaps in response to the advice given in the medical journals Langstaff read,[16] his use of calomel apparently declined – it was the fourth most commonly mentioned drug in the 1850s and one of the least-recorded drugs in the 1880s (mentioned once in two years). Nevertheless, Langstaff continued to use it in seemingly desperate situations until his final year of practice, and he recorded the toxicity of swollen gums in one of his patients as late as 1888.[17]

Jalap, another cathartic, nearly disappeared from the record between the first five years and the last decade of Langstaff's practice, when he occasionally prescribed it for intractable constipation. This drug had been a favourite of the pioneer physician-politician William 'Tiger' Dunlop (1792–1848), who counselled that it, together with calomel, should be given unstintingly to the new immigrants to ward off colonial ills.[18]

The numerous untoward side-effects of tartar emetic, including vomiting, painful diarrhoea, cardiovascular collapse, and death, had made it a controversial remedy for various fevers since its introduction in the sixteenth century.[19] Langstaff seems to have clung to this medication, despite its declining popularity elsewhere on the continent – it was the second or third most frequently recorded drug in every decade of his practice. He used it as a specific remedy for fever of any origin, especially in erysipelas and pneumonia. The dose was titrated according to the patient's condition; he advised families to continue if the patient was flushed and to stop if the patient became pale or cool. Vomiting and purging were accepted as anticipated signs of the drug's action, but occasionally he stopped the medicine when the patient vomited. He measured its benefits by slowing of the pulse and cooling of the skin. Langstaff gave minuscule doses to infants and children, with what he considered to be laudable results, even when he accidentally gave too much.[20] He sometimes observed improvement within an hour of administration.[21] Called at 11 p.m. to see Matthew Teefy's almost-three-year-old son, Baldwin, violently ill with fever, stiff neck, and vomiting – the ominous signs of meningitis – Langstaff prescribed tartar emetic. The next morning he reported that little Baldwin had 'vomited & purged severely,' but the child was convalescent; over the course of a month, during which the doctor made nineteen visits, he recovered completely.[22]

Bloodletting was an ancient technique that had enjoyed a certain revival in the late eighteenth and early nineteenth centuries, when it was promoted as a treatment for fever by influential physicians including Benjamin Rush and J.-B. Bouillaud.[23] Opponents of excessive bloodletting objected more to the removal of large quantities of blood than to the act of bleeding itself. Several techniques were used to let blood. First was venesection or phlebotomy, the method of extracting large quantities, usually from a vein in the arm, leg, or neck. Second, and equally ancient, was cupping, which allowed for the removal of small quantities of blood or the creation of a bruise through suction into heated, inverted jars placed over unprepared skin (dry cupping) or previously lanced skin (wet cupping). Finally was leeching, the removal of blood by the application of living leeches. This last method was almost negligible in Langstaff's practice. In Canada, leeches were difficult to obtain; the short supply was a source of complaint at the Toronto General Hospital in the 1850s.[24] Langstaff used leeches only once or twice in each decade and, in 1888, regretted that there were none available for a patient with an abdominal swelling.[25] On two occasions he applied leeches to ophthalmia (inflamed eyes), a common practice, since leeches would fit in awkward places around the swollen eye where cups could not.

Warner demonstrated a decline in all modalities of bloodletting in American hospitals and a decline in the practice as a whole.[26] Langstaff did not entirely conform to this trend. He bled his patients at a fairly constant rate of roughly twice a week; between 3.5 and 5 per cent of all his visits ended in a decision to let blood. Over the forty years of his career, however, there was a dramatic decline in phlebotomy as opposed to cupping (Table 4.3). In other words, the indications to bleed patients occurred just as frequently later in the practice, but the amount of blood removed in each treatment was less.

Nearly all Langstaff's bloodletting in the 1850s was by venesection, during which twenty ounces or even two quarts of blood were removed or the patient fainted, whichever came first. The patient was usually raised to a sitting or standing position to achieve the maximum effect with the least loss of blood. That venesection often produced immediate results tended to endorse its continued use. For example, in the case of fever, characterized by a rapid pulse and hot, flushed skin, venesection resulted in a slower pulse and a cool, clammy patient. There are many instances in which Langstaff found that it produced improvement. He also performed phlebotomy on cases of head injury resulting in loss of consciousness or seizures.

In the 1880s Langstaff preferred cupping; his choice seems to have been recommended by the 1866 textbook on surgery written by his fellow Canadian William Canniff.[27] Unlike his American colleagues, however, Langstaff clung to the value of bloodletting through cupping, which became the most commonly recorded therapeutic

TABLE 4.3
Average annual rate of bloodletting by venesection and cupping in Langstaff's practice

	1850s	1860s	1870s	1880s
Venesections/year	64.4	36	13	4.5
Cuppings/year	11	79	111	97
Total bleeding as a percentage of all visits	5.4	3.4	3.6	3.7

Source: All entries in Langstaff's daybooks for 1849–54, 1861, 1872–5, 1880–2

TABLE 4.4
Percentage of men, women, and children Langstaff treated by venesection or cupping

	1850s		1860s		1870s		1880s	
	Ven	Cup	Ven	Cup	Ven	Cup	Ven	Cup
Men	51	50.9	69.4	44.3	46.2	48.9	66.7	38.7
Women	32.6	32.7	13.9	19	35.9	30.9	22.2	53.6
Children	16.3	16.4	16.7	36.7	17.9	20.1	11.1	7.7
Total	100	100	100	100	100	100	100	100

Source: All entries in Langstaff's daybooks for 1849–54, 1861, 1872–5, 1880–2

manoeuvre in his last two decades, sometimes to be used several times in a single day. Nor did he totally abandon phlebotomy. As late as July 1888 he resorted to double venesection, first of sixteen ounces, then fourteen ounces, in the dire pneumonia of a woman, whose lips were blue from lack of oxygen and who had a temperature of 102.5 and a pulse of 122. After the bleeding Langstaff noted that her 'pulse got quicker for a time, but she felt a great deal better.' She appears to have survived.[28]

Langstaff seems to have used a physiological concept of heat-reducing and pressure-releasing to understand the mechanism of the action of bloodletting; he related it to the natural bleeding of menstruation and birthing. For a man with fever and headache, he wrote cryptically about 'determination of the blood to the head.' Following a birth he seemed not too concerned by 'a little flowing' of blood, because the woman's 'system was very full of blood.' A twenty-six-year-old married woman who had never had children consulted him for severe headache and 'convulsions'; she volunteered that she was

Figure 4.1 Langstaff's bleeding practice by decade, age, and sex (average no. of interventions/year)

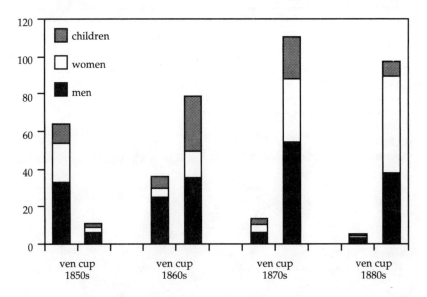

ven = venesection or phlebotomy
cup = cupping

'subject to' headache and scant menses, but that her headache was less when her periods were heavy. Langstaff made many visits to her home and noticed that when the headache was severe, her head was hot and her veins prominent. After sixteen days he decided to bleed her by applying cupping jars to the temple; incidentally 'a very small artery was cut and spun out' and the subsequent loss of three ounces of blood provided 'great relief.' Langstaff observed that the headaches recurred following 'her turns' in later months.[29]

Theories that seek to explain bloodletting include anthropological analyses that suggest it may have had a symbolic value as a form of artificial menstruation – a drastic intervention best suited for men.[30] Langstaff's practice tends to support this theory: he used venesection and cupping on patients of both sexes and all ages; however, he tended to phlebotomize men more often than adult women or children, and in his cupping practice also there was a slight predominance of treated males (Table 4.4 and Figure 4.1). His growing fondness for cupping seems to stand in contrast to Warner's findings for two large American hospitals, only one of which displayed a transient upsurge of the method during the 1860s; however, Warner studied male patients only and gender may have played a role in cupping too. Perhaps there was an additional cultural stimulus for the use of cupping; if, for example, it had been a more popular folk remedy in Canada than it was in the United States, then the doctor might have been more inclined to select it.

Manipulation of diet was an equally venerable aspect of therapeutics. The decline, in Langstaff's records, of the more aggressive therapies coincides with a relative rise in the importance of diet. For example, milk, cold or boiled, diluted or straight, was the second most cited 'drug' in the 1870s. Beef tea, chicken broth, and a beer and egg concoction were viewed as 'nourishing' supplements for patients wasted from diarrhoea or long-standing fever.

Langstaff also made use of plasters and poultices, sometimes medicated with irritating substances to cause a blister. Like cupping, these blisters were theoretically intended to pull the inflammatory substances away from the vital organ into the skin. The details are too sparse to determine his opinion in the controversy over the ideal position of blisters or cups on the same or opposite side of the body from the affected part. Mustard and cantharides (a powder made of 'Spanish flies') were among the most commonly mentioned preparations. Rarely, Langstaff used setons, by inserting 'linnen [sic] threads' through soft tissues like the scrotum to promote drainage of swelling.[31] As with other active treatments, records concerning blister-causing plasters were commonly mentioned in the 1850s but appeared only once in the 1880s.

Langstaff once wrote, 'fever cases in children are all disposed to cold feet.'[32] In the management of fever, especially in children, he relied on physical methods to cool the head and warm the feet. This was intended to prevent confusion and convulsions, which were common complications of uncontrolled fever. Thus, he shaved or clipped the hair to an inch in length, applied 'cold to the head' (with snow or ice), and put mustard plasters on the feet. This response was standard throughout his practice; however, there seems to have been a technological modification. In July 1871 he first spoke of 'showering' the head; in 1873 he specifically mentioned using a 'shower meter for about a half hour' in a child with a bulging fontanelle, an unmistak-

able sign of increased intracranial pressure, which for Langstaff indicated brain fever or meningitis.[33] Thereafter, the new technique was
a regular feature of Langstaff's fever management. Concerning one
recovered patient he wrote, 'showering was the main thing that saved
her.'[34]

Other old remedies appeared regularly in the Langstaff record,
including a wide variety of enemas and laxative preparations such as
aloes, asafoetida, castor oil (ricini), Chinese rhubarb (rhei), croton oil
(tigli), magnesium (Epsom salts), potassium bitartrate, and senna.
Although no single purgative was the most commonly cited drug, all
laxatives combined were mentioned as frequently as opium. A syrup
made from the bulb of the scilla plant was commonly used to favour
expectoration. For asthmatics and patients with tenacious sputum,
Langstaff prescribed the narcotic-like 'stramonium seeds,' to be
smoked like tobacco. He found that one dying patient could not 'do
without' his stramonium.[35]

Langstaff was an advocate of temperance, but he made liberal use
of alcohol as a medication. He and his contemporaries considered it
a stimulant and sometimes gave it to arouse patients slipping into
death-like coma. Gin, beer, cider, wine, whisky, rum, and above all
brandy appear in a variety of forms, often mixed with honey or milk
to form a punch. Once he used whisky as there was 'no brandy to be
had.'[36] On at least two occasions he used punch for cases of delirium
tremens.[37] If a patient became flushed or agitated, then the alcohol
was discontinued. The doctor saw these effects often, although he
once noted, 'some say it does not affect a sick man.'[38]

Disagreement with patients and other physicians over the indications for alcohol therapy occurred, but even Langstaff's most temperance-minded colleague, Dr John N. Reid, would resort to brandy
for the desperately ill.[39] Once Langstaff, normally so opposed to drink,
'drove up to [Victoria] Square and got a bottle of beer' for a man
dying of bloating and diarrhoea, even though he 'had the look of a
broken down drunkard.' 'Beer is his favourite drink,' the doctor wrote,
but before offering it to the sick man he mixed it with egg.[40] Was the
small shopping expedition designed to fulfil the patient's last wish
or the doctor's final prescription?

Langstaff was certain that in select cases alcohol was beneficial. A
little girl 'would have died but for giving the punch freely.'[41] Sometimes the anti-alcohol convictions of the patients or their attendants
outstripped those of the doctor and prevented the use of alcohol as a

remedy. For one man, Langstaff wrote, 'I ordered brandy but they would not give it and hardly make the punch strong enough to my notion.'[42] He wrote that a woman who 'got set against taking brandy' downed some of her mother-in-law's 'strong drink of currant preserve' and 'says she feels better, but all the symptoms [are] worse.'[43]

Patients' lack of compliance with medical treatment was not confined to the use of alcohol. The doctor was often faced with those who would 'not follow directions': from a little child with diphtheria who 'caught the medicine spoon and threw it on the floor' to an old man who, when cupped, 'cried out to have it off that he'd rather go to Kingdom come.'[44] Seeming to deny their illness, some patients refused to stay in bed: one man was 'determined to have his vest on and got up'; another insisted on 'walking out of doors and with bare feet on the floor.'[45] The old and sick sometimes refused care, Langstaff said, because they were 'childish' or exhausted.[46] Still others misinterpreted his motives: after he had carefully scraped caked-on secretions from the teeth of a young woman, he overheard her tell an attendant that he 'had tried to cut her throat.'[47] Langstaff's notes suggest some frustration, especially when he considered 'discontinuing as they do not go according to orders.'[48] Only for children did he insist that therapy be given: when an 'emaciated' child would 'not take any nourishment but potatoes,' he recommended the family 'put milk down it by force.'[49]

Some people in the community, like the woman to whom Langstaff provided her 'first doctoring in about 40 years,'[50] may never have felt a need to consult the doctor; others may have had an intrinsic fear of him and preferred their own medications. Folk remedies were reported in all decades, including the topical applications of quack plaster, carrot poultice, slippery elm, goose grease and onions, hen's fat, chicken weed, and weasel skin, as well as beverages of nature wine, mayweed, pumpkin seed tea, and cold cow's milk. Some preparations could be obtained for a modest price at Teefy's general store; in certain seasons, the postmaster seems to have done a roaring trade in liniment and gargling oil for the soothing of throats and the preservation of voice, the latter a commodity valued by Langstaff's lawyer, even in summer. Rarely did the doctor indicate his opinion concerning these practices; possibly he expected and condoned them or was simply resigned to their inevitable use.[51]

Despite his fondness for some older remedies, Langstaff did keep abreast of medical innovation. Evidence suggests that he learned about these remedies from the medical journals to which he subscribed (Table 4.5). His pharmacopoeia came to contain several drugs that were relatively new to orthodox medicine: anaesthetics, aconite, bromides, carbolic acid, chloral hydrate, digitalis, ergotamine, morphine, and salicylates. He also adopted electrotherapy. The dates Langstaff first recorded using these items allow measurement of the delay between discovery and his own inclination to apply innovations and suggest that he was somewhat hesitant; however, the delay between the original discovery and its presentation in the Canadian journals was almost always longer than the delay between the latter and Langstaff's first use. Comments in the daybooks about new remedies reveal a range of reactions, from enthusiasm to caution and even scepticism. (Anaesthesia and carbolic acid will be discussed in chapter 7, ergotamine in chapter 8.)

Digitalis, a derivative of foxglove, had been brought into orthodox medical practice in the late eighteenth century by William Withering (1741–99), who touted its value as a diuretic in relieving cardiac dropsy (now called heart failure). Withering had learned about its properties from proponents of a folk remedy based on the secret recipe of 'an old woman in Shropshire.'[52] Many nineteenth-century clinicians, including Laennec, remained unconvinced of the value of foxglove and were wary of its strong side-effects.[53] Langstaff seems to have been in this category. He mentioned digitalis only on rare occasions and, in almost every case, in order to draw attention to its dangers, some of which are no longer considered part of its toxicity. Once he noticed that a patient's blood was 'very dark from digitalis' and said that it 'seems to produce considerable narcotic effect.'[54] Records of the use of digitalis decrease from the original eight times a year in 1851 to once a year in the 1880s. The decline seems to be more than simply an artefact of his record-keeping and may represent his actual practice, as he claimed to have seen severe side-effects, including nervousness and convulsions. He also recognized the toxic effects of 'unequal pulse' and stomach upset, to which he seems to have been sympathetic to the point of discontinuing treatment.[55] Langstaff never overcame his apprehension about digitalis; even in the last decade of his practice, he criticized colleagues for prescribing 'heavy dangerous doses.'[56] One source of change in Langstaff's practice and his scepticism are apparent in his sarcastic account of a therapeutic choice for a man with severe tuberculosis: '[He is] taking digitalis equal to ten minims of the tincture every two hours. The other two medical

TABLE 4.5
Dates of innovation, appearance in Canadian literature, and first mention by Langstaff

	Approximate clinical début	Canadian literature	Langstaff's practice
Diagnostics			
Stethoscope	1816	1821	1849
(flexible)	1843		1865
Microscope	1830s	1860s	1879
Thermometer	1868	1860s	1878 (1881)
Ophthalmoscope	1851	1873	1886
Therapeutics			
Aconite	1830s	?	1858
Bromide	1857	mid-1860s	1869
Chloral hydrate	1868	1870	1872
Salicylate	1874	1876	1878
Electromagnetism	1820s	1861	1861 (1868)
Surgery			
Ether	1846	1847	1850
Chloroform	1847	1848	1857
Carbolic acid	mid-1867	1867 (Dec.)	1868 (Aug.)

men approve of it and as so many medical men are now advocating digitalis as a heart tonic, I submitted my judgment to theirs, thinking ultimate recovery about hopeless and wishing evidence for my own satisfaction. They held that it would 'slow that heart.' He died in the evening ... '[57] Despite an initial increase in pulse, the drug was ultimately so effective in fulfilling its physiological promise that it 'slowed that heart' to a stop. Digitalis was an innovation Langstaff did not adopt.

Morphine, a powerful opium derivative, was first isolated in 1806 and had been introduced prior to Langstaff's medical studies; however, it was slow to replace opium. As late as 1855, Toronto doctors were uncertain of the right dose – and their ignorance sometimes had tragic results.[58] Langstaff seems first to have used morphine powder in early 1851 and then only two or three times a year, reserving it for patients with intractable pain.[59] He once applied it to a case of hepatitis with jaundice,[60] a gesture that would now be considered inappropriate; however, most of the patients given this drug received it as palliation for terminal illness. For example, a young girl who suffered 'horrid pains' possibly from what might later be called appendicitis was given 'all the morphia she will bear.'[61]

Aconite, a 'powerfully poisonous alkaloid,' is derived from wolfsbane, a medicinal plant with a long and colourful history, from which the active ingredients were chemically extracted in the late eighteenth century.[62] This drug, which was thought to be narcotic, sudorific, and anti-inflammatory, could slow the pulse and was therefore known as a 'cardiac sedative.' Aconite was unusual in that it was adopted by homeopathic practitioners before it became popular with their regular counterparts; its origins may have accounted for the slowness of its rise to predominance between the early 1840s and the late 1860s.[63] Warner has shown that while it was used in two American hospitals in the 1830s and 1840s, there had been a resurgence in its popularity in the 1850s and 1860s through a reappreciation of its physiological properties.[64] Langstaff first used aconite as a specific remedy for rheumatism in March 1858. He reported that it 'had a powerful effect' on the first patient: 'she felt as large as a house' and 'looked strange,' but she recovered.[65] He encountered cases in which aconite 'almost entirely banished the pain,' or made 'cheerful' those in misery with arthritis, or 'began to tell on' (improve) hearts tainted with murmurs.[66] He recognized its side-effects, including 'prickling in the skin,' vomiting, and debility.[67] A recurrence of disease was attributed to a patient's having 'slackened' the dose because he had been 'unable to bear aconite.'[68] Langstaff expected aconite to work quickly: one child was 'running about' after only two days of treatment. Perhaps encouraged by their early symptomatic response, other patients continued to give themselves this medicine, even when the doctor told them to stop.[69] In severe cases Langstaff gave the drug at hourly intervals, expecting improvement within a day but continuing therapy in the absence of response up to four days later.[70]

Although reports of the effects of potassium bromide on animals can be traced to the early 1840s, its clinical use in epilepsy was first published in 1857.[71] It had appeared in American hospital prescriptions in the 1860s;[72] scattered reports about its applications and dangers appeared in the Canadian medical literature from the the middle of that decade. Langstaff used potassium bromide on rare occasions in the early 1870s, first as an analgesic and later for the treatment and prevention of convulsions, sometimes in women who had had seizures at earlier deliveries.[73] It quickly became one of the most frequently mentioned remedies in his record. Bromides later posed a serious problem to the general population as they were a component of patent medicines and could lead to addiction and serious side-effects. There is no evidence that Langstaff was aware of these potential dangers.

Chloral hydrate, another sedative, was synthesized by Justus von Liebig (1803–73) in 1831, the same year he synthesized chloroform, but its popularity soared after it was touted as a new hypnotic by Oscar Liebrich in 1868. It first appeared in American hospitals in the 1870s. Warner has suggested that, more than any other drug, chloral hydrate was both product of and 'harbinger for the fulfilment of experimental science's promise to bring about a therapeutic renaissance.'[74] In keeping with the stellar expectations elsewhere, the *Canada Medical Journal* broke its silence on the topic in 1870–1 with no fewer than eleven items in a single volume concerning 'chloral's' many applications.[75] Warsh has demonstrated that chloral hydrate prescriptions increased in Canadian institutions when the use of alcohol as medical treatment came under attack from the temperance movement.[76] Langstaff seems first to have used chloral hydrate in July 1872, in the same decade it appeared in American hospitals. He used it for analgesia as well as for sedation. It was among the ten most commonly mentioned drugs in the last two decades of his practice.

Salicylates, one of which is the familiar preparation called 'aspirin,' are derived from the bark of the willow tree. Such derivatives had been known to produce a soothing effect in antiquity, but the properties were rediscovered in the eighteenth century and promoted in chemically treated form in the late nineteenth. In 1874 a method was discovered for producing large quantities of salicylic acid.[77] Langstaff first mentioned using a salicylate ('of soda') for rheumatism in February 1878; on the second occasion, he thought it 'may not have checked' his patient's pain.[78] Throughout the last decade of his practice, this remedy appears only rarely, and exclusively for joint symptoms associated with rheumatism.

Various forms of electricity and 'galvanism' had been used in medical practice since the early nineteenth century, but the technique enjoyed a certain revival in the late 1860s. Although usually reluctant to employ new drugs, Langstaff seems to have been in the forefront of Canadian electrotherapy, since he purchased 'galvanic soles' and an 'electric machine' in 1861.[79] Special clinics were developed for this modality in the later nineteenth century, such as the 'Electro-Therapeutic Institute' on Toronto's Jarvis Street, which was operated from the mid-1870s to 1882 by Canada's first licensed woman doctor, Jenny Trout.[80] After his first application of the battery, Langstaff displayed a certain feeling of reservation, in writing that the patient's painful urination was 'not worse after jolting.'[81] Nevertheless, in the 1870s he used his 'galvanic battery' on just under one per cent of his patients, adults and children, for painful joints, neuralgia, and paralysis. In March 1867 he seems to have acquired a new model, for which he paid thirty-five dollars through his medical student William Comisky; but this instrument required repairs within the year.[82] He carried the equipment with him on house calls and occasionally left it at a patient's house.[83] In a single twenty-four-hour period he used the battery on four different people; the suggestion is that he may have made special 'electric rounds' on certain select cases.[84] Although the most common indication was joint pain, Langstaff 'electrified' his patients for migraine ('hemicrania'), sore eyes, torticollis, paralysis, and coma. Most people could bear the effects 'pretty well,' but one child started to cry and a woman whom he had treated 'pretty strongly' on the leg and hands felt tingling in her neck.[85] There was a slight decline in the records of electrotherapy, from 0.9 per cent of all visits in the 1870s to 0.2 per cent in the 1880s. For a few of the early patients Langstaff noted immediate relief,[86] but the later records do not reveal the outcome and display neither enthusiasm nor contempt for the method.

Langstaff believed in the value of his therapy, especially the drugs and bleeding, and he attributed most of his successes to them. 'She feels like another woman,' he wrote of a 'relieved' patient; occasionally he used phrases like 'I cured him twenty years ago by cupping.'[87] Many times he wrote that his medicine had 'acted like a charm' or 'entirely banished' symptoms. Occasionally he observed that when patients ran out of pills their problems returned: a woman was 'without the med last night [and her] cough was like to kill her.'[88] The controversial tartar emetic given to an unconscious man 'soon brought him to' and made a child with headache 'distinctly better' in less than an hour.[89] The family of a baby who had been 'blue' with bronchitis before receiving the drug 'wonder[ed] at the change.'[90] To the late twentieth-century reader some of these remarks resonate with grim irony: 'I got there in time to save her,' he wrote of an elderly woman bleeding from a cancerous bowel.[91]

The doctor's confidence in his ability to help the sick led him to blame the attendants if they did not call him as soon as they had promised should there be any change.[92] He was highly critical of 'Mrs Winslow's soothing syrup,' which in one case, he said, 'had something to do with' the death of a child, who 'just pined away.'[93] He also expressed annoyance when families altered or failed to give the drugs as he had prescribed, or when they administered other remedies without telling him. When he discovered that a father had been giving opium at hourly intervals to his sick boy, Langstaff wrote, 'no wonder he vomits.' Similarly, he criticized the medications other doctors had given: the man 'has been purged and puked severely,' he said of a colleague's care.[94] As these were medicines he himself used in other cases, it seems he may have been troubled more by the patient's lack of allegiance than by the choice of the therapy. These qualifiers usually appeared in records of cases with unhappy outcomes.

Just as he blamed the families or other doctors for giving certain treatments, he sometimes blamed himself for not doing so, or for not insisting. When one man died, Langstaff wrote that he had taken 'none of my medicine ... would not have happened if he had sedatives.'[95] He became increasingly diligent, especially in the second decade, about noting when he told the family to stop a drug; on several occasions he wrote that he had given no medication at all. In fact, orders to 'stop' medication increased slowly over the last three decades, until they appeared as often as the five most commonly prescribed drugs (see Table 4.2). This may have been a response to the numerous malpractice inquests in Toronto during the 1850s. In his last decade Langstaff recorded actually throwing medicine away when the family would not discontinue it.[96]

In the later years a few scattered comments about drugs and other therapies hint at an increasing therapeutic scepticism. Almost all such remarks are directed against specific treatments, especially innovations. He claimed that they 'did no good' or 'were to no avail,' or doubted the value of an intervention. Once, he prescribed nothing: 'let her sleep without med if she can.'[97] However, Langstaff seems always to have been certain of his intangible but therapeutic role in providing information, reassurance, comfort, and social order, even if there was no medicine to recommend. When a man began working harder to cough up phlegm, Langstaff wrote, 'Spits more, perhaps from my encouraging him to be on the sounder side.'[98] Often he noted, 'mother frightened' or 'father alarmed' or 'they think he is dying,' as if the anxiety of the attendants were a reason for his concern.[99] When he stayed all night in a patient's home, he knew his presence could be comforting: after attending a young girl who had been sick for weeks, he wrote, 'I lay down for an hour and she became easier and slept some while I did.'[100] He stayed till daylight twice with a young man who imagined 'someone [was] abusing his horses': 'I told him he was dreaming & he quieted down.'[101]

Langstaff often recorded 'improved' or 'good spirits,' as if this were one of his objectives. 'I managed to make him smile,' he wrote of a man with typhoid; and another 'soon smiled' after the doctor washed his face.[102] It is clear that some patients asked him about their chances and others conveyed their presentiments of death. 'She asks if she's dangerous,' he said of a young woman with an 'anxious countenance,' soon to die of bronchopneumonia.[103] Some nineteenth-century physicians kept bad news from their patients, fearing that psychological depression could damage their chances for physicial recovery; Langstaff seems to have differed. He liked to see his patients happy and recognized the negative effects of fear, but in most cases he answered their questions truthfully. 'It is understood there is great danger of life,'[104] he wrote of the household where a little boy lay ill; and for a young woman with consumption,' I gave her to understand she was not likely to live.'[105] Although the doctor seems not to have spent much time with cancer and tuberculosis patients, this may well have been due to a lack of summons, since palliation also appears to have been important to him. On occasion he went to patients simply 'to ease [their] dying.'[106] Since untended material concerns could be detrimental to peace of mind, Langstaff made sure that his adult patients put their affairs in order, became disturbed if they had not,[107] and several times helped 'draw' a patient's will.[108] 'Has said she is prepared to die,' he reported of a woman in extremis; clearly, his assessment of this composure applied to the patient's emotional, spiritual, and legal state as well as to her bodily decline.[109]

When there was a death, Langstaff sometimes went back to the house in the days that followed to tend the grief of the survivors.[110] Once he was asked to 'satisfy' a widow of the cause of her husband's death; on another occasion, to encourage a widow to eat. Virtually all such visits were to bereaved mothers and widows; none appear to have been made to men.[111] Here too his involvement was medical as well as social: Matthew Teefy, members of the doctor's family, and many other people in the community well understood that, like a painful and frightening disease, grief too could be lethal.[112]

Langstaff recognized the importance of psychological support for his patients, but he also relied heavily on drugs, bleeding, blisters, and other material treatments in all decades of his practice. Only tentative statements can be made about the frequency of his use of specific drugs, because he did not often record the names of the items prescribed. Nevertheless, analysis of the daybooks tends to suggest that he did follow the therapeutic trends of his era, with an apparent decline in the use of venesection and some strong drugs like the mercury-containing calomel, and with a parallel tendency cautiously to adopt some new remedies, like salicylate, aconite, bromides, and elecromagnetism, although he had little enthusiasm for morphine or digitalis. Langstaff seems to have been less hesitant about using new drugs than he was about using new diagnostic techniques, possibly because diagnostic innovations usually required the learning of skills in addition to the acquisition of a new instrument. His implementation of new treatments always followed a discussion of the innovation in the Canadian literature, a pattern suggesting that he read and learned from the medical journals he received. The continued presence in his records of drugs that were being displaced in other practices, such as tartar emetic and opium, implies that he was more ready to adopt new treatments than he was to abandon old standbys. Langstaff displayed confidence in most of his therapeutic decisions, but passages written in later years hint at some scepticism, especially about new pharmaceutical agents.

CHAPTER FIVE

Patients and Their Diseases:

Morbidity and Mortality in
Children and Adults

Sickness, injury, birth, and death were intimately woven into the social and cultural fabric of nineteenth-century Ontario life, and virtually all persons in the community – regardless of age, sex, or economic status – found they had need of the doctor at one time or another. In studying the diseases that afflicted any population, historians are not obliged to forget what they know now, but they must come to terms with the definitions and categories of illness used in the records of the past. Classification, or the grouping of diseases, tells us a great deal about the presumed causes of illness. Over the course of the nineteenth century, disease classification changed with increasing emphasis on the sciences of anatomy, physiology, and, later, bacteriology, but scholars have shown that social factors such as gender, race, and class have always had a profound influence on what was thought of as sick.[1] Nineteenth-century doctors were sometimes frustrated by the various possibilities for naming sickness and began to realize that the increasingly valued medium of medical statistics would have significance only when they could agree on what diseases were to be called. One of the first initiatives of the Ontario public health movement in the last decade of Langstaff's career was to establish a reliable classification and list of diseases that was to be applied to every death in the province.[2]

With the qualification that Langstaff lived in an era of shifting categories and that his name for a patient's condition might not correspond with our own, his record can be taken to be indicative of the pattern of diseases, or 'pathocoenosis,'[3] that characterized a rural Ontario community in the second half of the nineteenth century. The vast majority of diseases were febrile illnesses, recognizable, now if not then, as specific bacterial and viral infections; he also saw metabolic or degenerative diseases. The names Langstaff used in diagnosing these conditions are listed in Appendix F, but the classification he might have used for grouping diseases and possible changes in it cannot be derived from his record. The daybooks are written from the perspective of a doctor, but they do give some indication of what it was like to be sick. A blend of three methods will be used to examine his patients and the nature and severity of their diseases: first, analysis of the age and sex of Langstaff's patients; second, analysis of mortality and the causes of death; and third, presentation of some patient histories representative of various diseases. One striking aspect of this study is the great frequency of death and disease among children.

The number of different people Langstaff attended can be ascertained from a regrouping of the daybook entries from their original chronological order to alphabetical order by patient name (Table 5.1).[4] In the first decade, the number of people attended annually more than doubled, from just over four hundred individuals in 1851 to close to one thousand in 1861; thereafter, the yearly patient population was relatively stable, but not all patients were seen in all years and Langstaff was probably in a position to serve two to three thousand different persons at any one time. Most patients were descendants of the Scots and Pennsylvania German settlers. The prominent and well-to-do, like Colonel Bridgeford and W.W. Baldwin, were seen along with the poor, including unnamed shanty dwellers and fatherless children. Langstaff occasionally noted the presence of 'Indians,' Irish or English 'emigrants,' and 'blacks' or 'negroes,' but after the early 1870s, members of these groups were either no longer present or no longer remarkable.[5] Although he recorded the race of patients, he seems to have given non-whites the same attention as others.

The proportion of activity given to children, men, and married and unmarried women can be determined with some qualifications (Table 5.2). The doctor wrote the name of the head of the household only, as this was the person likely (or unlikely) to pay the bill for the sick

TABLE 5.1
Number of patients in Langstaff's practice in single years*

	1851	1861	1872	1882
Visits in the year	1,030	3,423	2,978	3,270
Individuals	410	940	954	1,046
Unspecified	26	3	0	0
Men	139	272	258	331
Women	144	342	351	400
Children	101	323	345	315
Average visits/person	2.5	3.6	3.1	3.1
Range of visits /person	1–20	1–118	1–45	1–58
Families	283	526	600	620
Anonymous	43	18	7	3
Family members	1–7	1–7	1–11	1–6
Average visits/family	3.6	6.5	5	5.3

* Based on individuals identified in the visits made during single years; the age and sex of some individuals could not be determined.

TABLE 5.2
Percentage of visits to men, women, and children

	1849–54	1861	1872–5	1882–3
Men	38.1	28.9	27.3	28.3
Married women	33.7	34.6	37.0	39.6
Unmarried women	6.8	4.1	6.9	9.7
Children	21.3	32.4	28.8	22.4

Source: All entries in Langstaff's daybooks for 1849–54, 1861, 1872–5, 1880–2.

relative. For example, 'Mrs Ben Jenkins,' 'Henry Miller child,' Watkin's ostler,' or 'Wilkie's negro.' He did record the sex of newborn infants, but the sex of other very young patients cannot be determined, since a little child was usually referred to as 'it.' Older children were referred to as 'boy,' 'son,' 'girl,' 'daughter,' or 'Miss.'

When the relative activity Langstaff gave to each of these groups, in both the first and the last decades, is compared with their percentage in the local population, it can be seen that married women consulted the doctor considerably more often than would be predicted; children and unmarried women, less often. The extra attention given

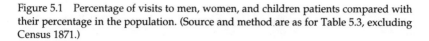

Figure 5.1 Percentage of visits to men, women, and children patients compared with their percentage in the population. (Source and method are as for Table 5.3, excluding Census 1871.)

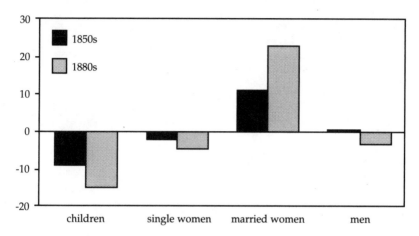

to women disappears when obstetrical activity is eliminated; the remaining visits to women are in proportion with their numbers in the population, a finding suggesting that women were just as likely as men to consult the doctor for non-obstetrical ailments. The proportion of visits to adult males was roughly the same as their proportion in the population (Table 5.3 and Figure 5.1).

Allegiance to a particular doctor may have constituted a statement about a doctor's method and style, but it was also related to genealogy and politics. Attention to friends and relatives made up a significant part of the doctor's early practice. He served all the Langstaffs, several in-laws in the Miller family, and the widow and children of the Reverend William Jenkins. He also assisted the wife of his old friend Benjamin Jenkins in her confinements; when her son, named James Langstaff Jenkins, grew to manhood, Langstaff attended his family too.[6]

In Langstaff's era the classification, diagnosis, and treatment of disease fell into the first of three branches of medical practice, called 'physic' or, more recently, 'internal medicine'; the other two branches

TABLE 5.3
Langstaff's activity for men, married women, unmarried women, and children relative
to their numbers in the population (in per cent)

	Men	Married women	Unmarried women	Children
1850s	0.3	10.3	-2.1	-8.6
1870s	-2.0	25.8	-3.1	-14.6
1880s	-3.4	23.2	-4.8	-15

Method:
[Percentage of Langstaff's visits to each group] - [percentage of each group in population]

Sources: All entries in Langstaff Daybooks for 1849–54, 1861, 1872–5, 1880–2; Census 1851 for York County (York East and York West combined); Census 1871 for York County (York East and York West combined); and Census 1881 for Richmond Hill, Vaughan, and Markham combined

were surgery and midwifery or obstetrics. From long before Langstaff's début in practice, doctors in Upper Canada were usually licensed in all three disciplines; specialists did not emerge until late in the century. Langstaff was licensed and practised in all three, but most of his activity was given to medical problems, such as fevers and specific epidemic or internal diseases. In Langstaff's career, medical care remained constant at nearly eighty per cent of his activity; surgical and obstetrical cases combined made up approximately twenty per cent of his visits, but over the forty years obstetrics increased slightly and surgery declined (Table 5.4). Langstaff's surgical activity, including the nature and extent of accidents and injuries, his obstetrical practice, including aspects of women's reproductive problems, and the cases of murder and infanticide will be discussed in chapters 7, 8, and 9.

A reading of the entire forty years of the Langstaff record uncovers information concerning the deaths of 535 patients, excluding stillbirths (see Figure 5.2). This number should not be taken to represent the true death rate, either in the community or in the practice: daybook entries for seriously ill patients sometimes simply cease, and deaths were not included in this analysis unless Langstaff had confirmed them by clearly indicating that the patient was actually 'dead' or 'sinking' or '*in articulo mortis*.' Some years saw much higher death rates than others; 'spikes' in the mortality curve appear approxi-

TABLE 5.4
Obstetrics, surgery, and medicine in Langstaff's practice (in per cent)

	1850s	1860s	1870s	1880s
Obstetrics	6.8	14.8	12.4	11.8
Surgery	10.7	7.4	5.4	6
Medicine	82.5	77.8	82.2	82.2

Source: All entries in Langstaff's daybooks for 1849–54, 1861, 1872–5, 1880–2

mately every ten years. These correlate with epidemics of scarlatina, erysipelas, and 'sore throat.' The last-named was probably the condition now called 'strep throat'; all three diseases are now known to be manifestations of infection by the streptococcus, a single bacterial group. In the year or two following those of high mortality, there was an apparent respite; perhaps survivors were resistant to further infection or perhaps virulent strains emerged at intervals.[7]

Of the 535 deaths, over forty per cent (218) were of children (Table 5.5). More than two-thirds of the paediatric deaths were caused by febrile illnesses, most the result of infections that can now be prevented by vaccination or cured with antibiotics. One-third were infections of the upper airway. After stillbirth, the second most common cause of death in children was diphtheria, which constituted nearly one-quarter of paediatric deaths. The three conditions now associated with streptococcal infection and its complications combined were third. Diarrhoea and unspecified fevers also claimed many young lives, but cancer, tuberculosis, and measles each took only one. Accidents, including trauma and poisonings, ranked fifth in causes of paediatric deaths. Four children of indeterminate age died suddenly without explanation, an observation inviting speculation that they may have succumbed to what is now called sudden infant death syndrome (SIDS).

As shown when the deaths are compared by decade, the most common cause of adult death was childbirth and its complications; pneumonia and pleurisy combined were second (Tables 5.6, 5.7). Deaths due to unexplained fevers, diarrhoea, and accidents were as common in adults as they were in children. No adults died in Langstaff's practice of diphtheria, croup, whooping cough, or measles; fewer than ten per cent of the streptococcal deaths were of adults. Deaths of children and newborns taken together with stillborns always constituted one-half to three-quarters of all the deaths recorded in

Figure 5.2   Deaths in Langstaff's practice, 1850-89 (excluding stillbirths). (Note that daybooks for part of 1854-5 are missing.)

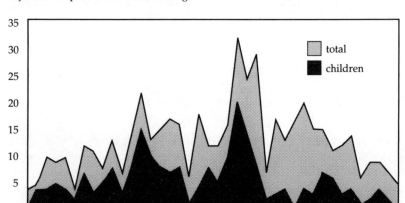

the practice. The single most common cause of death in every decade was stillbirth, which represented one-fifth to one-quarter of all deaths. If the annual paediatric death rate (childhood death and stillbirth combined) is expressed as a percentage of the average annual birth rate for the years analysed, it ranges between almost eleven per cent in the 1850s and 1860s to sixteen per cent in the 1870s and 1880s. Thus, a reasonably conservative estimate, based on these forty years of practice, suggests that one baby in six or seven did not survive childhood.[8]

Adult deaths comprised approximately half the deaths in Langstaff's practice in any given decade, but there was considerable discrepancy between the proportions of adults and children dying in the Langstaff records and those reported in the Canada Census for the years preceding 1851, 1861, and 1871 (Table 5.8): in the first two of these reports, the proportions of childhood deaths in Langstaff's immediate vicinity were even higher than those retrieved from the medical daybooks.[9] A search in the daybooks for visits to these persons shows that Langstaff attended an increasing proportion of all persons who had died in his region (from twenty-five to forty-eight per cent) and

TABLE 5.5

Causes of 535 deaths in adults and children, 1849–89 (excluding stillbirths)

	Adults	Children
Diphtheria, croup	0	52
Bronchitis	3	8
Whooping cough	0	3
Pneumonia, pleurisy, cough	32	11
Tuberculosis	19	1
Scarlatina, sore throat	1	27
Erysipelas	0	4
Fever	19	24
Diarrhoea	9	17
Other gastrointestinal (bleeding, vomiting, perforation of gut, liver disease, jaundice)	15	7
Obstetrical, toxemia, abortion	42	0
Meningitis	0	5
Accident	18	9
Heart	9	7
Alcohol	7	0
Suicide	8	0
Abscess/empyema	6	4
Cancer	11	1
Peritonitis	5	5
Renal, urinary	8	1
Typhoid	3	0
Stroke	10	0
Murder, infanticide	3	1
Iatrogenic*	5	3
Other or unknown	84	28
Total	317	218

* Some appear in other categories

Source: Langstaff's daybooks, 1849–89

a more rapidly increasing proportion of deceased children (from 13.6 to 40 per cent).

The change in these figures seems to reflect the community's rising trust in the doctor and the parents' increasing tendency to invite the doctor to attend their sick children. This trend may perhaps have been due to the impact of new attitudes towards childhood: certainly, a medical summons was tantamount to a financial commitment.[10] Comparing the incidence of childhood death in this practice

TABLE 5.6
Deaths in Langstaff's practice by age and sex

	1850s	1860s	1870s	1880s
Deaths (n)	49	17	99	42
Annual average (n)	9.8	17	33	21
Stillbirths (%)	20.4	17.6	16.2	23.8
Children (%)	36.7	47.1	36.4	26.2
Women (%)	26.5	11.8	22.2	30.9
Men (%)	16.3	23.5	25.3	19.1

Source: All entries in Langstaff's daybooks for 1849–54, 1861, 1872–5, 1880–2

TABLE 5.7
Causes of death in Langstaff's practice by decade

1849–54 Cause	(n)	1861 Cause	(n)	1872–5 Cause	(n)	1882–3 Cause	(n)
Stillbirth	10	Stillbirth	3	Stillbirth	16	Stillbirth	10
Fevers	8	Fevers	3	Fevers	9	Fevers	7
Pneumonia	7	Rheumatism	2	Obstetrical	9	Obstetrical	5
Obstetrical	6	Obstetrical	2	Diphtheria	8	Pneumonia	4
Diphtheria	5	Accident	1	Pneumonia	7	Scarlatina	3
Accident	3	Abscess lung	1	Diarrhoea	6	Diphtheria	2
Diarrhoea	3	Bronchitis	1	Peritonitis	5	Stroke	2
Kidney	1	Diarrhoea	1	Haemorrhage	5	Haemorrhage	2
Alcohol	1	Diphtheria	1	Accident	4	Heart	1
Sudden	1	Suicide	1	Liver	4	Cancer	1
Haemorrhage	1			Scarlatina	3	Diarrhoea	1
Heart	1			Cancer	3		
				Phthisis	2		
				Suicide	2		
				Rheumatism	1		
				Stroke	1		
				Smallpox	1		
				Heart	1		
Other or unknown	2		1		12		4
Total	49		17		99		42
Autopsies	3		3		5		0

Source: All entries in Langstaff's daybooks for 1849–54, 1861, 1872–5, 1880–2

TABLE 5.8
Deaths in the census for Langstaff's district and the proportion he attended*

	1851	1861	1871
Total deaths in regional census	36	16	31
Deaths/1,000 population	6.2	6.2	10.6
Children (%)	75**	81	48.4
Adults (%)	25	19	51.6
Deaths in census attended by JML	8	5	15
Percentage of all census deaths	22.2	31	48
Percentage of census child deaths	13.6	21	40
Percentage of census adult deaths	37.5	33	50

* 1881 Census deaths not available
** Includes stillbirths

Sources: Census 1851, c 11759–60, Vaughan Division II and Markham Division I; Census 1861, c 1088, 1089, Vaughan Division II and Markham Division III; Census 1871, c 9967, 9969, Vaughan Division II and Markham Division II; and Langstaff's daybooks, 11 Jan. 1851 to 11 Jan. 1852, 13 Jan. 1860 to 13 Jan. 1861, 2 April 1870 to 2 April 1871

with that reported for the local Census in the same years suggests that in the 1850s not all sick children received Langstaff's attention and that by the 1870s he was invited to attend terminally ill children almost as frequently as he was called to dying adults. Lending further support to this apparent difference in attendance on children and adults in the early period is the fact that he did attend the delivery of two male infants who died several weeks after their birth, according to the 1861 Census, but did not record having seen these infants in their last illnesses.[11]

Langstaff witnessed the death of approximately 0.5 to 2.5 per cent of his adult patients each year, but the risk of dying in any given year among Langstaff's child patients was always higher and ranged from 1.8 to 3.3 per cent (Table 5.9). This figure may reflect the fact that children succumbed more often and more easily than adults, but it could also indicate that families waited until the situation was relatively more desperate before consulting the doctor for their sick children. In other words, Langstaff's child patients may have been sicker than his adult patients.

The Langstaff daybooks offer an unusual glimpse, focused at a

TABLE 5.9
Approximate risk of dying among Langstaff's patients

	1850s	1860s	1870s	1880s
Children	1/35	1/40	1/30	1/57
Adults	1/70	1/100	1/40	1/64

Source: Derived from numbers of patients seen in each year and average annual death rate (Table 5.1 and 5.6)

tiny point in time and space, into biological and social aspects of the relationship between children and at least one adult.[12] Because the doctor's presence was determined by the parents or guardians and because he relied on such persons to effect his recommendations, a few other adults figure in his description. Children were important to the rural family economy and financial concerns may have determined whether or not they were given medical attention; however, this doctor and these parents were also aware of children as individuals, whose emotions they perceived and valued. As the son of a schoolteacher, an active Reformer, and a physician in a position to benefit monetarily from paediatric consultation, Langstaff may have started practice already committed to the new change in the status of the child, from an economic asset to a financial liability.

Langstaff seems to have been strict about his orders and stern with his advice, but he was not unmoved by the suffering of his small patients. He recorded their restlessness and certain ironies of behaviour: a young child who had been passing blood and shrieking took its medicine 'as if quite rational'; a child who had just had a seizure stretched and rubbed its eyes.[13] He listened to children and took their comments seriously. When one little girl 'would not have her tooth pulled,' Langstaff did not insist; of another he wrote, 'says she is better,' a contradiction of his clinical impression he apparently considered worth recording.[14]

The doctor spent time at the bedside and, if he could not remain, returned four or five times in a single day. He noticed an 'involuntary start' while he sat with a little girl.[15] He heard the content of children's fantasies and fears and documented their courage and their cries for mother. A little girl screamed because 'she fancied she saw snakes.'[16] Another had been terrified by a nightmare of a mad dog under the bed; Langstaff sat with her and 'persuaded her to sleep.'[17]

A confused little boy, who 'did not know his mother' and had 'struck his father in the face,' kept visualizing a 'rabbit popping out' from a crack in his ceiling; he eventually recovered.[18] Another 'hearty lad ... tried to whistle' through his scarlet-fever-induced delirium; Langstaff wrote, 'his face had colour to the last.'[19]

Testifying to poignant moments in the experience of the doctor are those recorded instances of eye contact with sick children. She 'held out her hand & looked anxiously into my face,' he wrote of a little girl, who died; of another, who also died,[20] 'she gave me one distinct intelligent look & fell at once again into the stupor.'[21] In writing about yet another little girl, whom Langstaff declared to be 'dying,' he said, 'she looked back over her shoulder at me'; these last words hint at how pleased the doctor might have felt when, three weeks later, he reversed his opinion and pronounced her 'convalescent.'[22]

Langstaff was frequently surprised by the resilience of his young patients: a baby who had been 'cross ... [now] lies in the cradle and smiles and seems comfortable'; a little boy who had suffered a 'great fever' was found 'sitting up in bed looking over his marbles'; another child made an 'astonishing' recovery and was 'running about with his playthings'; a baby whom the doctor believed would die slowly improved and looked 'bright and playful and smile[d].'[23]

Diphtheria was the most lethal and dreadful of all the grim diseases that attacked this community. An infectious disease now known to be caused by bacteria, it localizes in the nose and throat, where it forms a layer of pus and tissue called a 'false membrane,' which leads to an inability to swallow and thus to death by dehydration and suffocation. In Langstaff's experience, diphtheria came most commonly in the winter months, from late fall to early spring, but not in every year. In bad seasons affected families could lose one child after another. Langstaff witnessed the deaths of three or more children from diphtheria in each of the years 1859, 1863, 1866, 1873, 1874, 1879, and 1887. Other outbreaks, with apparently less mortality, occurred in 1860, 1861, 1873, 1876, 1880, and 1884. There seemed to be a respite in the one or two years following severe diphtheria outbreaks suggestive of naturally induced immunity; for example, in 1865 and from 1867 to 1869, no children died of this condition.

Langstaff based his diagnosis entirely on clinical appearances; there seems to have been considerable overlap between diphtheria and croup that sometimes extended into the diagnoses 'cough' and 'bronchitis.' The latter was supposed to be due to inflammation of the trachea (cynanche trachealis), identified by a characteristic barking cough. Thus, one sick child had 'croup,' while another in the same family had 'diphtherite,'[24] and the doctor once diagnosed 'croup following diphtherite.'[25]

Langstaff put children with croup or diphtheria to bed and insisted that they be kept warm. When a little boy with diphtheria went to the barn, he 'was sent right back'. The doctor's annoyance was apparent when he arrived to tend an affected family and found one of the patients 'running out in the snow.'[26] Both parents in this family also fell ill, as did seven of their children, four of whom died in the spring of 1863. Langstaff viewed early intervention as vital. When he observed a false membrane forming, he used a feather to apply iodine or a 'caustic' agent, such as silver nitrate, to 'scarify' the throat. If an abscess formed, he lanced it. He concentrated on alimentation, milk and other fluids, and gave the drug tartar emetic (antimony potassium tartrate) to those with high fever. In later years he began to use carbolic acid mouthwashes and only twice attempted tracheotomy (see chapter 7); otherwise, his fairly conservative approach to treatment seems to have changed little over the four decades of his practice.

Diphtheria could progress to 'closure of the larynx' and death by 'suffocation,' usually within five days.[27] Langstaff saw some little children die after only two days of sickness;[28] and the terminal illness of one infant lasted only twenty hours, four of which he spent at her side.[29] He attended these young patients up to five times a day by dropping in on them at the beginning and end of his day and by making quick visits as he passed near the home on his rounds. When members of a family sickened one after the other, the doctor became a frequent visitor in the home for weeks. Always on the lookout for favourable signs, he noted that these children could be hungry; he wrote how one little girl, who died three days later, 'asks for food but can't eat.'[30] Langstaff sat all night with a small boy and 'dropped a little cream into his mouth when asleep with his mouth open'; in the morning the child looked 'bright' and could 'sit up,' but he would take only cold water. He died that afternoon.[31]

In desperation family members gave their own treatments. Langstaff had been making regular visits to little Barbara for several days, paying special attention to her 'nourishment and warm drinks.' The family had asked him 'if she was past the worst,' but her illness continued. Langstaff tried to clear her choked airways by irrigating the upper passages with a syringe through a gum catheter inserted in one nostril. He arrived the following morning to find she had 'had a bad spell getting out deposit from [her] throat.' Langstaff's horror at the father's response was apparent in his note: 'he gave her a dose of COAL OIL! he said it would take rust off iron. I told him not to give it again. Great discharge of ropy mucus, mostly from nose, I think, as she sits up with her head back. Pulse still full & face a little flushed. Continue senna & drinks. She is drowsy today.' The girl died the following morning, of 'suffocation not debility,' Langstaff wrote, absolving the father of blame, but he added that she 'suffered greatly.'[32]

Ten days later Langstaff was still making regular thrice-daily visits to the same house to attend Barbara's older sister, Caroline, whose throat was 'very sore' and 'greatly swollen.' At first she had been strong enough to 'walk to the window to have her throat inspected,' but after the family sent for him in great haste claiming 'that she was choking to death,' the doctor found her 'black in the face.' Langstaff stayed two hours; he cauterized (or seared) her nostrils with silver nitrate and syringed her nasopharynx with 'one spurt' of warm water, while she held her breath. He came back later that day through a 'heavy rain' to repeat the measures and stay all night. Early in the morning her 'voice still ha[d] tone,' but there was a 'foetid' and 'adhesive mucopurulent discharge' from her throat and 'swelling had set in around her jaws settling towards [her] larynx.' She was dead before noon.[33] Two other children in the family survived the illness.

In a community already tense with diphtheria outbreak, anxiety rose in all family members, young and old, after a death. Langstaff viewed these fears, together with patients' premonitory feelings, as having an important effect on the outcome of sickness in people of any age. After seeing one family with diphtheria, he wrote that a child was 'near dying' and 'wants the lamp lit.'[34] He was called by a colleague to help care for an eight-year-old boy with diphtheria whose brother, he wrote, 'was buried today of same.' Over the following days Langstaff made regular visits, carefully titrating the dose of medicine for the child's age and fever, but when he arrived on the fourth day, the boy was dead. 'From fear partly,' the doctor wrote. 'He dreamed last night that he was dead. They asked him if he was ready to go. He reached out his hand & bid them good bye & died soon after.'[35]

For every child that died there were several others who survived;

only once, early in his practice, after spending all night beside a little boy, did Langstaff write that he 'gave up as [case is] hopeless.'[36] In time, he saw the recovery of children whom he had described as 'sinking' or 'cold and blue.' Once, with the 'mother frightened' nearby, he examined a little child with a pulse of 160 beats a minute, respiration of 85, and the death rattle in its throat. Whether by art or nature and defying all expectations, this child lived.[37] After nearly forty years in practice, that a case might appear to be 'hopeless' no longer seemed a reason to give up.

'Protect us, O God, from diphtheria,' one author wrote, had been the daily prayer of those who witnessed the grim parade of coffins filing past their homes in epidemic times.[38] All too familiar, the images of suffering and struggle against the spectre of this dreadful disease fostered and explained the zeal, without excusing the excesses, of the public health reformers who turned their attention to the schools in the decades following Langstaff's death.[39]

Like diphtheria, the conditions called 'scarlet fever,' 'scarlatina,' 'erysipelas,' and 'sore throat' were recognized purely by their clinical symptoms. Langstaff conceived of each of these conditions and each of their after-effects as separate entities; there is no evidence that he recognized any common cause for them or their sequelae, which are now called 'post-streptococcal' conditions and include rheumatic heart disease, chorea, and nephrotic syndrome. Langstaff did identify the after-effects usually as separate diseases and sometimes actually noticed the sequential relationship; for example, he wrote, 'dropsy with protein in the urine' or 'rheumatism ... following scarlatina.'[40] Once again there was considerable overlap in the diagnoses and sometimes hair-splitting distinctions were made between them; however, for the purposes of this discussion they will be grouped together. Post-partum fever could also be added to this list, as it is frequently caused by streptococcal bacteria, but it will be dealt with in chapter 8.

Outbreaks of these streptococcal infections could occur in any season. They affected more individuals than did diphtheria, but the mortality seems to have been slightly less. The year of greatest mortality was 1871, during which six children died, but four died in early 1872 and four in 1882. During the 1871–2 epidemic some unfortunate families suffered multiple losses; as in diphtheria seasons, fear reigned.

A rash was the distinctive identifying sign, but headache was also

a prominent feature of scarlet fever and some children suffered confusion and convulsion. Langstaff recorded the complaint of one little
child who moaned, 'O my head ... poor head.'[41] He noted that another little girl, who 'knows enough to ask for a drink ... washes [her]
face as accustomed [and] her mother seems to understand her.'[42]

Langstaff was summoned to see a little girl with scarlatina for a
symptom the doctor later considered may have been due to the drug
she had been given: 'They thought she was dying about 4 p.m. She
had been flushed in the face and they gave her 2 doses of [tartar
emetic] one after the other. She turned dark in the face, blue. They
did not say anything about the med[icine] & did not suspect it, but
she has been better ever since.' Despite the brief improvement that
followed this over-enthusiastic use of medication, the girl died thirty-
six hours later. Then 'all in the house,' including the hired girl, went
on to develop 'sore throat.' Two weeks after the first child's death
Langstaff was attending her little brother, whose mouth was 'very
sore.' The doctor wrote, '[I] asked if he had had scarlet fever'; the
inevitably frightened child answered, 'I have it now.' This patient
improved, but another sister died two days later.[43]

When the throat was involved, appearances could resemble those
of diphtheria. One little girl, among several sick in a single family,
became 'entirely unable to swallow.' Langstaff gave her a spoonful
of syrup; 'it seemed to go into the back of her throat & nearly strangle
her, but [he] turned her on her face & there was a slimy discharge
from mouth. [He] held her sitting in a chair & a large quantity of
mucus ... came from throat & ran down upon [the] floor.' Two days
later she was still alive, but 'croup' was 'setting in' and her feet were
'getting cold'; Langstaff tried 'feathering' her throat with lunar caustic, 'but it did no good.' The outcome is unknown, but it seems
unlikely she survived. Less than a month later Langstaff returned to
the home to assist her mother in the birth of a baby girl.[44]

Soft tissue inflammation could spread to the face, as in the case of
a child who lay 'apparently stupid, one eye partly open & dirty &
the other closed by swelling of lid & face.' She then became 'very
restless, rolling & throwing [her] hands about nearly half the time.'[45]
This little girl died, but her older sister recovered. The inexorable
cycles continued in this family too: a month later the mother gave
birth to a son.

Scarlatina visited the Teefy family in the autumn of 1856 and affected eight-year-old John, five-year-old Clara, three-year-old Louise

Adelaide ('Louie'), and Miss Dowling, the servant. The girls recovered quickly, but John was particularly irritable, picking at the rash
on his face near his nose and the corners of his lips and refusing to
allow the doctor to feel his pulse. He developed an abscess under his
chin, which burst spontaneously leaving a 'hole' that enlarged 'greatly'
and became an ulcer with a foetid discharge extending to the boy's
ear, although at first the 'flesh [was] clean as if dissected.' He looked
pale and weak and Langstaff worried that his appetite was failing;
however, over the course of two months, with a laxative every morning, dressings made of rags soaked in alcohol, a little light cautery,
and at least forty-six visits from the doctor, the ugly sore healed. Six
years later the Teefy household may have been worried when
scarlatina returned to afflict eighteen-month-old Armand, but he recovered quickly without after-effects.[46]

Chorea, or St Vitus dance, a movement disorder that sometimes
follows these conditions, appeared from time to time but did not vex
Langstaff greatly. Although it has a spectacular appearance, he seemed
to recognize 'well marked' cases as having a benign course and rarely
made more than one visit after making the diagnosis. He saw one
person with chorea in 1872 and an annual maximum of four cases
appeared in 1883; both years followed scarlatina epidemics.

Rheumatic fever, however, was a source of great morbidity in this
practice; Langstaff followed some patients with joint and heart problems for many years. His own nephew, John Langstaff's son Charlie,
developed severe rheumatic fever with pericarditis. Langstaff saw
him twenty-five times in six weeks during the spring of 1873. The
boy seemed to recover slowly, but the following year his heart failed
again: he lay 'partly on his breast, eyes partly open, easier from
opium, still suffering from want of breath, face puffy, feet and legs
cold.'[47] He died that night.

When scarlatina progressed to acute rheumatism, the consequences
of a single epidemic could plague a family for years. In November
1856 four children in Johnathan Shell's family developed scarlet fever. Langstaff made twenty-one visits to the household before the
end of December. The sickness was aggravated by five intestinal
worms in one child. Two boys likely developed the kidney complication of glomerulonephritis, because they began to show scant and
'intensely albuminous' urine, but one of these children, the doctor
said, was 'cheerful and says "I'm well."' A girl and a boy died, the
rest seemed to recover. Two and a half years later, however, one son

was suffering from severe 'cardiac tumult' and pain in his wrists and fingers. Langstaff saw him repeatedly until his 'very easy' death more than four years after the original infection.[48]

Many children were sick with febrile illnesses that cannot be specifically identified. Convulsions were common and terrified the attendants, though Langstaff seems to have viewed one or two seizures to be of little significance. Some children suffered repeated convulsions. A few others, especially infants, displayed signs, such as a bulging fontanelle, sufficient to suggest a diagnosis of meningitis – although Langstaff rarely used the word, most often calling the condition 'acute inflammation of the brain.' With fever, a stiff neck, and vomiting, Baldwin Teefy was one of the few children said to have 'meningitis,' but the little boy recovered completely after six weeks and twenty-three visits from Langstaff, who gave him tartar emetic.[49] In May 1864 four children in different families were seen for febrile convulsions, a record suggesting an epidemic of a specific infectious agent. A similar situation arose in April 1874. In a few post-mortem examinations Langstaff noted pus or 'greatly engorged' congestion of cerebral vessels and thickening of the membranes around the brain.[50]

Whooping cough was common in 1864 and 1874; minor outbreaks, confined to several members in one family, occurred in 1861, 1876, and 1888. The spectacular 'paroxysms' of coughing often left patients blue and exhausted, but it appears that this disease claimed only three children in Langstaff's practice.[51] Measles was apparent in all decades except the 1870s, but only one child died of this disease, when it was aggravated by bronchitis.[52] In 1868 and 1869 there were more cases of measles than usual, allowing for generalized immunity to explain its relative absence in the early 1870s. Langstaff identified measles by the rash, which might be 'out thick,' but he also noted complications such as laryngitis and bowel haemorrhage, which in one patient he attributed to 'measles in the rectum.'[53] Mumps epidemics occurred in 1869 and 1879; at least twice Langstaff recognized the related swelling of the testis called orchitis.[54] Chickenpox, though mentioned in all decades except the 1850s, caused very little morbidity: when six-year-old Baldwin Teefy, who had suffered meningitis three years earlier, developed chickenpox, Langstaff went to see him only once.[55] Smallpox was infrequent, but it was deadly and greatly feared; a small epidemic in 1880 had devastating effects on Langstaff's personal and political life (see chapter 9).[56]

Accidents were a frequent cause of childhood death, and many other traumatic events became surgical problems (see chapter 7). Some cases, like that of the child who swallowed glass, defied intervention; most poisonings fell into this category. Langstaff saw one child die of an accidental opium ingestion; another, from swallowing lye.[57]

Parasitic and fungus conditions, including 'worms,' 'taenia,' 'ascarides,' 'ringworm,' 'scabies,' and 'lice,' were mentioned in all decades. Langstaff noted when children passed live worms or 'worm seeds.' He was ready with vermifuges, powders, lozenges, and lotions to treat these conditions, which he associated with unsanitary living – even in early years. When the children of a family named Hogg developed scabies, the doctor wrote, 'Hogg children = pigs.'[58]

Langstaff saw several babies born with congenital ailments such as spina bifida, harelip, club-foot, congenital hip displacement, and morbus caeruleus (or congenital heart disease). Some were treated surgically when they were older, but he did not return to visit infants with heart disease. Perhaps he had cautioned families that there was no treatment and the prognosis was poor. He also saw children with convulsions unrelated to fever. In one child he attributed the condition to the heat of the sun.[59] A little boy who had been hit in the head by a fork suffered multiple minor 'fits' daily, but, the doctor observed, he was 'lively' and managed to avoid dropping the wood he happened to be carrying during one of his seizures.[60] In the later years cases of epilepsy in adults and children were managed with bromides and other sedatives.

Diarrhoea was common, especially in the late summer. Langstaff used a variety of names for it: 'dysentery,' 'purging,' 'summer complaint,' 'enteritis,' and 'cholera infantum.' It could be deadly for adults, but more than half the lives it claimed belonged to children. Other studies suggest that childhood mortality was highest in those less than two years of age.[61] Mary Ann Langstaff's little nephew died in this manner, with his limbs 'blue black'; purging may have been responsible for the loss of Langstaff's own baby daughter, Isabella who died near the same date.[62] Three children died of the 'summer complaint' in 1871; five in 1872. One family lost a child in the first epidemic, 'screaming and clawing her hands about her face,' only to lose another in the second.[63] There were outbreaks with less mortality in 1864, 1873, and 1874. Langstaff sometimes recorded seeing a rash of 'petechiae' or 'purpura' with diarrhoea, suggesting a diagnosis of typhus (see below) or perhaps the vascular condition now called Henoch-Schönlein purpura.[64]

The accompanying dehydration and fever frequently produced neurological symptoms. One eleven-year-old boy, purging 'like pea soup,' was delirious and 'did not know his mother.' Two days later Langstaff wrote, 'he knows me,' but two brothers, a sister, and the father were now ill. The daybook describes the scene: 'one or the other is talking most of the time during the night'; the boy 'looks like an old man but is ravenous.' The whole family recovered.[65]

Langstaff recognized the danger in loss of fluid or nutrition and encouraged his patients to drink 'beeftea,' 'gelatine,' and milk boiled and/or spiked with alcohol. The notes reveal that children who died of diarrhoea were in a state of severe dehydration, with sunken eyes and stuporous staring. Complications such as prolapsed anus and progression to haemorrhagic diarrhoea, 'bloody flux,' were not uncommon. One six-year-old girl suffered miserably for three months following diarrhoea with intractable abdominal pain and ascites. When the greatly wasted child finally died, Langstaff performed an autopsy and discovered multiple adhesions and a bowel perforation near the caecal valve.[66]

Diarrhoea was almost as deadly for adults as it was for children. It was this disease that had carried off Mrs Elizabeth Brett, Sr, the mother-in-law of John Langstaff, Jr.[67] It spread rapidly through families and its effects on Langstaff's in-laws illustrate its impact in the community. In 1865 Langstaff was summoned to his own mother-in-law, Mrs Henry Miller, Sr, whom he had known since his schooldays. She was very sick with vomiting, abdominal pain, and bloody bowel movements. Nothing could control her symptoms she felt hot and uncomfortable. He 'hoist the window & let the cool breeze blow in her face,' called in two colleagues for a consultation, and spent all night at her side. Hourly doses of opium and boiled milk were prescribed, but she became unable to swallow, gagged, and 'said "no" in answer to whether she would have her lips wet.' After ten days of this suffering, she expired.[68]

Three years later, in the same epidemic that likely killed Langstaff's baby daughter and his wife's nephew, the Miller family was again visited with diarrhoea. Mary Ann's younger sister, twenty-five-year-old Eleanor, had recovered from measles six months earlier, only to develop severe 'vomiting and purging' two weeks after the nephew's death. She was 'half comatose' and 'seemed to be sinking'; the Reverend Mr Dick was summoned. In this case Langstaff was annoyed that the family gave her opium every hour instead of every two hours, but the diarrhoea continued unabated. He stayed after midnight on several nights until she died, six days from the onset of her illness.[69]

The following morning another sister-in-law, Mrs Henry Miller, Jr, mother of the deceased baby nephew, began to experience uterine contractions though she was only three-and-a-half months pregnant. Possibly she too had contracted the summer complaint, known to be dangerous for pregnant women since the time of Hippocrates. Langstaff attended her frequently for purging and vomiting; one week later she was convalescent, but she had miscarried.[70]

Pneumonia could occur at any time of year, but it was most common between October and March. Langstaff occasionally saw this disease spread between family members, but he considered it to be the result of exposure to cold air: one man with pneumonia 'took cold' going to Toronto; another developed the illness after he had 'rushed out of the house without even a shirt on; a company of men found him singing in a clump of pines about $1/4$ mile off.'[71] This disease, which often complicated other illnesses and injuries, affected children as well as adults. Three or more people died of pneumonia in each of 1857, 1862, 1874, and 1882. There were other years, such as 1853 and 1854, in which it also seems to have been common, but with lower mortality. Vigorous people and children often recovered, but pneumonia in the old and weak was, as Osler wrote much later, the 'friend of the aged': relatively painless yet deadly.[72] An elderly husband and wife fell ill with pneumonia and, despite Langstaff's ministrations, died within a week of each other.[73]

The disease usually began with abrupt fever, chills, pain in the chest, and breathlessness; one patient had 'all the windows and doors open for want of air.'[74] Illness could be severe for two weeks and recovery often took a month or more. With percussion and auscultation Langstaff could determine which part of the lung was affected and follow its progress. He would add pleurisy and pericarditis to the diagnosis, if the stethoscope confirmed it. Blueness of the lips and face or a dark black colour of the blood were danger signs. A few cases progressed to abscess of the lung or empyema. Langstaff's sole contribution to medical writing was an observation concerning the physical diagnosis of pneumonia with involvement of an entire lung.[75] The little girl who had been the subject of this report was treated with cupping and tartar emetic and recovered as Langstaff had predicted, but not without developing an abscess in her chest that drained spontaneously eight weeks later.[76]

Some of the ambience of illness was created by the doctor and his treatments. In a pneumonia case, for example, Langstaff would have entered a darkened room, possibly smoky from stramonium, to attend his breathless and often blue patient, confused from fever, wet and bald from showering and shaving of the head, and lying nearly motionless so as not to disturb the mustard plasters on her feet. Several of Richmond Hill's most prominent citizens died in this state. The wife of politician Amos Wright, member of the Canada West legislature, survived a severe attack in 1857, only to suffer a fatal recurrence four years later.[77] George Soules, the town baker, died after a protracted illness, as did the Presbyterian minister, the Reverend James Dick, for whom James and Mary Ann Langstaff had named their last-born child.[78] But, to Langstaff, the most important pneumonia case he attended may have been that of his own father.

John Langstaff, Sr had stayed on the homestead property. From at least 1861 he lived with the large family of his second son, John, Jr, his wife, Elizabeth, her mother Elizabeth Brett, and a domestic servant.[79] Mrs Brett had died of purging in 1862, but the family had grown to seven children with another on the way as illness struck the nonogenarian father. Langstaff had treated him for a carbuncle in the past,[80] but in February 1865, when the old man developed a high fever, he diagnosed pneumonia of the right lung and offered the usual medications and bleedings. Sixteen days after the onset of the illness, the doctor found him eating 'toast with relish' and pronounced him 'convalescent.' Nevertheless, in early May after many visits he had to admit his father was 'getting weaker.' In this interval Langstaff assisted his own wife in the birth of their son Rolph and attended his sister-in-law Elizabeth for a miscarriage with profuse bleeding. On 14 May, a few days after the miscarriage, John Langstaff, Sr, died. The doctor saw only three other patients that day, but on 17 May, the day of 'father's funeral,' he saw six patients and attended a complicated delivery at six o'clock in the morning.[81]

When old people had pneumonia, they knew the time had come to put their affairs in order. John Langstaff, Sr, obeyed this rule. His cash and mortgages, worth nearly $5,000, were originally to be divided among the sons (excluding Miles); however, two days after he developed his pneumonia, he wrote a codicil. One third of the money was bestowed on his daughter-in-law, Elizabeth, who had sheltered him in his final years and, though herself mothering, pregnant, and sick, had nursed him in his last illness.[82] The timing and directions of the codicil are significantly related to the old man's pneumonia.

Another patient, an elderly woman suffocating with pneumonia in both lungs displayed a similar understanding about the implications of the diagnosis. Langstaff wrote, 'She became of a leaden hue, quite sensible to within half an hour when she became comatose & died without the least struggle. She bid all good bye, [and] said "I am dying."' The day before Langstaff had noted that he 'could hear her heart beat about 8 feet away.'[83]

Tuberculosis (also called consumption or phthisis) is thought to have been one of the most important causes of death in the nineteenth century; the Canada Census listed it as the major cause of death in the years studied.[84] Therefore, it should have been a great source of morbidity and stress in the community, but the Langstaff daybooks are disappointingly cryptic on the subject and indicate that 'phthisis' was responsible for only twenty deaths. At most, even when all cases diagnosed as phthisis are combined with those that are suggestive of it (e.g., coughing of blood), it ranks third as a cause of adult death. For personal or cultural reasons the doctor may have had some inhibition about actually naming it; thus, the low mortality figure could be artefactual.

Despite the relatively low number of deaths attributed to phthisis, Langstaff did see many patients with the disease; yet he seems not to have spent much time treating them. Once families were aware of the nature of the problem, they may have chosen not to call on the doctor, perhaps because the prognosis was known to be poor even with treatment. Sometimes, after a single visit to a given patient, Langstaff wrote simply, 'dying' or 'far gone' in phthisis.[85] Occasionally the notes indicate that the person had been sick for over a year and that it was only near the end, when the situation had become desperate, that the doctor had been called.[86]

Women are said to have been more susceptible to tuberculosis than men; their greater vulnerability is thought to have given biological support to the idea that women were more frail and has been related to the nature of their work or their relative lack of nutrition.[87] Langstaff's own experience differed from that described by the late-century statistics. In his practice, men died more often of tuberculosis than women and were suspected of having the disease more frequently. Of the twenty deaths attributed to this condition, sixteen were in men, three in women, and one in a child. Similarly, a survey over all the years of the daybooks revealed eighty-two people in whom Langstaff suspected tuberculosis: fifty-one men, twenty-five women, and six children. Could this finding suggest that a society already somewhat loath to consult for phthisis was even more hesitant about consulting the doctor for this disease in a woman or a child? Or does it suggest that the disease was actually more prevalent in men in this community?

According to family tradition, the disease Langstaff suffered near the end of his stay in England may have been tuberculosis. The records lend subtle credence to this story: for example, he considered it significant that a young man who displayed 'all the appearance of a consumptive' had 'just returned from Scotland.'[88] The diagnosis in this person, and in all patients in whom he suspected 'consumpsion [sic]',[89] rested on a careful examination of the chest. If there was evidence of dullness or cavity 'beneath the clavicle' in the top of the lungs, he considered the condition to be 'threatening,' but he rarely named the disease, either directly or euphemistically. He let the record stand with a description of the ominous physical finding and without the word 'phthisis,' although he may have kept his suspicions to himself for years. One exception to this rule was the case of Matthew Teefy's thirteen-year-old daughter Clara, whom Langstaff had seen for a left upper lobe pneumonia three years earlier. Perhaps because he had been pointedly asked or because she now displayed trouble in the opposite lung he confidently wrote 'apex phthiscal,' but he was probably pleased to find over the course of fifteen more years before her marriage that the lung changes he had heard did not turn into an active form of consumption.[90]

Interpretation of the stethoscopic findings in early tuberculosis was a diagnostic challenge requiring skill and sophistication. Once, without knowing that two other consultants had preceded him, Langstaff was called in to resolve a diagnostic conflict. Although he confirmed the disappointing presence of phthisis in the patient, he seemed pleased to have been told later 'that [my assessment] agreed perfectly with [Dr] McMaster.'[91] Some patients requested chest examinations because they were afraid they had tuberculosis. The doctor relied on his skill with the stethoscope when he reassured a man who 'says he has consumption' that his illness was pleurisy instead.[92]

Fever, wasting, night sweats, the coughing of blood, and breathlessness were signs of advanced disease. One young woman had had 'company and afterwards [could] hardly get her breath.'[93] Rarely, the disease presented with sudden death due to rupture of a pulmonary blood vessel and copious coughing of blood.[94] Deliberately or inadvertently, Langstaff may have labelled some consumptives as having 'pleurisy' or 'hydrothorax' or 'pneumonia.' One elderly women was said to have 'chronic pneumonia perhaps kept up by tubercles.'[95] Extra-pulmonary manifestations of tuberculosis involving kidney, bone, and skin do appear in the daybooks,[96] but except for a single case in which an autopsy revealed 'tuberculosis of the liver,'[97] there was rarely any indication that a tuberculous condition localized outside of the lung had been recognized as such.

Rest and nourishment were the mainstays of therapy in the few consumptives the doctor was charged to follow closely. He saw one man fairly regularly for six and a half years, from his first attack of coughing blood at 2 o'clock one morning until his lingering death, with the 'family hopeful' each time he 'rallied' to sip his 'beer and egg.'[98] Another man was seen almost daily for six months; although no diagnosis was written, the sparse comments suggest that he too died of phthisis.[99] The doctor's continued visits in these cases seem to have been in response to the family's wishes.

Typical of tuberculosis management was the care given to Frank Boynton, whose family Langstaff had treated since 1856, when Boynton had sustained a severe injury to his thigh. Through three decades Langstaff had attended the births of their children, helped Mrs Boynton with mastitis, presided over fatal diphtheria in their twins, and set the fractured leg of one of their sons. In June 1884 Mrs Boynton took the doctor aside and showed him 'about 6 oz of pus and blood' that her husband had coughed from his chest. Langstaff recommended a nourishing diet; a month later the patient was eating three pounds of beef a week but still having coughing spells that left him exhausted and hungry. By fall he was 'losing appetite and strength & ... had some pain with gradually increasing resp[iration]' of thirty or more breaths a minute. Boynton now had a low-grade fever and was beginning to feel shooting pains in the lower part of his chest and numbness in his limbs; he still coughed but no longer brought up sputum. To keep him comfortable, Langstaff prescribed sedatives and painkillers, including chloral hydrate, opium, hyoscine, and inhalations of chloroform as often as once an hour. Within two days Boynton felt better, his pains had lessened, and his breathing was easier, but he still displayed ominous signs, increasing chills, and diarrhoea; he continued in this slowly declining state until his death at the end of January.[100]

Once only, a patient, whom Langstaff attended for many months, seems to have recovered from active tuberculosis, although her long-term prognosis may not have been good. He first saw this young woman in October 1884 and found a low-grade fever with signs of 'deficient respiration' in the upper part of her lungs. By December she was 'extremely thin' and 'so hollow between her ribs' that the doctor could not place his stethoscope properly in order to listen to her chest. After a great deal of medicine and nine months of frequent visits to her home, more than five miles from his, he found her 'gaining distinctly in weight but ... a skeleton still. Her mother lifted her out in the rocking chair and she sat and rocked & talked. Her hair is growing & looks well. She takes rum & raw egg.'[101]

Unspecified fevers that were not localized to any part of the body and not given any diagnosis are numerous in this record, making assignation of incidence rates next to impossible. When young Armand Teefy reached the age of twenty-one, he contracted such an illness. His case was typical of any number of other unnamed febrile complaints: Langstaff gave him medicines but did not specify what they were, and visited him daily for four days, then every two or three days for a total of eleven visits over the course of three weeks. Some people died of diseases like this, which can only be character-ized as 'fever,' but it is easier to focus on varieties of fevers that may have been less common but are diagnoses on which Langstaff and late twentieth-century physicians would probably agree: cholera, ty-phoid, typhus, malaria, and venereal disease.

Cholera epidemics began in 1832, with recurrences in 1834, 1849 to 1854, and 1866.[102] There is little evidence of these epidemics in the daybooks, although Langstaff considered cholera in two people in August 1852 and diagnosed it in four more in August 1853. His use of the words 'rice water stools' and his description of cold, blue skin in the context of purging suggest that he was on the lookout for it.[103] The word 'cholera' appears fairly often in the record from 1852 to 1888 and seems to have been almost interchangeable with the words 'purging' and 'dysentery.' The summers of 1863, 1865, 1868, and 1884 seem to have had more than the usual number of cases. Langstaff did not indicate that any of his patients died from cholera, although it does seem possible that some of the other dysentery or purging deaths may have been related to it. For example, Langstaff recorded seeing a woman 'who lost her child of 8 months this afternoon. She has had vomiting and purging, cramps, cold surface for last 4 days, very like epidemic cholera.'[104] Sometimes he specified 'sporadic' or 'infantile' cholera to distinguish it from the deadly 'Asiatic' variety that had so heavily taxed the ill-prepared resources of Toronto and district. Once he attributed a child's diarrhoea to 'cholera' from eating cheese. He diagnosed 'cholera' in himself, 'from having eaten buckwheat, pork, and gravy.'[105]

Langstaff diagnosed typhoid fever on infrequent occasions from at least 1857 to 1882; he thought it could be an unnecessary result of unsanitary conditions. There may have been some hesitancy in actually naming the disease, as he wrote 'in a typhoid state' or 'seems like typhoid fever,' or mentioned only the characteristic symptoms such as 'rose spots' or 'pulse not so quick' to indicate that he was considering this diagnosis.[106] The fever could produce severe delirium and debility. When Langstaff arrived to see a man with typhoid, he found him kneeling on the floor unable to get back into bed. 'He thought he was dying,' Langstaff wrote. Six weeks later the man was still sick, but he seems to have recovered slowly.[107]

Less fortunate were three women considered to have died of the disease, whose stories show that Langstaff seems to have thought that typhoid, like peritonitis, had a predilection for the menstruating or post-partum woman. One fell ill during a heavy menstrual period; another had given birth to a baby only one month before she died, feverish, disoriented, and deaf; and the third died just two weeks after her baby was born, while the post-partum flow of 'lochia [was] going on.' Langstaff described her last moments: 'She tried to swallow a teaspoonful of water for me this morning, blood & slime running out of her mouth. Abdomen tumid but quite soft. She died at 7 A.M. about half an hour after I arrived.'[108]

Typhus, a disease transmitted by lice, ravaged the impoverished immigrants who travelled to Canada in the crowded holds of ships. Its mechanism of propagation was not understood; despite quarantine rules, it spread to the mainland through harbour cities.[109] Aside from the suggestive cases of diarrhoea with petechiae, there were few instances (under ten) in which Langstaff actually named this disease – all occurred between 1856 and 1864. He seems to have diagnosed typhus with confidence, since he wrote that it was 'quite distinct' in one patient and, in another, that it was 'setting in.'[110] In 1856, three people in one family were said to have typhus,[111] but no deaths were ever attributed to the disease.

Malaria was common in Upper Canada, where the early traveller

Anna Jameson complained of mosquitoes that 'came in swarms, in clouds, in myriads, entering our eyes, our noses, our mouths, stinging till the blood flowed ... as pretty and perfect a plague as the most ingenuous, amateur sinner tormentor ever devised.' Like so many of the early settlers, Jameson also contracted malaria or 'ague': 'I shiver through the day and through the night ... my teeth they chatter, chatter still'; at intervals, 'I am burned up with a dry hot fever.'[112] Malaria vanished from Ontario in the second half of the nineteenth century for a variety of reasons, including the steady progress of land clearance and drainage of the mosquito-infested swamps.[113]

Recognized by periodic fever and chills, 'ague' caused considerable morbidity in Langstaff's early practice, especially in the late summer and early fall. Quinine was a specific and effective remedy and the most commonly named drug from 1849 to 1854. When the fever came irregularly, he called the illness 'dumb ague.' Some patients had attacks for more than a year and could be quite weak; nevertheless, no one seems to have died of malaria, although it is impossible to know if the few but deadly cases of jaundice and hepatitis were variations of this condition. Certain signs suggest that incidence of malaria declined slowly in this practice: the last diagnosis of 'ague' was made in 1879; during 1882 and 1883, quinine was prescribed only three times as a strengthening tonic together with iron; and in 1883, on the last occasion Langstaff mentioned the disease, he wrote that a man had 'had an attack like ague.'[114] His reluctance to name 'ague' may have been greater than its actual scarcity: for example, in 1888, he described another patient as having a 'chill every other day, but not regular.'[115]

Five deaths can be attributed to either jaundice or hepatitis, but one of the patients concerned was found at autopsy to have 'tuberculosis of the liver.'[116] Pain, tenderness, and enlargement of the liver accompanied by yellow skin, dark urine, and blood were the features Langstaff usually called 'jaundice' or 'hepatitis.' Once he palpated an enlarged gall-bladder, which condition suggests an obstruction of the common bile duct due to a gallstone or cancer of the head of the pancreas.[117] Another case of hepatitis had been provoked, he claimed, 'by passage of [a] gallstone.'[118] Late in his practice he revealed awareness of the relationship between biliary function and digestion of fats when he wrote that a man 'ate some pie which caused a relapse' of his jaundice.[119]

Langstaff left indications that eight of his patients, all males, suffered from either gonorrhoea or syphilis.[120] His terse notes about them were usually written in Latin. Since half the cases were seen in the first five years, it seems possible that other cases may not have been recorded at all. Therefore, on the basis of Langstaff's papers, little can be said about the relative incidence of these problems. Other sources, however, suggest that venereal disease was present and that doctors viewed patients so afflicted with a certain mistrust. For example, the 1875 fee schedule for the North Ontario [County] Medical Association recommended a higher fee for visits to such patients and that payment be sought in advance of treatment.[121]

Peritonitis, which is inflammation of the membranes of the abdomen, was a relatively new and not infrequent diagnosis, based on the clinical setting of severe pain in the stomach or lower belly.[122] Langstaff used the term in an unrestricted manner to describe otherwise inexplicable abdominal pain. He seems to have thought women were particularly susceptible to peritonitis during or after their menstrual periods; he attributed the susceptibility to 'exposure to strong wind during menstruation' or to 'getting wet just after [her] courses.'[123] The doctor diagnosed peritonitis in himself, as he had cholera, but his relative lack of incapacity shows that he understood the condition to be somewhat milder than present definitions would allow: he managed to see seven other patients that same day.[124] He also recognized peritonitis as a result of abdominal trauma in a young man who had been pierced in the belly by a pitchfork.[125] Ten deaths, five of them in children, were attributed to peritonitis. Because the pain was localized to the right lower quadrant, at least four of these may have been due to appendicitis; in one little girl the diagnosis is almost certain, since an autopsy revealed 'pus very abundant from behind the bowels.'[126] In Canada no surgical interventions were made for appendicitis until at least 1883.[127]

Bleeding from the gastrointestinal tract accounted for twelve deaths and frequently complicated 'diarrhoea' and 'peritonitis.' Langstaff made little attempt to establish the cause or the site of haemorrhage, although three autopsies were on patients who had passed blood per rectum. Excessive bleeding at other sites, nosebleeds, bruises, and the coughing of blood suggest problems with blood clotting. Langstaff recorded three such patients, who had previously been well. They may have had an underlying diagnosis of leukaemia, especially a little girl who had pain at her sternum and highly 'buffed' blood.[128]

In the early 1870s, the Canadian medical journals published discussions of leukaemia, which had been described by Rudolf Virchow in 1845;[129] however, if Langstaff was aware of leukaemia as a clinical entity, there is no discernible trace in his daybooks.

Non-infectious conditions also occurred in Langstaff's practice, although they were far less frequent. One of these was 'chlorosis': formerly called the disease of virgins, it was named for the supposed greenish cast of the skin. Chlorosis is no longer diagnosed, but is usually thought to have been similar to the condition now known as iron-deficiency anaemia.[130] Langstaff also used the word 'anaemia' to describe pallor and weakness, but from 1851 to 1886 he saw at least eighteen patients with chlorosis, all of whom were young women: only one was married, and none seem to have been seriously ill, although one had ceased menstruating. A cluster of three cases occurred in 1867 and five cases in 1870; there appear to have been only four cases in the last twenty years of practice. Was this because the condition was becoming less common, perhaps for reasons of improved diet, or was it that chlorosis had been supplanted in the mind of the practitioner by other diagnostic categories?

Strokes and threatened strokes (transient ischaemic attacks) were recognized approximately once a year; at least ten patients died of them. Langstaff usually described the deficit, be it loss of consciousness, movement, or speech, blindness, drooping eyelid, or paralytic 'palsy'; this last he sometimes called 'hemiplegia.' Stroke affected only adults, most often those in old age. With perhaps a reversed attribution of cause and effect, he diagnosed hemiplegia in a ninety-five-year-old man, 'from fall full length on the ground.'[131] In one patient who could hear a throbbing, Langstaff made the practical assessment that he thought she could hear her own carotid arteries from her ears being 'stopped.'[132] One man 'fell insensible in the field ... they raised him up and poured cold water freely over his head and carried him in.' When Langstaff saw him ninety minutes later, he was 'disposed to turn his head and eyes over his left shoulder... In about two hours he was able to walk ... but could not yet speak.' Five months later while 'sitting at tea, all at once he could only see half, i.e. one side, of his wife's face.' The doctor wrote, 'I found he was quite changed in manner being exceedingly cheerful, laughing, and speaking loudly & suddenly, "Langstaff is that you?" [he said] when he first opened his eyes after I arrived.' The doctor recalled that the man had had a 'brain attack like a sun stroke while in the field last summer,' and encouraged him to take his medicine, but the patient died a week later on Christmas Day.[133]

Sudden death suggestive of heart attack was quite rare; only two cases answer the description.[134] Other abrupt deaths that Langstaff attended are suitably attributed to pulmonary embolus, choking, stroke, or haemorrhage, although he usually did not offer much explanation. The history of a 'great pain down the left arm' in one man is suggestive of angina, but the fact that Langstaff said 'half his chest seems to move when his heart beats' indicates the origin of this pain may have been aortic valve deficiency rather than atherosclerosis. Most of the 'heart disease' that Langstaff recognized was the result of rheumatic fever; equally common in children and adults, swelling of the legs or 'dropsy' he attributed to 'heart disease'; and occasionally he named 'endocarditis' as a particular cause. From the outset of his practice Langstaff appears to have been able to use his stethoscope to recognize various heart murmurs; he distinguished 'mitral regurgitation' from 'aortic systolic bruits,' commented on aortic 'whifs' (or insufficiency), but did not mention mitral stenosis. An inability to lie flat or blueness of the lips was a danger sign, and he reported palpitations and irregular heartbeats. Once he noted that a young woman's heart 'gave a strong beat then two light ones.'[135]

Langstaff observed cancers in at least thirty-five people over the forty years of his practice. Breast cancer represented nearly one-third of all malignancies; eight of the patients concerned underwent surgery. Some women treated themselves secretly with folk remedies and dressings for a long time before the doctor first visited; for them, surgery was out of the question (see chapter 7).[136] Langstaff understood the ominous significance of a retracted nipple, creased skin, and lumps in the armpit; he seems to have considered as benign the multiple small tumours in a young woman's breast.[137] Some women lived for many years with breast cancer, but patients with other malignancies do not appear to have fared so well. Langstaff attended four people with stomach cancer diagnosed in a terminal state. He also saw malignant growths involving lip, bowel, liver, ovary, testis, throat, neck, finger- and knee-joints, uterus, and possibly lymphatic glands. Cancer was entered as part of the family history in two patients with unexplained chronic illness. He resected tumours of the lip and lymphatic glands, but most internal malignancies were gravely advanced at the time of diagnosis; except for those with breast cancer, he rarely made more than one or two trips to patients with this disease. When called some distance to consult on a colleague's patient with cancer of the throat and palate, he arrived to find the 'man with tumour dead and buried ... no charge.'[138] Terse notes on the single visits to four other patients reported 'cancer,' but the site of origin was not named.

Langstaff's third brother, Dr Lewis Langstaff of nearby Springhill (now King City) in King township, probably suffered from cancer or the equally gloomy tuberculosis. The men were close colleagues as well as brothers; Langstaff had taken over the care of their sister's orphaned children in order to facilitate Lewis's study of medicine. The daybooks are circumspect about the specific diagnosis that caused him to spend many days with his brother, but they offer some insights. Lewis first fell ill in 1868 at age forty-eight, when he suffered a massive haemorrhage from some part of his chest. Langstaff wrote: 'haemorrhage 6 a.m. fearfully spouting a stream like a goose quill about 2 inches up from his breast part of blood coming from the sac itself most likely. I put on a graduated compress, meal pad, and smoothing iron about 8 lbs. It stopped at once completely ... I have been there almost constantly for the last week.'[139] The lesion bled again, the pressure bandage caused 'sloughing' at the 'edge of the orifice,' and Lewis suffered fainting spells, but he convalesced.

Ten years later there was a visible growth on Lewis Langstaff's neck, which may or may not have been related to his mysterious bleeding 'sac.' James Langstaff and his son assisted Dr Hillary in 'removing a tumour from the neck below the jaw ... the size of a hen's egg.'[140] In six months the 'tumour' had regrown and Lewis was vomiting and failing. Langstaff saw no more than three other patients each day for the two weeks before and after Lewis died. He helped arrange the funeral and settled the other affairs of the widow, Annie, and her seven children. In the years that followed he seems to have supported Annie financially, by making mortgage payments to her and employing her sons, Alva and Herman, at his office and farms.

Occasionally patients passed kidney stones, which Langstaff called 'calculus' or 'gravel.' He recognized the characteristic pain of renal colic that moved 'down the back from the hip forward into the spermatic cord.'[141] This pain sometimes appeared in young women, an observation suggesting that their underlying problem may have been renal tuberculosis. One young lady who had severe pain and bloody urine 'became easy,' Langstaff wrote, 'when I suppose the stone passed into the bladder.'[142]

Bright's disease, a kidney ailment characterized by swelling and familiar to any former student of Guy's Hospital, appeared in the record three times. In all three cases the diagnosis was proven by protein in the urine; one case was complicated by pericarditis.[143] Bright's disease was yet another condition that Langstaff diagnosed in himself. It seriously restricted the last six months of his practice before it took his life. The family retained a memory of the distinction between this condition and diabetes. Many years later Langstaff's daughter-in-law wrote: he 'was a very hard working physician – old style – had kidney ailment – albumen, not sugar, but fatal.'[144]

Much has been written about the dangers of the nineteenth-century pharmacopoeia; historians have been fond of suggesting that doctors killed more people than they saved. Their drugs were indeed powerful, but these statements rarely take into account the fact that the patients were already sick and had appealed to the doctor for help; moreover, doctors were aware that medicines could be poisons. Langstaff thought that some of his patients, both children and adults, had died of iatrogenic causes, in other words, that their deaths had been hastened or caused by their doctors. Two women had apparently sought abortions (see chapter 8); one child he attended with Dr Geikie had been taking an abundance of 'stimulants,' including brandy, prescribed by someone unknown; and three men and a child, all of whom had underlying illness, were considered to have been victims of treatment given by Dr Hostetter. Langstaff occasionally blamed himself for not providing a treatment, but if he considered himself guilty of causing a patient's death, he did not record it. We do not know how often Hostetter was given an opportunity to blame a patient's demise on his rival Dr Langstaff.

Langstaff's patients included men, women, and children. At all times women patients occupied a greater proportion of his activity than their numbers in the population would predict; the increased attention seems related to problems of childbearing. Children were seen slightly less often than their numbers in the population would predict, but severe illness and death in children were always common and indicators suggest that the doctor was summoned more often to care for children in the 1880s than he had been in the 1850s. Most of the sickness and death in Langstaff's practice was the result of infectious fevers with distinct patterns of presentation and prolonged recovery periods, but he also attended persons with cancer, diabetes, and stroke. Tuberculosis was present, especially in men, but it seems to have been less common, less dangerous, or less worthy of medical attention than is implied by its reported prevalence in the general population.

CHAPTER SIX

Lunatics, Dreamers, and Drunks

❧

Over the course of the nineteenth century, physicians increasingly viewed mental illness as the product of 'moral' or emotional causes, amenable to 'moral' or emotion-based therapy; specialized hospitals or asylums were founded to provide such treatment. In the past, historians of medicine portrayed these changes as laudable, but recently others have challenged this assessment. Taking their lead from Michel Foucault's revisionist analysis of insanity and without necessarily embracing all his interpretations, the newer studies suggest that the impulse to 'medicalize' (i.e., diagnose, isolate, and treat) the mentally abnormal may have been neither benevolent nor effective.[1] Most of these studies have been based on the records of large institutions and the prominent alienists who operated them; therefore, the existence of an ordinary doctor's daybooks affords an opportunity to re-examine the new theories concerning the changes in nineteenth-century medical attitudes towards the mentally ill.

Langstaff is difficult to situate in the larger history of psychiatry, since he was relatively cryptic about his patients with mental illness. Indeed, it is perhaps a misnomer to refer to his care of the mentally ill as 'psychiatry,' since he himself seems to have viewed it as an aspect of general medical practice. Why his comments are so sparse is unknown, but the silence itself may be revealing: of a lack of interest in cases he viewed as non-medical or hopeless; or of an interpretation of professional ethics; or of a manifestation of his inability to master the new psychiatric concepts and jargon.[2]

Mental illness was stigmatizing and placed a considerable burden on families, who accommodated their often violent or suicidal relatives, sometimes in complete seclusion.[3] These patients were incapacitated for work, yet they had to be fed, clothed, and sheltered for years. If families were unwilling or unable to offer support, the sick were left to the mercy of the community. It appears that this mercy was sometimes strained: Langstaff once described an unnamed man as 'insane and starving.'[4]

Between 1830 and 1833 the government of Upper Canada enacted legislation to provide for the destitute insane, but since there was no proper facility, these people were housed in a Toronto gaol. The Provincial Lunatic Asylum opened in the early 1850s, but in just a few years it was crowded. Committal required a written certificate signed by two physicians, as specified by the Lunatic Asylum Act of 1853, based on an English law of 1828. Potentially dangerous persons could also be received through the courts on a warrant. No provision was made for the separation of the insane from the criminally insane or the mentally retarded.[5]

In his forty years of medical practice Langstaff encountered twenty-nine persons – fifteen men, thirteen women, and one little girl – whose thought patterns were pervaded by a complete break with reality and who could probably be considered 'psychotic' using today's terminology. He also saw another fifteen who might be considered 'neurotic,' eight who committed or attempted suicide, and fifty or more who suffered predominantly psychiatric symptoms as part of another physical disorder. Nine of the thirty 'psychotic' people – three women and six men – were seen with one or two other physicians for the express purpose of certification.[6] Other physicians sometimes arranged the encounter, but Langstaff indicated that family members and the community had also appealed to him for this service. In his daybooks he referred to these patients as 'lunatic,' 'insane,' or 'crazy,' but the only words he used for diagnosis of mental disorders were 'chronic brain disease,' 'delirium,' 'hysteria,' 'insanity,' 'lunacy,' 'melancholia,' 'mental derangement,' 'moral insanity,' 'nervousness,' 'puerperal mania,' and 'religious delirium.' His daybook entries were brief, but he wrote more on the official papers possibly to improve the chances of admission: in one case he wrote, 'took history to get her into the hospital,' as if he expected his narrative would influence the outcome.[7] Nevertheless, Langstaff seems to have prefered description of behaviour over identification and avoided using psychiatric terms. If any of those certified were people with mental retardation, it seems that he, like many of his colleagues, failed to distinguish their problem from other mental disorders.[8]

The Toronto asylum records have been traced for five of the nine persons whom Langstaff certified: all were male, two were single, and the other three each supported a wife and five or more children (Table 6.1).[9] Certification occurred if three physicians agreed that the patient was a danger either to himself or to others; indeed, while in the asylum, one of these men attempted suicide, slitting his throat into the trachea; another escaped, and a warrant was issued for his arrest, although the register claimed that he had been discharged to his family against advice.

Neither Langstaff nor the other certifying physicians supplied a psychiatric diagnosis on the admission history, but another doctor at the hospital read their reports and inscribed a diagnosis, together with the presumed cause, in a general register. In three of the five men Langstaff had seen, masturbation (or a cryptic 'M') was given as an inciting cause; however, Langstaff himself did not name this as a cause in any of the cases he helped to certify. Alcohol was considered to have been a factor in two other cases; and in one, the cause was said to be 'religion,' which referred to a patient's excessive guilt feelings over masturbation. Once only was a possible syphilitic origin mentioned (in conjunction with alcohol abuse), but the words were qualified as 'incipient general paresis.' The adjective 'incipient' may have been added to ensure admission, since patients with either full-blown tertiary syphilis or the mentally retarded ('idiots') were theoretically inadmissible.

Langstaff's first two certificates were signed within two days of each other, in September 1859. At that time certain improvements in the care of the insane were on the horizon: the Toronto asylum was almost ready to open a new branch; centralized inspection of prisons and asylums was to be implemented; and the building of a specialized asylum for the criminally insane at Kingston, Ontario, had been authorized.[10] It seems there may have been some relationship between the promise of these reforms and the families' decisions to release their relatives to institutional care. Langstaff had met at least

TABLE 6.1
Five case summaries of Langstaff's male patients in the Provincial Lunatic Asylum*

Marital status	Children	Diagnosis	Cause**	Admission duration and outcome
Married	6	Monomania	A; GP	21 months; discharged to friend
Single		Chronic mania	M	35 years; died of pneumonia
Married	7	[None given]	H	8 weeks; discharged at wife's request
Single		Melancholia	A; M	2.5 years; discharged; suicide attempt in asylum
Married	5	Mania	M; R	6 weeks; escaped, captured but not returned at wife's request

* Only five of nine patients certified could be traced
** Cause attributed by asylum doctors
A = alcohol; GP = general paresis (syphilis); H = hereditary, M = masturbation; R = religion

Sources: Langstaff's daybooks; Archives of Ontario, Provincial Lunatic Asylum, Admission/Discharge Warrants and Histories. RG 10 Series 20-B-1, registration nos. 2183, 2967, 5246, 5413, 5611

three of the Toronto asylum superintendents, Primrose, Telfer, and Workman, but there is no evidence that he ever visited the institution.

The admission form in 1859 required that the three referring physicians examine the patient together at one time and sign a single document. Perhaps the logistics of arranging such a meeting between three rural practitioners may have been too complicated, because this practice was changed. The revised admission form allowed each of at least two physicians to make his own statement. Hence, three of these cases offer the exceptional opportunity to compare Langstaff's assessment of a patient with that of a colleague. His statements differ in that he wrote only what he observed and rarely stated a diagnosis or a cause. His colleagues seem to have been less verbose, but also less hesitant to diagnose and interpret. Typical of all Langstaff's meticulous record-keeping, his remarks were made in sentences complete with punctuation. For example, concerning one patient he wrote: 'I observe that he is tied in bed & has his hands wounded & swollen from striking the doors & furniture of the house which I see wrecked. His conversation is disconnected and absurd. He sometimes bursts into boisterous laughter without cause & suddenly changes to screams etc. He last night made an attack upon his family & would have killed them but they blew out the lights & escaped from the doors & windows, as stated by the wife in presence of a company of neighbours. 25 Dec. 1881.'[11] Two other doctors wrote notes on the same patient: both described the violent behaviour rather than the evidence for it, although they had not witnessed it; their point-form jottings were less than half the length of Langstaff's prose.

For a second patient seen by another doctor, Langstaff wrote: 'he is labouring under great trouble of mind as to his future prospects; is subject to fits of excitement; has a great deal of absurd talk; seems unable to distinguish what belongs to himself & others. From what has been told me, he is dangerous to himself & others, has threatened his own life & the lives of his family.' Two days earlier his colleague Dr W.J. Wilson had written the following about the same patient: 'He admits being a masturbator for years & thinks that he can never receive divine pardon for the act. He says he is strongly tempted at this & admitted being tempted to suicide his wife states he has several times attempted suicide once with a razor when he had it to his throat but was prevented by his wife snatching it from him & throwing it into fire. He has attempted to hang himself or at least got the rope to do so. At present he want [sic] to go out from house & take a butcher knife in his pocket. He threatened to kill his wife & children.'[12]

On the admission form of another patient, at the line marked 'Cause,' Langstaff had entered, 'Do not know, was studying *hard* when first taken'; his more confident colleague, temperance advocate Dr John N. Reid, scratched out Langstaff's words and wrote 'self abuse.'[13]

Certification could lead to prolonged incarceration. The last-mentioned young man, who Reid decided had become deranged through 'self abuse,' stayed in the hospital until his death from pneumonia thirty-five years later. His file contained letters from family members asking the doctors about his welfare, if he had liked his Christmas gift, and how much he had suffered when he died. Brief but reassuring replies were always written, but sometimes four or five months had elapsed before they were sent. Contact with family and friends was usually preserved: four of the five patients traced were eventually released to those who had kept in touch with the asylum and been responsible for paying the sizeable bills generated through lengthy admission at the exorbitant rates of three or four dollars per week (for those who could pay).

Aside from the individuals who were 'certified insane,' at least one other 'insane' man may have been sent to the asylum, since there is no record of his having been treated or seen again.[14] The remainder seem to have been tended by their families, but the doctor also gave them medicine, including narcotics, sedatives, iron, and blisters. The absence of fever was an important factor in making a diagnosis of 'lunacy' or 'insanity,' but it seems that Langstaff shared the opinion of Joseph Workman, superintendent of the Toronto asylum, that insanity was 'never purely moral' and may have been partly organic.[15] Indeed, several of the so-called insane and hysterical patients had physical problems. It is equally possible that behind some 'psychoses' that did appear to be 'purely moral' lay as-yet-unrecognized medical problems that can mimic psychiatric disorders, such as auto-immune and hormonal diseases.

Langstaff saw the insane who were kept at home more frequently than those in institutions; their stories can be partially reconstructed. Their precise diagnoses, however, must remain obscure, since there is nothing in the document to allow the assumption that Langstaff's application of the various terms would correspond with our own. He no more used the newly evolving terminology to describe cases treated at home than he did on documents bound for the asylum.

Hysteria was named as a diagnosis in eleven patients, including one man and two married women; the rest appear to have been daughters still living at home. Like that of chlorosis, another disease that had been associated with the biology of young women (see chapter 5), the frequency of hysteria declined in his records: five cases were seen in the 1850s, three in the 1860s, two in the 1870s, and only one (the male) in the 1880s. Pain or difficulty breathing and eating ('hysterical phthisis,' Langstaff once wrote) were the most common symptoms; none seemed to have suffered paralysis. Two felt the classic inability to swallow or 'globus hystericus': a woman who developed her 'hysteria' after giving birth and a girl with repeated 'fits.' The man with hysteria was seen in consultation in 1883. Unfor-

tunately there are few details about his case. Langstaff commented
on the menstrual status of only two patients with hysteria and managed most of them conservatively, either with no medicine at all or
with small doses of opium, sometimes combined with a laxative. He
usually made one or two more visits to make sure the patient had
improved or the medicine had 'checked the attacks'; most recovered
completely.[16]

In these cases, doctors tried to determine whether or not there was
an organic basis for the trouble, but their task was not easy. Langstaff
disagreed with Dr Eckhardt, who had consulted him about a young
female patient who he believed was 'beyond hope from heart disease'; Langstaff thought her rapid breathing was 'hysterical' because
her pulse was slow and her chest clear, but she was given a small
dose of iron.[17] Langstaff himself once thought a patient seemed to
have an organic problem, although he later decided she had hysteria.
Called in haste to this young woman, who was suffering from continuous convulsions and choking, he immediately performed a phlebotomy of twenty-five ounces, but he noticed the blood was only
'half-buffed' and did not have the appearance of inflammation. The
next day she 'took a fit' while Langstaff was there: her head rolled
rapidly from side to side for several minutes, while the rest of her
body was still; he prescribed strong laxatives and stayed for three
hours until the drugs had an effect. The next day she was better and
he gave her a bromide sedative. It was not until the third day that, in
the absence of physical signs and perhaps owing to her brother's
having been sick with rheumatism, he wrote, 'there seems to be a
little hysteria.' He added that 'her turns were on her,' perhaps because he saw the natural evacuation as an explanation for her improved condition. Nevertheless, the family was convinced she was
dying and Langstaff returned a dozen times in as many days to
observe the nearly mute patient, who 'sometimes reache[d] out or up
with one hand'; but he gave no more strong medication and she
eventually recovered.[18]

Another young man was considered by his attendants to have
'hystericks [sic]' and they sprinkled him with water, but Langstaff
thought his severe pain was due to a fracture. Twice only did he
diagnose 'melancholia,' and not until 1885, when he consulted on a
male patient of his nephew Dr George Langstaff at the newly opened
Hawthorn Mineral Springs Residence.[19] Only once did he specifically
name 'puerperal mania'[20] and 'moral insanity.'[21] Of a single young

man who was shaking, he wrote, 'admits of the masturbation.'[22] This behaviour loomed large in the aetiological formulation of many nineteenth-century alienists, but its significance in Langstaff's own concept of mental disease is less clear: he saw this patient once only and the brief record contains the ambiguous words 'inquired after [masturbation] at first,' like an apology or explanation for mentioning the word, suggesting that the nervous man may have raised the subject himself. 'Idiocy,' the nineteenth-century term for mental retardation, does not appear in this record, but four children with probable retardation can be identified by the reported delay in their learning to speak or walk; in one case Langstaff commented on the child's 'somewhat idiotic expression.'[23]

Thus, the majority of the 'psychotic' and 'neurotic' patients are identified for this study by their persistent delusions and aberrant behaviour in the absence of any other identifiable physical ailment. Langstaff attended one possibly autistic child over the course of two years, beginning with care for a fever and cough. She screamed in terror when she experienced hallucinations of snakes, when she was moved, or when strangers entered the house. Otherwise, she ate well and 'seemed cheerful.' Once she lay still without speaking for over a week. She complained of 'flying pains.' Her family was 'alarmed about her. They think she is dying,' he wrote, early in her illness, but she lived on, having strange 'fits' and attempting to bite herself. At first Langstaff prescribed medication for this child, including bromides, iron, hyoscine, electromagnetic stimulation, and laxatives. As the case wore on, he appears to have given no treatment, but he visited the family regularly, even on Christmas Day. Seven years later her attentive mother lay deathly ill of pneumonia: answering a telegraphed summons, Langstaff found that another doctor had not administered the medication properly; he wrote, 'I asked her if she would get better & she said she would,' but she died eight hours later.[24] The little girl's outcome and her reaction to the loss of her mother are unknown.

A few other people seem to have been fortunate enough to be attended at home for months and years, even though their illnesses might have warranted certification. The families may have been devoted to their well-being or ashamed of their lunacy. Most seemed resigned to the situation, but Langstaff saw one man who had consulted 'seven or more doctors' for his 'chronic brain disease' suggestive of dementia.[25] The continued residence of these patients in

Langstaff's community offered him the opportunity for making frequent observations; sometimes he witnessed improvement. For example, he pronounced one young woman to be 'insane' but three months later concluded that 'her reason was returning.'[26]

On two occasions the doctor was called to attend women who had wandered away from home. The first was a patient he had known for a long time: in the spring of 1861 she had been 'out of her mind' and 'unruly'; later that summer she fainted while he treated her son for a painful bladder condition; and a month later she miscarried. Six years later he wrote, 'she has stolen out in her night clothes. Found her down the hill behind the Ritter house,' and the next day, 'she has not spoken since sometime before [she left the house,] only looks down will not speak.' This woman remained in her home and apparently recovered from this incapacity. Langstaff noted seeing her two years later; in a gesture that seemed obligingly to acknowledge some concern of dubious origin, he placed a cup above her left breast, 'where she has felt the pain for years.' Much later he gave her electrostimulation treatments and pronounced her 'cured,' but of what he did not say.[27]

Another young woman wandered many miles one summer night, seemingly obsessed with guilt over small financial matters. Langstaff saw her three days later, after she had been sent home, and he described her journey: '[She left the house at 11 p.m.] stealthily with only her night dress, polonais [an over-dress], shoes & stockings, nothing on her head. Went over to Buttonville, called at Thompson's storekeeper, woke them up, asked to be forgiven for not having paid two cents; passed north to Fierheller's old place as she had not paid ... for an exhibition ticket, woke Miss Fierheller up, talked to her at the door but would not come in. She then passed over to Unionville by the sideline ... to the fifth, then down to a lane to the village ... where they were unable to capture her. During rest of night she walked down [the railway] track to Toronto which she did not reach until afternoon. Early evening she was taken by policemen to the Haven on Seton Street.[28]

Guilt played a similar role in the case of a young hired man who, according to Langstaff, kept pacing 'back and forth across the floor,' saying, 'I will never get better. I have been very foolish.'[29] When the doctor returned the next day, the young man 'had just left for home.' Another man, who had a serious physical ailment, was also apparently consumed by guilt: he was found 'praying noisily' and Langstaff watched by his side with the local minister.[30] Similarly, an older man who was 'very hard of hearing' had been 'seeing things like in delirium tremens [and] seemed to be trying to pray muttering loudly.' Langstaff stayed four hours with him.[31] These particular disturbances seem to bear some relationship to the brief illness of a man who had a wakeful 'religious delirium' and was treated with the electromagnetic battery before his recovery.[32]

Suicide occurred in Langstaff's practice, but it is impossible to know if it happened any more or less often than in other communities.[33] At least nine people in Langstaff's practice tried to commit suicide; most were successful (Table 6.2). Three others may have been intending to kill themselves, as they sustained injuries suspiciously like self-inflicted wounds.

The only suicidal person whom the doctor seems to have attended prior to death was the patient in whom he diagnosed 'moral insanity.' She was receiving care in a neighbour's home; he gave her the newly promoted bromides, iron, opium, aloes, and electrostimulation. How she killed herself is not known, but the coroner called an inquest and Langstaff recorded that the husband 'blamed the coroner' for the autopsy and the intrusion into their privacy.[34] Adopting an attitude of inevitability, the local newspaper seemed to agree that the investigation was 'unnecessary,' but it published her name and the details: 'everybody acquainted with her knew that she had been suffering from depression of spirits ... friends had been uneasy about her for several months ... we heard melancholy tidings and we confess we are not surprised.'[35] Neither physician nor society appears to have displayed any sense of responsibility for such seemingly unpreventable deaths.

Most, but not all, suicides were similarly investigated by the coroner (see chapter 9). For those patients who survived the immediate attempt, the doctor's attentions were necessarily directed to repair of the physical injury; no mention was ever made of the antecedent emotional problems that had produced them. Sometimes his attentions failed. A man who had cut his throat refused to cooperate with the doctor's plans to introduce a feeding catheter and died.[36] Another, who had taken an overdose of laudanum, died after twelve hours of being marched about and fed coffee, the therapy Langstaff had enjoined the family to give.[37] Other patients survived. A young man who tried to hang himself was found 'just after he had kicked over the bench ... black in the face' and vomiting, but he recovered.[38]

TABLE 6.2
Suicides and attempted suicides in Langstaff's practice

Date	Sex	Method	Outcome
12 Feb. 1857	M	Stabbed	Died
30 Aug. 1859	M (murdered wife)	Cut throat	Lived
8 Oct. 1861	M	Laudanum	Died
12 March 1870	F, 'moral insanity'	Overdose?	Died
18 Sept. 1872	M	Cut throat	Died
14 April 1873	M*	Cut wrist	Lived
11 July 1874	M	Cut throat	Died
17 April 1875	M*	Stabbed, drunk	Lived
21 Aug. 1876	M*	Drowned	Died
26 July 1878	M	Cut throat	Died
21 Jan. 1879	F	Hanging	Died
24 April 1879	M	Hanging	Lived
14 July 1884	M*	Alcohol, laudanum	Died

* Suspected suicide identified by circumstances, but Langstaff did not use the word

Source: Langstaff's daybooks

A widow who had taken, probably deliberately, an overdose of morphine was successfully revived; Langstaff was paid for this triumph by the sale of a horse.[39] It is not known if these people chose to continue living when the doctor had discharged them from care.

In the case of a twenty-four-year-old disabled man, the word 'suicide' was not mentioned in the daybooks or in the newspaper, although it may have been whispered. The press referred to him as 'a cripple ... with a spinal complaint,' who could 'walk only with crutches.' The inquest concluded that he had fallen off a fence beside a pond, was stunned, and 'accidentally' drowned. The crucial question, why had he tried to climb such a strategically located fence, remained unanswered; indeed, it was not asked.[40]

Among the patients who might qualify for a diagnosis of neurosis were a few with so-called nervousness. Just as Langstaff believed that fear could have a detrimental effect on pre-existing physical illness, he seemed to think that excessive anxiety could *cause* debility and vomiting. In the case of a nervous young girl who was 'growing very fast' he adopted the corollary that physiology gone awry could produce mental symptoms.[41] His experience with a multitude of febrile patients only endorsed this view.

Langstaff saw many patients with psychiatric symptoms induced by severe illness, especially fever. He indicated they were 'raving,' 'out of [his/her] mind,' 'wandering,' and having 'fancies.' He seems to have taken a special interest in the content of their dreams and hallucinations, since he described them in his records. He commented that one man 'fancies he is three persons and has to bear the sufferings of all three.'[42] A woman who had lost several of her children to diphtheria a few years before was convinced she had 'swallowed a living creature.'[43] Indicating the drastic extent of another man's confusion, Langstaff observed that when the dedicated Presbyterian minister dropped in to visit, he 'thought Rev. Mr Dick [was] a Catholic priest.'[44]

These rather detailed notes contrast markedly with the cryptic entries for the more deeply and more permanently disturbed persons Langstaff sent to the lunatic asylum. Did he think, in some pre-Freudian conception of the unconscious, that in their mutterings these patients would let slip a key to unlock the mystery of their disease? Certainly some early nineteenth-century European physicians, including the influential Maine de Biran, had cited the importance of dreams.[45] Was it simply shocked fascination or amusement?

Bemused fascination with the altered states that heralded death may explain Langstaff's record of the confused ideation of a young man who refused treatment for his fever. The doctor wrote that he found his 'intellect bright ... I asked him repeatedly to let me give him an enema. He said "Who are you?" As I left he said, "Make the chips fly."' The next day the doctor found him silent and dying.[46] Similarly, he wrote about the 'dreamy night' of a man who 'thought he saw eatables & dreamed of eating trees, lamps etc. & gave an amusing account of the fine scenery he witnessed during the night.' Two days later the man was 'excited just like delirium tremens [and] talking incessantly on imaginary occurrences. "Fifteen to twenty men down in my cellar manufacturing the same goods advertised in Chicago."' Langstaff gave this man morphine and opium, with laxatives to counteract the side-effects, and he 'sat on bed with him and stroked his forehead.'[47]

The doctor distinguished between visions (or delusions), which occurred in a waking state, and dreams, which occurred during sleep. Some dreams had sinister, premonitory connotations, if only in retrospect. A man with fever dreamt about his financial problems and about 'goings on' with the Americans. He died four days later.[48] A young woman told the doctor she had dreamt that she was 'falling off a house'; a young man thought someone was abusing his horses; and a little boy who dreamt he had died, did so on the following day.[49]

❦

Alcohol was often cited as a cause for mental illness; it was frequently abused in nineteenth-century Ontario, where it was both an important commodity and a serious problem. According to the vivid memories of Langstaff's brother John, liquor caused many tragedies and was far too readily available in the numerous taverns that 'cluttered' the country – 'two per mile' along Yonge Street.[50] The problem of drinking to excess was not thought of as an illness so much as a personal weakness that could eventually bring poverty, violence, and illness. Physicians, such as Langstaff's teacher John Rolph, were among the first supporters of the early temperance movement, which also included political Reformers and members of several Protestant denominations, among them Presbyterians. The Dunkin Act of 1864 (Canada West) and the Scott Act (or Canada Temperance Act of 1878) created the so-called local option, making it possible for municipalities to set their own standards about liquor sales.[51] After this legislation, medical enthusiasm for temperance waned, as the movement set its sights on the extreme of prohibition and began to rely on the support of alternative practitioners, such as homeopathists and eclectics.[52] Alcohol as a medication for the insane came under attack in the Ontario legislature in the late 1870s, but most doctors continued to use it, as a stimulant and as a source of nutrition in treating other diseases, and despite scientific evidence that it was neither.

Throughout Langstaff's life, his attitude, like that of his colleagues, appears to have been somewhat contradictory: he opposed drink as a social evil and used it often as a medication. For him, however, there was no contradiction: the proper use of alcohol was to be decided by qualified medical practitioners; alcohol was a drug and, like the other remedies he used, could be dangerous. Langstaff collected newspaper reports on alcohol consumption, editorials attacking Canada's irresponsible involvement in the 'licensed groggeries,' and poems satirizing drink; he pasted the clippings in his daybooks.[53]

Matthew Teefy also kept clippings about alcohol; however, he and the doctor, with whom he so often agreed (and almost always voted), seem to have parted company on matters of temperance. Teefy sold liquor from his general store; a survey of his records shows that it may have been one of his greatest means of livelihood. In the twelve months between June 1854 and June 1855 he bought and presumably sold no less than 1,785 gallons of whisky. He replenished his stock in two- or three-barrel quantities every few weeks and sold it to his thirsty customers by the quart or the gallon – a torrent of Amazonian dimensions to have flowed from a single source into a village of some three or four hundred souls served by several other stores and taverns. My survey was confined only to whisky and did not include the postmaster's impressive trade in porter, gin, and cognac.[54]

Teefy's own collection of newspaper clippings on alcohol reflects his dual concerns, first, as an upright magistrate and village clerk in an age of increasingly stringent legislation against liquor and, second, as a law-abiding merchant loath neither to sell nor to take a drink. One excerpt from the *Whitby Chronicle* told how a magistrate's judgment under the Dunkin Act had been overturned on a technicality; the village clerk had failed to sign his municipality's own copy of the law, thereby making it invalid. The author warned that 'magistrates have to act with caution ... many – and perhaps that is the safest course – refuse to convict under [the Dunkin Act].' As a careful magistrate who prided himself on never having a decision reversed, Teefy pasted this item near the title page of his book on the duties of justices of the peace.[55] Perhaps it was to serve as a reminder for some future time when he might be confronted with the clerical task of registering legislation distasteful to village shopkeepers; an absent-minded village clerk could be an asset to a law-abiding magistrate tolerant of both the needs of merchants and the foibles of human nature, especially when merchant, clerk, and judge were one and the same.

Teefy's preoccupation with getting around the anti-drink legislation may have turned into amusement over his doctor's attempt to see a new law upheld. Late one Saturday night in July 1859, a fight broke out in Lemon's tavern; in the middle of the night a young man came to Langstaff needing attention for thirteen cuts on his head and some bruises. The outraged doctor knew alcohol was to blame and laid charges against the tavern owner for having sold liquor after 7 p.m. on a Saturday 'contrary to the law passed last session.' Liquor had indeed been sold, but magistrate R. Marsh said that, as the buyer 'had put his horse in the stable, he came under the denomination of "traveller," which Dr Langstaff disputed'; travellers were exempt from the law. The tavern owner made peace and avoided a conviction by offering to pay all costs, but it was agreed that the law needed clarification. In spite of Lemon's offer, Langstaff paid a court cost of fifteen shillings and saw no returns for his midnight dressing, while Teefy, pleased with finding a new loophole, pasted another clipping in his book.[56]

Drunkenness and its consequences – fighting and injury – appeared regularly in Langstaff's practice. A significant proportion of his surgical cases and coroner's inquests involved people who directly or indirectly had been victims of alcohol. He attended nearly twenty attacks of delirium tremens in fourteen different men. Some of these patients lay ill in taverns, where the doctor came to prescribe narcotics and sedatives. A single, uncontrollably violent man who had 'the horrors' was sent, 'bound hand and foot,' to the hospital in Toronto.[57] One man suffered four episodes of delirium tremens over the course of five years. His illness was marked by the gentle quality of his behaviour: Langstaff wrote, 'he fancies a baby along side him in the bed ... [and] said how funny it seemed with his arms off. He fancies many absurd things.'[58] Another, who had been 'drunk and fighting his family,' seems to have been removed from his home for months.[59] Occupational predisposition is apparent: patients with drinking problems included one hotel-keeper and three doctors.[60]

In 1858 Langstaff described confabulation, the classic dissembling banter of alcohol-induced confusion: the man, he said, was 'disposed to talk cheerfully [and] it is a little while before his wandering is noticed.'[61] So familiar was the doctor with the characteristic features of alcoholic delusions that they became the standard by which all other perceptual disturbances were measured. Indeed, because families often dosed their sick with spirits, it was difficult to determine to what extent alcohol was responsible for symptoms in *any* medical case, unless the patient 'smell[ed] strongly of whiskey.'[62]

Thus, the man who mistook his pastor for a priest had a condition 'just like delirium tremens.' He had been drinking beer and bleeding from his intestine; which of his problems came first in this obscure illness is not clear to the reader and was probably no more obvious to the doctor. Langstaff reported that the patient was singing 'Johnny come home & we'll all get stone blind,' but he ordered him to drink more beer (mixed with egg, of course) and buttermilk. 'Two [men] have to sit and almost hold him,' the doctor wrote, and 'his brother keeps quietly rubbing his hair.' This man died at the end of two weeks.[63]

The long-term ravages of alcohol abuse were also familiar to Langstaff, but the fact that they were far less frequent than intoxication, delusions, and injury suggests that such patients died of accidental death before they developed cirrhosis or the dangerously dilated esophageal veins called varices. The doctor attributed enlargement of the liver, jaundice, ascites, and debility to drink; after caring for one such patient he wrote the aphoristic statement 'old drunkards sink readily.'[64]

All patients with delirium tremens were male, but Langstaff was aware that women could be drinkers too; occasionally he saw children accidentally poisoned with alcohol. He was summoned to prescribe for a little girl who 'drank a bottle of whiskey'; when an infant died one hour after birth, he noted, 'the mother drank.'[65] The doctor adjusted his therapy for a young girl with altered sensorium, because she was 'used to taking six glasses of beer a week.'[66] The general availability of alcohol fostered suspicion of surreptitious ingestion: when a sick woman felt 'suddenly worse,' the doctor observed that 'she motioned for the brandy.'[67]

Treatments could be given for intoxication and for the physical changes induced by alcohol, but there was no real medical therapy to stave off the impulse to consume: doctors simply instructed their patients not to drink. To prevent alcoholism, Langstaff and physicians like him could do no better than set a dry example and support organized temperance. In fact, the first temperance society in the region had been founded by Dr Lucius O'Brien of Thornhill.[68] The zeal of Dr John Reid, Sr, was captured in his written vow of total abstinence in the daybook Langstaff acquired with the practice.[69] Reid's son, John N. Reid, also of Thornhill, conspicuously promoted the merits of prohibition in the years between the 'local option' legislation; his activities earned him a semi-literate threat on his life, which was duly published by the local press.[70] Curiously enough, Reid, Jr, and Langstaff were often at odds over the use of alcohol in medical cases; in this setting, sometimes Reid advocated brandy when Langstaff did not.

Quietly, but consistently, Langstaff used his position as a prominent Presbyterian citizen to take a political and social stance on booze. Above all, he did not drink alcohol, though he was offered many opportunities; from time to time, given the hardship of his work and his faith in the nutritive and restorative powers of alcohol, he may actually have been tempted. After a thirty-mile journey in the dead of winter to attend a patient at Mount Albert, he wrote that the 'tavern keeper pressed me to take rye but I stayed with cold water and was the warmer for it.'[71]

Alcohol problems appear to have reached an all-time high in Langstaff's practice in the early 1860s and may have been a motive for the doctor's seeking a position on the Vaughan township council in 1864. At the end of his first year as a councillor he moved that the township respond to a petition and pass a by-law to prohibit the sale of intoxicating liquor; there is no evidence that the by-law was passed. At another meeting soon after, Langstaff moved that the fees for tavern licences be raised from fifty-three to one hundred dollars. This decision carried and the fees were raised, but it was quickly protested by those whose livelihood depended on liquor consumption, and the council backed down.[72]

Belying the evidence in Langstaff's daybooks, Richmond Hill prided itself on its relative calm. The local press made it plain that the contrasting rowdiness of Thornhill, three miles south, had a great deal to do with the dissolution of drink, prevented in Richmond Hill by the edifying presence of a vigorous Protestant Sunday school, a Mechanics Institute, and above all an active Temperance Hall.[73] For many years Langstaff was landlord to the Mechanics Institute and the Temperance Hall; he even read an essay, the content of which sadly has been lost, at a Good Templars' meeting in 1871.[74] Five years later, in a gesture that might be interpreted as the result of a flagging interest in the cause, he converted his Temperance Hall to 'dwellings'; however, the account books make it clear that the Independent Order of Good Templars had rarely possessed sufficient funds to pay their rent. Nevertheless, the town quickly raised money to build a replacement building.[75]

Langstaff also attended the many 'Temperance and Educational Entertainments' that passed through Richmond Hill. He witnessed performances of the famous moralizing plays 'The Bottle' and 'Ten Nights in a Bar-Room.' The reporters found the latter 'most fastidious,' with 'nothing to offend the eye,' and confidently predicted that the 'civilized portion of the globe will check intemperance.'[76] Langstaff also subscribed to *Grip*, a satirical weekly of social criticism inspired by temperance and Protestant values, and he may have attended the Richmond Hill 'chalk talk' of its caricaturist-publisher, J.W.

Bengough.[77] The doctor was present at Good Templar reunions and noted going down to rowdy Thornhill, necessarily 'excited' over the temperance question, to hear the lecture of D.I.K. Rine, a reformed alcoholic and ex-convict whose brief tour through Canada came to an abrupt end a few months later after he was tried and acquitted on a charge of indecent assault.[78] When temperance advocate J.B. Gough went to meet his maker, the Protestant clergy of Richmond Hill gave a triple sermon in his honour at the request of the community temperance organizations; Langstaff was in the congregation.[79]

The doctor was also in the right place at the right time to have participated in two other related events, but the daybooks allow only for speculation about the extent of his involvement. During the 1860 tour of Canada of the Prince of Wales, he wrote, 'Toronto in & saw the Prince of Wales,' having been disappointed three days before when the events were cancelled owing to rain.[80] As Langstaff was no lover of the monarchy, it may be possible he was with the temperance demonstration: the *Globe* reported that a group of 'disappointed teetotallers' had been caught in the same rain that had thwarted Langstaff. Three days later, when the doctor did manage to see the royal visitor, the Prince received a deputation from the temperance societies as he inaugurated Queen's Park.[81] The other apparently close connection came in conjunction with the Centennial Exhibition of Philadelphia, which Langstaff attended in early October 1876, arriving during or just after a special conference held there by a group of physicians who founded a new journal to engage in medical combat against drink.[82]

Langstaff seems to have stood on the prohibition side of the temperance movement, as his 1864 motion to prohibit alcohol sales in Vaughan township certainly suggests. His position may have been slightly more extreme than that of his medical colleagues, although other Toronto physicians, especially those who were active Reformers, did support temperance. The lavish annual dinners of the Toronto School of Medicine, presided over by W.T. Aikins, were conducted on the 'strictest temperance principles': the Queen and numerous others were toasted with water.[83] In 1874, at one of these banquets, Langstaff met Canada's leading intellectual, Goldwin Smith, an advocate of true temperance rather than prohibition. Smith's presence at the dinner tends to imply some medical concurrence with his views: moderate drinking was fine, but cheap whisky was the bane of the country because it was accessible to the poor, who had the greatest need for oblivion.[84] Indeed, Langstaff's support of the hike in tavern licence fees ten years before had been an action designed to raise the price of alcohol beyond the means of those most likely to abuse it.

Perhaps influenced by his colleagues and illustrious associates, Langstaff may have softened his stance, from prohibition to moderation. If so, his attitude would have moved in concert with the generally accepted shift in medical allegiance that became increasingly evident in the decade after his death.[85] Unfortunately, the record is too vague to be certain: in later life he made only one small remark that hints at a turn away from total prohibition. During an 1885 Presbyterian conference Langstaff heard lectures pertaining to 'Religion in the home' and 'Temperance' and wrote that the speaker, the Reverend Mr MacDonnell, 'objects to teetotalism being called temperance ... [he] approves of a little sherry.'[86] The local paper took away the same impression of MacDonnell's attitude but did not condone his view.[87] Was the ageing Langstaff marvelling at creeping decadence? Or was he musing on the potential merits of a little sherry? A definite answer to these questions cannot be found in his records; and regardless of any subtle changes in his later stance on temperance, he did not abandon the cause. In later years the movement was championed by his second wife, who relied heavily on the doctor's monetary support; and, it is clear, the doctor gave generously (see chapter 9).

Langstaff was sensitive to the psychic state of his patients and believed in the interdependence of mind and body, but his records, together with documents he completed for the lunatic asylum, suggest that he had only a tentative awareness of or confidence in the new medicalization of psychiatric illness. He was strongly opposed, however, to the public use of alcohol, believing it to be a medication with stimulating properties capable of altering both the minds and the bodies of those who abused it. While he seems to have been sympathetic to people with psychic disorders, he appears to have been somewhat intolerant of people who drank, and he supported legislation and social action to abolish the problem. In later years his personal commitment to this cause through political and public channels would be increasingly apparent.

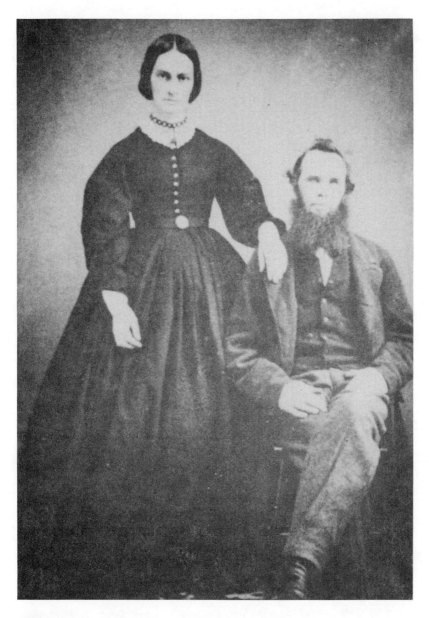

James Miles Langstaff with his first wife, Mary Ann Miller (1835–79), circa 1865. The couple had eleven children, only three of whom survived infancy. Langstaff attended Mary Ann during nine of her deliveries and through her final illness in 1879.

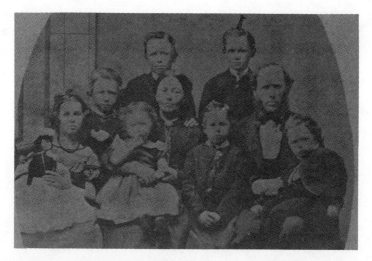

The doctor's older brother John Langstaff, Jr (b. 1819), and his wife, Elizabeth Brett Langstaff of Thornhill, shown here with their children, circa 1867. James Miles Langstaff attended Elizabeth during the births of six children and at least one miscarriage. The three oldest sons, George, Elliott, and Garibaldi, became physicians and practised briefly with their uncle.

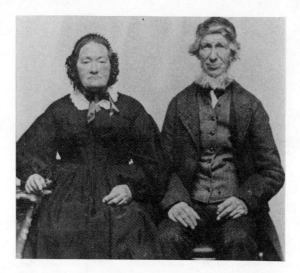

Henry Miller (b. 1797) and his wife, Mary Kennedy, were neighbours of the Langstaffs and the parents of James Langstaff's first wife, Mary Ann. Langstaff was often summoned to care for members of the Miller family. He treated his mother-in-law during her final illness in 1865 and his father-in-law during his, nineteen years later.

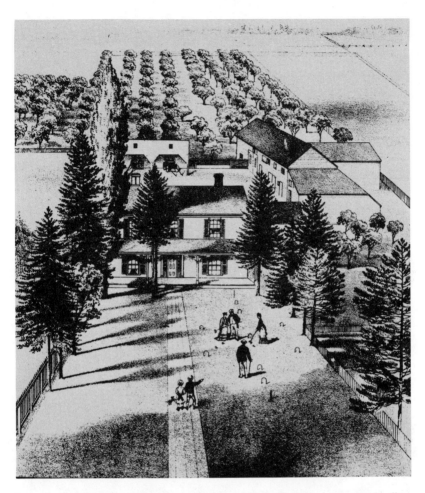

James Langstaff's house was built of squared timbers in 1849 as a one-storey dwelling facing Yonge Street, but it was expanded in the 1850s, and various additions and porches were added in the following years. The elegant lawn, drive shed, stables, and apple orchard are visible in this 1878 illustration. Both Langstaff's son Rolph and his grandson James Rolph practised from this house, which is still the residence of the latter.

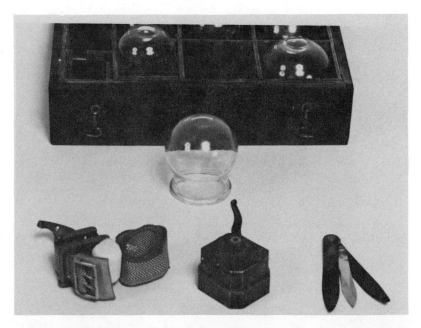

Instruments similar to those used by James Langstaff. At top: a cupping jar and case; at bottom from right: a vaccinating lancet, a scarificator to cut veins for phlebotomy, and a tourniquet

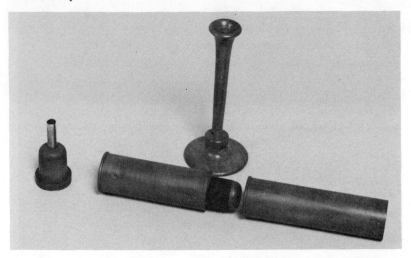

Rigid stethoscopes similar to those used by Langstaff until 1865, when he purchased a flexible stethoscope. At bottom: the three pieces of a replica of the original Laennec model of 1826, made by Bob Marvin of Woburn, Quebec. The doctor placed one end of the instrument on the patient's chest and listened at the other.

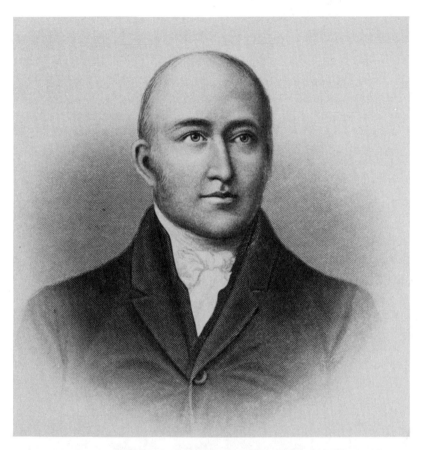

John Rolph (1795–1870) was a lawyer, politician, and physician who had trained at Guy's Hospital in London, England. He was exiled for his involvement in the 1837 Rebellion, but he returned to Toronto, where he founded a proprietary medical school in 1843. James Langstaff was a pupil in Rolph's School in 1844–6 and continued his studies at Guy's Hospital.

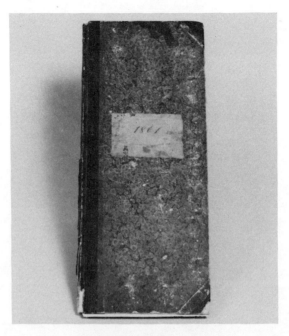

Langstaff's daybook for 1861

Detail from Langstaff's daybook showing the entry for 3 October 1864, discussed in the opening of chapter 1. All daybook pages were kept in this neat and legible script.

Typical page from one of Langstaff's account books, showing the medical debts of a few families whose names began with the letter 'B' for the years 1879 to 1884. On the upper left the record indicates that Francis Boynton paid some of his doctor's bill with a cow and oats.

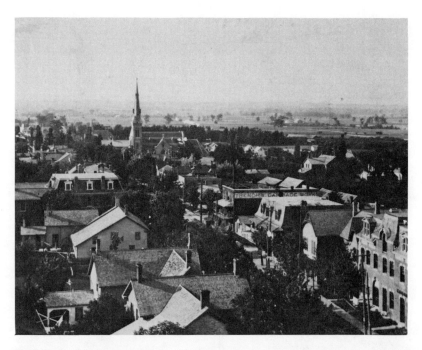

The village of Richmond Hill, as seen by one looking north from the tower of the Presbyterian Church (circa 1900). The community was situated on Yonge Street and was surrounded by prosperous farms in Vaughan and Markham townships. It was incorporated as a village in 1873; its population hovered around 1,000 for most of Langstaff's career. The doctor served on school boards, on township councils, and as the fourth reeve in 1880.

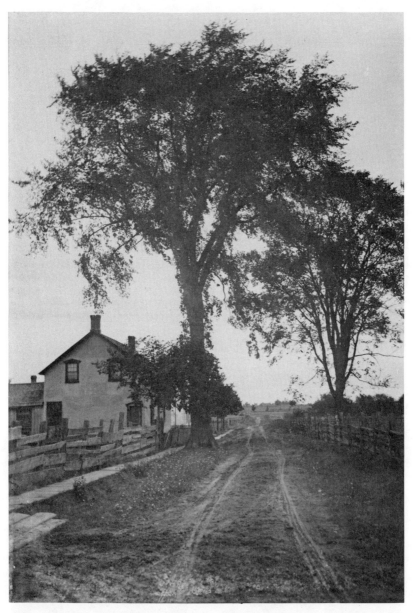

Unidentified road near Richmond Hill. Langstaff frequently saw injured travellers, and he became an advocate for road maintenance.

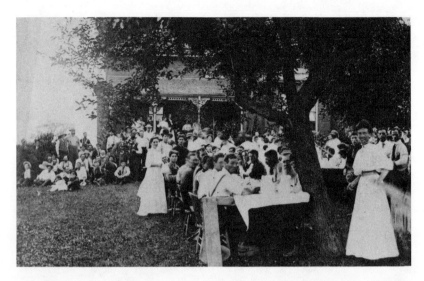

Supper at Harry Rumble's barn raising, 1908. Picnics, teas, concerts, plays, and fairs were an important part of the social fabric of Langstaff's community. The doctor's presence at such events was often noted in the newspapers, especially if he had provided emergency care to accident victims.

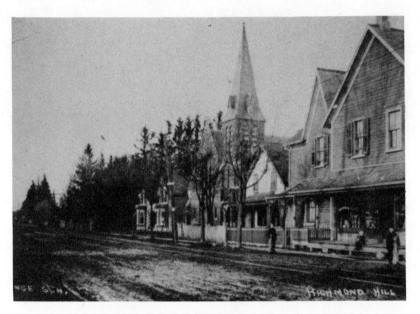

Yonge Street in the town of Richmond Hill, late nineteenth century

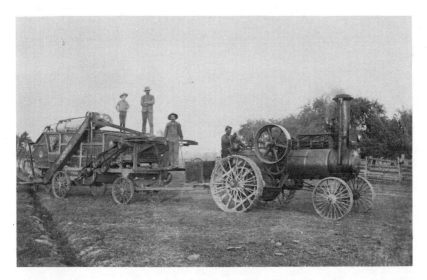

Men of the Richmond Hill region with steam-powered farm machinery, which had appeared in the community by 1879. Note the exposed belts and pulleys, which would now be viewed as unacceptably dangerous. Langstaff was called to attend many accidents caused by the new technology on the farms and on the railways.

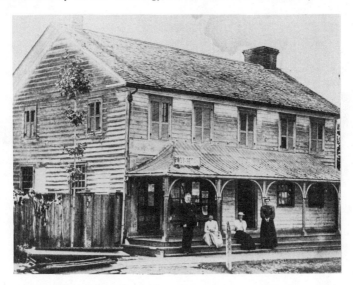

Matthew Teefy with his three daughters, Clara, Louisa, and Mary Alice, in front of the Richmond Hill post office. Teefy was postmaster from 1850 until his death in 1911, and he served as village clerk and treasurer for thirty-one years. Langstaff was the family physician.

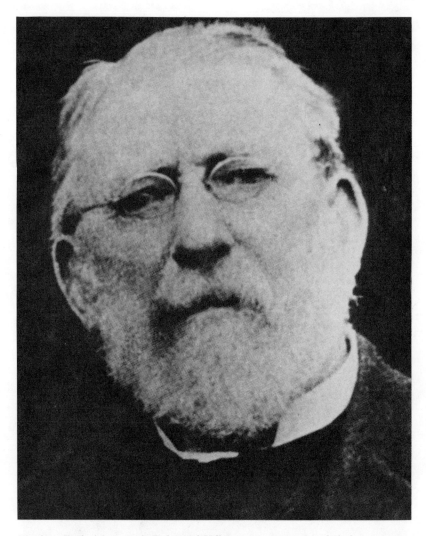

Matthew Teefy (1822–1911), Richmond Hill postmaster, municipal clerk, magistrate, and merchant, was the father of nine children, six of whom survived infancy. His political opinions were often similar to those of James Langstaff; however, the two men differed on the matter of alcohol.

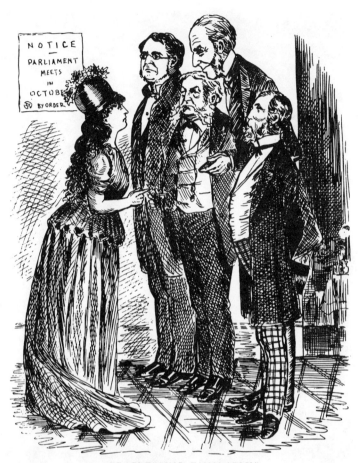

"PROGRESSING FAVORABLY."

MISS CANADA (ANXIOUSLY).—"DOCTORS, HOW DO YOU FIND THE POOR DEAR PREMIER?"

DR. B—N (FOR THE M.D.'s).—"MADAM, WE'VE JUST HAD A CONSULTATION; THE SYMPTOMS ARE HOPEFUL—WE BELIEVE
HE CAN'T SURVIVE OCTOBER!"

An anti-Conservative caricature by J.W. Bengough for the satirical magazine *Grip*
(4 October 1873), a favourite of Liberal (Reform)-minded readers, including James
Miles Langstaff. The Liberal politicians Blake, Cartwright, Brown, and Mackenzie are
portrayed as doctors confidently prognosticating to Miss Canada the impending demise
of Prime Minister John A. Macdonald. Langstaff knew both Blake and Brown, and he
spent many days in caring for Alexander Mackenzie, who was stricken with a sudden
illness while campaigning in Richmond Hill in June 1882.

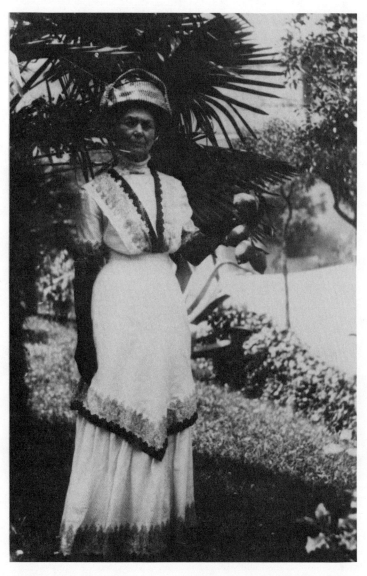

Langstaff's second wife, Eleanor Frances Louisa Palmer Langstaff (1851–1934), was a high school teacher twenty-seven years younger than her husband. She was obliged to resign from her job at her marriage in 1882 and had some difficulties with the doctor's adolescent children, who had been her pupils. She gave birth to four more children and was attended at delivery by her husband. She is shown here circa 1905, sixteen years after the doctor's death.

EXTENSIVE
CREDIT SALE!
——OF——
HORSES, COLTS, CATTLE, ETC.

The undersigned has received instructions from
DR. JAMES LANGSTAFF,
To Sell by Public Auction at the
PalmerHouse, RichmondHill
—ON SATURDAY,—
FEBRUARY 28, 1885,
The Following Valuable Property :—

1 Span Heavy Dark Dappled Grey Horses 5 years old.	1 Bay Mare, Draught. aged.
1 Span Draught Horses. 6 years old.	1 Bay Colt rising 2 years old, (General Purpose.
1 Chestnut Horse, Heavy Draught, aged	1 Small Driver, 5 years old.
1 Roan Mare, Light Draught, heavy in foal.	1 Colt, 9 months old, General Purpose.
1 Black Mare, 8 years old, General Purpose.	8 Heifers rising 2 & 3 years old.
	3 Steers, rising 3 years old.
	1 New Milch Cow.
	2 Cows supposed to be in calf.

All the animals will be sold separately.
Sale to Commence at 12 O'Clock.
TERMS:
All Sums of $50 and under, 8 months' credit ; all sums over
$50 one year's credit. 8 per cent per annum off at
any time for cash.

The above animals are owned by Dr. J. Langstaff, and are independent of his
driving horses and colts.

SALEM ECKARDT, Auct.
Richmond Hill, Feb. 16th, 1885.

Announcement of Langstaff's credit sale of 1885. The owner of several farms and abundant livestock, the doctor was one of the most prosperous citizens of his region, but he was frequently short of cash. After his second marriage, he made renovations to his home and donations to charities. This credit sale may have been part of an attempt to improve his cash flow.

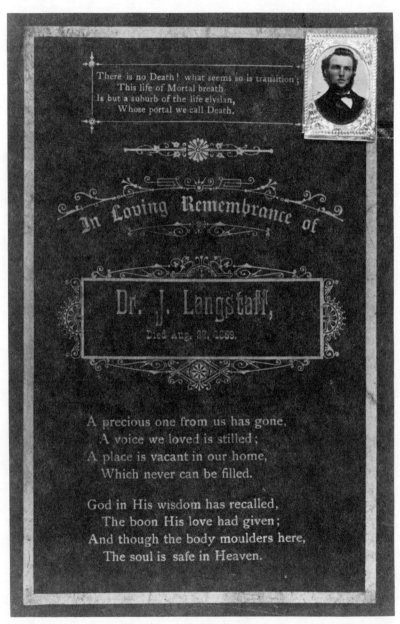

There is no Death! what seems so is transition;
This life of Mortal breath
Is but a suburb of the life elysian,
Whose portal we call Death.

In Loving Remembrance of

Dr. J. Langstaff,

Died Aug. 22, 1889.

A precious one from us has gone,
A voice we loved is stilled;
A place is vacant in our home,
Which never can be filled.

God in His wisdom has recalled,
The boon His love had given;
And though the body moulders here,
The soul is safe in Heaven.

Announcement of the death of James Langstaff with a poem and image of the doctor as a young man

CHAPTER SEVEN

Accidents, Injuries, and Operations:

Langstaff's Practice of Surgery

Surgical advances of the second half of the nineteenth century led to several changes in the practice of medicine, including increased specialization and a shift in the role of the hospital. The advent of anaesthesia in the late 1840s and antisepsis in the late 1860s fostered these changes by making it possible to perform previously inconceivable operations on the thorax and abdomen, without pain or fear of infection. The resultant flurry of surgical activity led to an increase in the rate of operative intervention and to the heady optimism that would characterize early twentieth-century medical endeavour.[1] The Langstaff records provide a special opportunity to observe exactly what the surgical needs of a rural community were and how these achievements came to affect an individual practice.

About ten per cent of Langstaff's daily activities were devoted to what can be called 'surgery': the treatment of injuries, fractures, wounds and lacerations, minor procedures, such as the insertion of urinary catheters, tooth pulling, and some operations (see Table 7.1). After the first decade this activity declined slightly to approximately six per cent of visits, where it remained for the next thirty years. In all decades most of Langstaff's surgical work was devoted to repairing fractures or dressing wounds, not performing operations – a

TABLE 7.1
Langstaff's surgical practice

	1850s (5 years)	1860s (1 year)	1870s (3 years)	1880s (2 years)
No. of surgery visits	791	256	613	326
Percentage of all practice	10.8	7.4	5.8	6
Total accidents	40	23	71	23
Yearly average	8	23	23.6	11.5
Yearly fractures	6.8	17	11	8
Type of activity (percentage of surgical visits)				
Dressings	36.6	36.9	34.8	45.8
Tooth extraction	28.8	18	20.9	24.8
Injuries and fractures	18	17.8	24.2	10.7
Operations	13.7	21.6	14.5	11.7
Cautery	1.9	1.6	4.1	4.6
Catheter	1	4.1	1.5	2.4

Source: All entries in Langstaff's daybooks for 1849–54, 1861, 1872–5, 1880–2

pattern typical of surgical and general practices elsewhere.[2] By the end of his career Langstaff had recognized and implemented some of the principles of anaesthesia and antisepsis.

Anaesthesia entered medicine at the same time as Langstaff. In 1848, only months after chloroform was introduced, he had witnessed its effects during operations at Guy's Hospital in London; both ether and chloroform had been used in Canada by the time he returned.[3] Langstaff did few operations in the early years; although he once noted having given a patient wine and laudanum before a procedure,[4] he never used ether for surgery. In the 1850s he did have patients inhale it from a handkerchief for the relief of discomfort caused by medical conditions such as asthma, delirium tremens, and palpitations; twice he claimed it had 'no effect.'[5]

Langstaff's first record of chloroform anaesthesia for a surgical procedure came during his eighth year of practice, in May 1857, when he put a little boy to sleep in order to remove a scar from under his toes and straighten his foot.[6] The second administration occurred more than two years later in the delicate catheterization of a little girl with a chronic leaking fistula between her bladder and her vagina, the result of a laceration caused by a fall upon a ladder one year before.[7] By this time a Toronto death had been blamed on chloroform anaesthetic that had been administered by J.H. Richardson, Langstaff's colleague and fellow Rolphian.[8]

Perhaps because of the known risks, Langstaff's surgical use of chloroform was exceeded by his medical use of the drug as a pain-killer in terminal illness until the mid-1860s (Table 7.2). If the patient so desired, he would occasionally leave the anaesthetic and instructions with the family. For example, a patient suffering with abdominal pain and vomiting 'asked for the chloroform to inhale. I left a bottle and showed [her husband] how to use it.'[9] Surgical use, especially in dentistry, increased slowly; eventually anaesthetic sleep was induced prior to treating fractures or dislocations and before most major elective operations; sometimes, however, he wrote that the 'chloroform did not take effect.'[10] On rare occasions after 1870, he gave anaesthetic to birthing mothers (see chapter 8).

Langstaff's community never ceased to generate accidents to which his surgical skills could be applied. Because of their patterns of work, men seem to have been most at risk for violent injuries, but children were often hurt too (Table 7.3). The doctor sutured, dressed, and splinted a litany of accidental and deliberate wounds, the recitation of which evokes the increasing mechanization of nineteenth-century Ontario. The most common source of injury was the horse that kicked, bit, threw, ran away with its riders, and sometimes fell on top of them. On at least three occasions Langstaff was called to attend severe fracture dislocations of elbow, clavicle, or shoulder in men who had been holding horses that shied because of a barking dog or 'on account of the steam cars.' On a hot day in 1869 he saw three different people who had been kicked by horses: one with a fractured jaw, another with blood in the knee-joint, and the third with a badly bruised thigh.[11]

The associated saddles, gigs, buggies, cutters, sleighs, wagons, and reapers contributed to the carnage. One man's ribs were crushed by the tongue of the wagon; another was dragged upside down with his foot in his stirrup; some people were run over. Racing teams of horses created great fear and serious injury, especially when their passengers were tossed onto stones or fence posts.[12] These injuries could lead to instant death,[13] especially if the horse fell on top of the victim, but death could follow even minor wounds if gangrene or tetanus set in. A man by the inapt name of Ritter suffered an excruciating crush injury to the genitalia turning his penis and scrotum 'black & as big as a mare's head'; despite successful catheterization, he died.[14]

TABLE 7.2
Applications of anaesthetic recorded in Langstaff's daybooks

	1850s (5 years)	1860s (1 year)	1870s (3 years)	1880s (2 years)
Ether	5	2	0	0
Chloroform	0	13	33	31
Yearly average	1	15	11	15.5
Number of times an anaesthetic was mentioned for each purpose				
Dentistry	0	2	18	20
Operations	0	3	4	2
Obstetrics	0	0	1	4
Pain relief	5	10	10	5

Source: All entries in Langstaff's daybooks for 1849–54, 1861, 1872–5, 1880–2

TABLE 7.3
Accidents and injuries in men, women, and children

	1850s (5 years)	1860s (1 year)	1870s (3 years)	1880s (2 years)
Men	22	9	39	12
Women	5	1	8	4
Children	13	13	24	7
Total accidents	40	23	71	23

Source: All entries in Langstaff's daybooks for 1849–54, 1861, 1872–5, 1880–2

Langstaff also witnessed the 'perfect *ris sardonicus*' (the ghastly but classic 'sardonic smile') of a man doomed to die of tetanus following an insignificant wound sustained when he was thrown from his buggy one week before.[15]

Bad roads, aggravated by rain and snow, were almost as dangerous as skittish horses. Thirteen-year-old diarist Sophia MacNab described tumbles, near accidents, and the 'dreadful state' of the snowbound or 'muddy roads'; when the sleigh carrying her 'poor old vicar' overturned, the man was 'unable to move' until Sophia's sister and the driver 'managed to clime [sic] over the side of the sleigh' and 'assist the poor gentleman out of the snow.'[16] Late in life Langstaff would become a crusader for improved roads, perhaps in the interest of his own health as well as that of his patients (see chapter 9).

Children and women also suffered horse-related injuries. One little boy fell under 'a waggon loaded with manure.' Langstaff described the horror of the father, who 'looked down & saw him crossways under the wheel' as it passed over his abdomen; 'the print of the child's back & hips was in the mud,' but he survived.[17] A woman broke both arms when her horse 'threw her back against the sill of [a] tavern, [and] ... her daughter fell on top.'[18] Another mother, thrown from her buggy when the horses ran away, sustained a severe head injury because, Langstaff wrote, she 'held her child safe & let her own head strike.'[19] The doctor was obliged to attend his own lively daughter Nelly after she was thrown from her mare and bruised her hip.[20] The public laid some responsiblity for these accidents on the riders: Miss Langstaff and her horse had been in trouble for terrorizing children in a holiday crowd once before, and at that time even the Toronto paper had made it plain that she and equestrians like her had a moral obligation to safeguard the welfare of others.[21]

Other animals also caused injuries, by biting, kicking, and goring. Langstaff sutured and dressed face wounds caused by dog bites in five children and saw wounds caused by cattle and pigs. One man lost two teeth when a cow's horn 'hooked his mouth' and passed out through his cheek just below the bone.[22] The doctor explained how another patient broke his collar-bone: 'a yearling bull got him down and would have killed him if not for Jo Bond's boy.'[23] Yet another lad was 'attacked by a bull ... as if only in play' and was found 'insensible' with 'horrid gashes' to his face that healed slowly and scarred.[24] In the late 1860s the doctor attended knife wounds sustained in butchering a pig and a cow; he noted that one of the butcher's cuts was 'poisoned' and a spotted rash was spreading.[25]

Infrequently, Langstaff was called to attend burns. A child was seen after swallowing scalding water that produced '100 blisters the size of a turnip seed' on the tongue.[26] A boy with a rheumatic hip was burned by a relative, whose hand had slipped during the dutiful execution of Langstaff's order to pass a hot smoothing iron over the aching joint covered in thick flannel.[27] Another man badly seared his hands and the top of his head when he tried to save grain from a barn fire, a little girl died at a fireworks party, two boys were injured in an explosion of powder, and the high school inspector's daughter suffered minor burns when a bottle of ammonia exploded in her face and eyes.[28]

The press was interested in injuries and often mentioned the role of the doctor; on slow days the reporter may have exaggerated the situation. When a little girl at a village picnic 'was struck on the temple by a swing,' the paper viewed Langstaff's presence as 'fortunate' and reported that he 'immediately attended to her' and that 'under his care ... she is recovering rapidly.' Casting some doubt on the accuracy of the paper, the daybook mentions only a single visit to a little girl of a different name, with a minor 'scalp wound at picnic.'[29]

The mid-nineteenth century advent of machines brought its own special surgical problems. Between 1851 and 1854 the Northern Railway was laid just west of Richmond Hill and extended north to Collingwood. Langstaff attended men injured during the construction. In the following years he saw other people hurt by passing trains or by stumbling on the rails.[30] One man lost his life, another his arm, from intoxicated sleep on the railway track.[31] The trains frightened horses, further aggravating the damage the animals already caused: Langstaff's physician-nephew George nearly died of head wounds when his horses reared and threw him on the 'hard pavement' of Yonge Street at a railway crossing near Yorkville.[32]

To some extent, trains could be avoided, but the farmers, lumberjacks, and sawmillers could do little to escape the axes, drums, blades, buzz-saws, and threshing machines that lacerated their flesh, claiming digits, limbs, and lives. Axe wounds resulted in deep cuts and Langstaff was always wary of the lethal inflammation that favoured dirty wounds. The doctor managed cuts conservatively, with washing, suturing if necessary, and dressing with dry lint and, later, carbolic acid. Saw injuries, if they did not result in amputation, were usually cleaner and less ragged, but when extensive they could be fatal too. When David Troyer was killed in his sawmill, the local newspaper reported that he died with his 'head injured, back broken, leg smashed, and breast broken in.'[33] The figures are too small to make generalizations; however, serious axe injuries appear to decline (from four in the 1850s to none in the 1880s), while those caused by circular saws and planing buzz-saws remained relatively constant throughout the four decades (at one or two every ten years). The mills brought other forms of injury even to bystanders: two little boys were crushed to death by a falling sawlog.[34]

Langstaff tended his first threshing-machine accident in 1860, about nine years after the machines first appeared in Ontario and just as they were becoming commonplace.[35] These machines, powered first by horses on a sweep or treadmill and later by steam, consisted of a spinning cylinder covered in spikes into which grain was fed and a tumbling shaft where the chaff was separated.[36] At first there were few safety devices to prevent limbs being drawn into the rotating drum; Langstaff saw several injuries of arms, hands, and even legs and feet.

Threshing-machine injuries could be fatal. Langstaff saw one man three days after he had been caught in the tumbling shaft and had suffered a compound fracture of the lower third of his leg. Two other doctors had decided to suture and bandage the wound rather than amputate, because there was still a pulse in the foot. When Langstaff was called in he found the limb plagued with gangrene: 'sooty black & foetid and fine crepitation in the thigh along the outside of which is a broad red band of erysipelas up to the hip.'[37] This man soon died. The following year, despite safety modifications, another man 'caught bottom of his pants ... in [the] tumbling shaft; smooth joint, no bolts at joint, they thought it could not catch ... tore his foot clean off except dingling [sic] by a few cords; knee twisted around ... head cut and blood oozing out of each ear; fracture of base [of skull], comatose, & prostrate, cold, pulse thready.' Five days later he too was dead.[38]

In Langstaff's practice threshing-machine accidents peaked in the late 1870s; he was called to only one such injury in the last eleven years of his practice.[39] 'Who will be next?' the newspaper demanded after the first accident of the 1879 season. A movement to legislate safety standards received the attention of the government.[40] It is not known whether the decline observed in this practice resulted from improved equipment or the advent of specialist surgeons, who effectively removed such cases from Langstaff's sphere.

Gunshot wounds were quite infrequent. Langstaff saw only four in his entire practice. All but one were self-inflicted and accidental. The first occurred in 1860 when a young man, out hunting, shot himself just below the nipple. Langstaff saw him three hours later at his mother's home, where he had been carried on a stretcher faint from bleeding. Detecting 'no chest symptoms,' he managed the case conservatively, making regular visits and removing seven shot pellets while the wound healed over the following six weeks.[41]

The only deliberate shooting was of a widow by her supposedly 'feeble-minded' male employee, because she refused his offer of marriage. He used a 'double barrel shotgun' loaded with 'heads of horse-shoe nails.' The newspaper predicted her death, but Langstaff extracted two nails from her hip and two from her side and judged the wound to be 'not fatal.'[42]

Most other fighting was done with bare hands; the doctor was called to six major fist fights. In the aftermath he dressed cut faces and hands, sometimes of pugilists on both sides of the dispute and once of an innocent bystander who had been hit by a flying stone.[43] A patient recuperating from a brawl in Durose's tavern the week before died suddenly at breakfast, possibly of a clot on the lung.[44] Hale young men were not the only victims of aggression: a pauper was brought to Langstaff with his thigh broken because of 'manual violence,'[45] and the doctor witnessed and suspected the beating of women on several occasions. 'Supposed to have been struck by sleigh tongue,' he wrote of a woman's broken arm.[46]

Accidental falls from scaffolding, hay lofts, hay wagons, apple and cherry trees, and down 'sellar' [sic] stairs were responsible for considerable morbidity in Langstaff's patient population. Objects struck on the way down, including a chisel, a washtub, a hot stove, and, once and most improbably, 'a large apple,' only served to aggravate the injury. Dr Geikie asked Langstaff to consult on a man who had fallen out of a wagon and broken his neck: a 'partial fracture at the bottom of cervical vertebrae' that had left him partly paralyzed on the right, completely paralyzed on the left, and unlikely to survive.[47]

Falls from a height were very dangerous because of the irreparable internal injuries they could cause. When confronted with an unconscious patient, Langstaff often opened a vein to let blood. He was concerned for the kidney function of one little boy who fell to the barn floor: 'vomits; no urine,' he wrote.[48] He was equally concerned when a man fell from a loft, fractured three ribs, and 'spat blood,' a symptom suggesting damage to the lung.[49] Another man was thrown from a load of hay against a fence and sustained injuries to lung and kidney. Langstaff attended him three or more times a day and stood with him as he 'sat on the edge of bed & signed his will.' He improved briefly, but died in pain twenty days after his accident.[50]

Some people survived against remarkable odds. Eight-year-old Baldwin Teefy fell from a loft and opened a large cut at the side of his nose next to his eye, but walked away in good spirits; the next day Langstaff found him convalescent. When James Langstaff Jenkins, son of the doctor's old friend Ben, 'fell 22 feet to the bare barn floor,' he lost consciousness, but he was assisted to the house and 'used his legs to support most of his body.' Three days later he was better, with just a few 'numb & prickly' sensations.[51]

Fractures were common and not all resulted from overtly violent activity. Early one morning, while making breakfast, a middle-aged woman broke her tibia and fibula 'in turning upon the floor – her son upstairs in bed and her husband in bed in the next room heard it snap.'[52] Another younger woman dislocated both condyles of her jaw from vomiting; a man fractured his arm during an epileptic seizure.[53] The majority of broken bones, however, were caused by animals, falls, machines, and fights – the type of trauma described above. More fractures seem to have occurred in the 1860s than in the other decades, a finding that invites speculation on the relationship between recent industrialization and society's facility with it (Table 7.1). Over the forty years of his practice Langstaff was called to set or dress at least one break of almost every bone in the body.

Langstaff sometimes arrived at the scene of an accident too late to see the victim alive, but an earlier arrival rarely would have made any difference. This was the case when a man was hit by a falling well bucket that caused a 'dislocation of the neck near the head' and instant death.[54] A child who had been scalded was already dead when the doctor appeared; thus, he listened to the distraught father tell how 'it had seemed quite lively' but suddenly 'looked wild and twitched.'[55]

If the patient survived an accident long enough for Langstaff to attend, he would establish a plan for dressing the wounds. Since antiquity, wounds had been washed, dressed, and bound with various substances and in various manners. When Langstaff began practice there were several recommended recipes for dressings. These agents were thought to act by promoting healing rather than by killing bacteria; some may actually have had antiseptic properties, but this action was not understood until later in the century. Langstaff mentioned the use of simple bandages, solutions, and poultices, commonly containing zinc compounds and silver nitrate, but he also referred to several special substances, such as flour, snow, iodine, slippery elm (*ulmus americana*), 'chickenweed' (possibly *alsine media*), lead acetate, alum, and suet. Silver nitrate was recognized as a caustic agent and was used, instead of heat cautery, in situations requiring the searing and sealing of a wound; flour and starch were applied to burns. Langstaff mentioned 'astringent,' 'caustic,' or 'sooth-

ing' as the reason for his choice of wound dressings. Mostly, however, he gave only scant details until the late 1860s. For example, an
elderly man was seen forty-eight times during the year 1850–1 for
dressing an ulcer on his leg, but the substances used were never
described.[56]

Illustrative of his early management of wounds is an exceptional
note about a young man cut by an axe in the knee 'across the liga-
ment patellae but perhaps not reaching the capsule.' In haste the
doctor 'removed clots, but not to bottom of wound for fear joint
might be opened & thinking there would be less chance of
haemorrhage. Put 4 or 5 sutures in and placed a compress of lint
across the lips, roller tightly across & above patella & elevated the
foot.' He ended this entry with an experiential pearl of wisdom:
'Pressure upon femoral [artery is] better than tourniquet.'[57] During
the next month Langstaff dressed the wound regularly, but the functional outcome was not described.

Langstaff's approach to wound dressing changed dramatically with
the introduction of specific antiseptic dressings, nearly two decades
after the advent of anaesthesia. Following the 1867 publication of
Joseph Lister's successful experience with carbolic acid, Canadian
practitioners did not immediately accept or understand the principles
of antisepsis, and, intentionally or not, they made modifications.[58]
Langstaff began to use carbolic acid in the same year as reports appeared in the medical journals to which he subscribed.[59] His applications were even more diverse than those recommended in the literature; the suggestion is that he may have relied on his students or his
colleagues to keep himself informed. His first recorded use of carbolic acid was in mid-August 1868, when he employed it in dressing
the stump of a man's thumb blown off by a gunshot.[60] In January
1869 he injected a weak solution into the rectum of a child with
diarrhoea,[61] but by 1870 there was a hint of scepticism: a child had
'begun to improve [from febrile diarrhoea],' he wrote, 'before either
carbolic or i.e. [infusion erigeron] were given.'[62] A few months later,
however, he seemed more convinced of its powers: he treated a compound fracture of the tibia, which contained 'considerable dirt and
sand,' with irrigations of carbolic; in two weeks the 'bone [was] bare
& as white as snow but lying well down in the wound'; two months
later the leg was 'nearly healed.'[63]

After 1870 Langstaff used carbolic acid in a few but by no means
the majority of dressings following injuries or operations. As with

his contemporaries, there is little evidence that he adhered to Listerian principles.[64] Carbolic acid became a component of enemas,[65] lotions, and washes, as 'carbolized water,'[66] 'carbolized milk,'[67] and 'inhalations.'[68] It was used to irrigate the uterus 'through a large gum catheter' and was sprinkled on the bedclothes of an incontinent patient with severe diarrhoea.[69]

In December 1873 Langstaff used carbolic acid to manage the severe laceration of the arm of fifteen-year-old Albert Brown, who had been tending the belt of an engine in Jerman's cabinet and planing factory when he was thrown beneath a piston rod, which struck and tore his forearm. The other doctors present clearly did not agree with Langstaff, who wrote: 'Drs Doherty and Black wanted to take the arm off, but it is only a severe flesh bruised wound crosswise of ... [the muscles], radial artery all right, skin lacerated for about a foot. I put in two stitches at outer end upper margin of wound, applied a little carbolic solution to deepest part of wound then wrapped lint around arm & poured on tinct benzoin comp freely, elevated shoulder & arm & flexed them to bring wound together some. Other Drs made no objections or argument, [they were] 'mum' – at which I was surprised.'[70]

Langstaff then made regular visits to young Albert in Markham Village over a six-week period. At first he kept the wound covered with 'linnen [sic] wet with weak solution of carbolic acid and lukewarm water & oil silk on top.' Three wĕeks later the 'numbness' had resolved, 'a slough' had entirely separated, and 'active granulation [was] going on,' indicating healing. However, the boy developed a bent arm or contracture. One of the doctors who had disagreed with Langstaff's courageously conservative management went public with his criticism, either in print or in person, complaining that the boy's health had been undermined and he had missed nine months of school.

An undated manuscript draft of Langstaff's angry reply to 'two letters' apparently written by Dr Black and addressed to an 'editor,' possibly of a medical journal or a newspaper, is the only document testifying to this controversy. In his rebuttal Langstaff said that it was better to have a disabled arm than no arm at all: '[the boy can] carry a stick and uses it to buckle his skates on and take them off [and] enjoys about as good health as he ever did.' He also poked fun at his colleague's mixing of metaphors derived from biblical and classical sources and said Black 'reminds me of a crazy man I once knew. He sometimes thought he was a deity and again would think himself a worm.' He continued, 'Dr B would cut a little boy's arm off and save a few months of schooling and then, if he did not die from the operation as many have after a severe injury, he could go to school with the stump ... I think that in all cases if there is any chance of saving a limb it is the surgeon's duty to try it, whether the case turn out successfully of not ... Any butcher can cut off a limb.'[71] Perhaps Langstaff recalled his student days at Guy's Hospital, when he had seen Key and Syme successfully treat an injured arm, although 'some high authority' had said that the limb could not be saved; perhaps he had read of Lister's similar case published just six years before.[72] He likely felt vindicated when the April 1875 issue of one of his medical journals published an article on the importance of conservative surgery.[73]

In Albert Brown's situation Langstaff thought he had been right, but he readily acknowledged mistakes when he believed he had been wrong. In one of the most spectacular blunders of his career, he accidentally stabbed a patient while dressing an arm, broken and punctured by the tines of a threshing machine: he wrote, '[I] ran a sharp jack knife into [the lower] abdomen ... [I] think it penetrated.'[74] He recommended rest and prescribed opium, but since he did not see the patient again, the outcome is unknown. The family likely found a different physician.

In managing fractures Langstaff would splint the limb, sometimes with 'pasteboard', and bind it with 'starch bandages' or 'factory cotton,' if the fragments were in good alignment.[75] He did not mention plaster of Paris, although it had been brought into practice in the late 1850s.[76] In the case of dislocations or if the alignment was poor, Langstaff would set the bone or joint, sometimes using chloroform to ease the pain and facilitate manipulation. He was careful to measure the length of a broken leg in his daily visits and insisted on the use of weights if splints were insufficient to keep the correct position. When he found a little boy had taken off his splints and the leg had shortened, Langstaff 'sewed smoothing irons to the bottom of the bandage' to ensure proper alignment and perfect compliance.[77] He instructed Dr Wright and the family of an older woman with a broken leg to 'pull down occasionally and firmly' on the limb.[78]

Langstaff took pride in managing dislocations. 'Duncan Wilkie's negro ... put out [his shoulder] at 3 a.m.'; Dr Hillary 'failed' to correct it in the afternoon and, the next day, 'could not be found.' Langstaff wrote that he had 'set [it] in 3 minutes,' after he fixed the 'apparatus for extension at right angles to the body, pressing the acromion towards the side & head of humerus and towards it.'[79]

Treatment of dislocations required some originality. On the same day that his daughter Nelly had fallen from her horse, another horse and buggy ran away with the 'Deputy Reeve of Vaughan.' Langstaff was called to attend the man's dislocated shoulder. Working outside, as he often did, Langstaff 'laid him on his back, put right arm through straps and fastened counter extension through window, put pry against cistern pump and tightened ropes passing from the straps before prying with *forkhandles* for a lever; then gave chloroform till he felt easy, then moved handle about six inches till it bent some and head of bone went in, in about $3/4$ minute.'[80]

There were other original solutions for dislocations and Langstaff was open to suggestions from his patients. One old man 'leaned on his cane as a crutch & ... forced shoulder into place better than bandages.'[81] The doctor used two assistants and chloroform to help reduce a man's complete dislocation of both elbows 'caused by his holding a horse' that 'suddenly reared up.' With the man seated on a chair and both attendants on their knees, one behind holding the arm firmly above the elbow, the other in front pulling strongly at the wrist, Langstaff 'clasped [the] elbow with both hands' and 'with sudden, determined force crushed [the bones] into place with a crack'; he then put the arm in a sling.[82]

To bandage fractures in the early years, Langstaff used splints, lint, and straps of linen. He used 'figure of eight bandages' for fractured clavicles – once called 'Sayre's method.'[83] Broken legs were immobilized in 'fracture boxes,' which were long containers with only bottoms and sides: an ostler's broken leg was placed 'in fracture box surrounded by bran' to keep it immobile;[84] a child's sore was covered with a pepper box to allow a scab to form.[85] Later in his career he seems to have given up on fracture boxes; he accused a rival of choosing over-dramatic treatment for a small fracture of the ankle simply to deter Langstaff, who had been invited by the patient: 'Hostetter put on starch bandage & put it into a great box lest I should attend him. He put a pair of splints on yesterday after I was there.'[86]

The first mention of starch seems to have been in late October 1861, one month into the management of the fractured tibia and fibula sustained by Rob Stephenson, when his wagon upset in the ditch as his team of horses raced home from Toronto. Langstaff 'bound the leg in pasteboard and starched the bandage' in an attempt to construct a cast that would allow the man some mobility without displacing the limb. Stephenson slowly improved and by Christmas was able to walk with crutches. Then, to everyone's dismay, a horse fell on him, breaking the leg in the same spot, and the long process of dressings and visits began all over again. The leg 'seemed solid' by the end of January, but he continued to wear bandages into February, not with starch, since the 'hard starch bandage hurt ... his skin.'[87]

For most fractures Langstaff followed the patient for six weeks, but special injuries, like Stephenson's or a fractured patella,[88] required eight weeks or more of regular visits. Even after the bone had healed, mobilization was a problem partly from weakness of the atrophied muscles, partly from contractures, and partly from the patient's fear of disturbing the union. When one young man rose from a month of bedrest for his fractured lower leg, he experienced a 'deathly feeling' and summoned Langstaff, who 'stayed till morning as they were greatly alarmed.'[89] Little in the doctor's approach could prevent these complications, although he described a bandage for an arm fracture in 1870 that would 'put into action the teres major and latissimus dorsi [muscles].' Once in 1880, he recommended 'passive motion,' presumably to prevent contracture, for a boy who had broken both the humerus and the radius of his arm.[90]

A leg fracture could be disastrous, not only because the risk of sudden death from haemorrhage or clots, but because the immobilization favoured pneumonia and other infections and could lead to permanent disability and financial ruin. A man developed severe pneumonia one spring, ten days after he broke his leg. Four and a half months later Langstaff found him in a weakened condition and, even though autumn was advancing, recommended that the family 'lead him out each day that it is fine.'[91]

Similarly, Langstaff had first attended David Hart to treat his dislocated elbow in 1868: 'I put my knee in hollow of elbow,' he said, and 'pried against the foot of bed & it soon went in.' A year and a half later Hart sustained a fracture of his thigh that extended into the hip joint. Langstaff anaesthetized him with chloroform and noted that 'drawing off his boot helped to set leg as he was thoroughly under.' The thigh turned green and the bandages 'were galling' for the patient, who was plagued with fainting for a long time. Three months after his injury he could not sit on the edge of the bed without feeling he would pass out; two years later and still disabled, he caught pneumonia and his wife fell ill too. When Langstaff looked in on them two days later, he found 'both worse, cold last night & they let the fire go out.' They were very weak, 'almost sinking,' and Hart began to refuse nourishment; however, six weeks later they had both improved.[92]

With the exception of two women who watched or helped with operations, 'nurses' do not appear in the surgical record (see Appendix B2). Virtually all other care was given by the family and friends of the patient.[93] The situation may have been bad for those who had inexperienced people to look after them, but it was worse for those on their own. When a man broke his leg as he arrived 'at the northern station,' Langstaff set the fracture on the scene, 'lent him $5 and he went back to Toronto.'[94] No one would tend the ostler whose leg had been placed in a box of bran, so Langstaff resolved 'to send him to hospital.'[95]

Minor surgical procedures included catheterization and cautery. Several times a year Langstaff was called to catheterize patients, most often adult males with urinary retention caused by an enlarged prostate gland or urethral stricture. There were a few cases involving children and women who had sustained trauma to the bladder, such as the little girl to whom Langstaff gave anaesthetic in trying to repair the vesico-vaginal fistula caused by a fall the previous year. Without chloroform, Langstaff had passed a bistoury, or metal instrument with a curved blade, along the closed track of the urethra; as it 'entered the bladder urine shot out about a yard.' He was optimistic that she would be 'as well as before the injury,' but in the days following he noted that she was 'suffering greatly' with extreme pain. Since the female catheter was too large and she was unable to retain a silver probe, he 'used chloroform and passed a larger sized catheter into bladder while she was asleep. She woke in about 10 min.'[96] After several weeks of visits, during which she intermittently required a catheter, there was no further mention of the case.

Catheters were passed usually without difficulty; once, however, Langstaff deplored the action of a colleague who had 'tried several times' without success to catheterize an uncomfortable man and then 'left him with his bladder full to [the] navel.'[97] Langstaff easily drained this bladder, but he was not always so successful. Another patient had undergone surgery to open the bladder from below. Langstaff unsuccessfully tried to pass a catheter, first via the rectum, then via the urethra, but the patient 'gave a start & I withdrew it & blood followed.'[98]

One man, with urethral stricture, came frequently over the course of two years to have his bladder emptied. He was given a 'gum elastic catheter' to take home, but lost it and had to return to the doctor.[99] Not until nearly twenty years later did the doctor trust another patient with a catheter.[100] He understood that an empty bladder in a patient with a clamped catheter was of grave significance, since it meant the kidneys were not functioning, and he recognized that the easy passage of increasingly large catheters could imply that the stricture was 'spasmodic' rather than anatomical.[101] He used catheters to introduce medication into other body cavities such as the uterus and the back of the nose.

Like catheterization, cautery with heat or caustic chemicals was a technique Langstaff employed between five and ten times each year throughout his entire practice. On several occasions he cauterized sores in the mouth and throat, ringworm, and moles; less often he managed haemorrhoids or prolapsed anus in this manner. During 1869 he treated at least five women for uterine bleeding with caustic substances introduced through a catheter (see chapter 8).

Operations were a small but interesting part of Langstaff's practice (Table 7.4). Some were essential, unavoidable procedures, such as the completion of amputations begun by an accident or the draining of pus or fluid from infected wounds. Others, such as the correction of birth deformities or the removal of tumours, were elective – the product of a choice made by the patient, the family, and the doctor. Elective procedures seem to have increased into the third decade of Langstaff's career and then tapered off after 1880. The rise in surgical intervention may have been related to Langstaff's increasing ease with the techniques of anaesthesia and antisepsis, but only ten per cent of Langstaff's operations (excluding tooth extraction) were recorded as having been done under anaesthesia. Sometimes the operation was so quick that anaesthetic was probably not given; on other occasions he may simply have neglected to mention it, especially in the later years, when he seems to have been accustomed to his patient's being 'chloroformed.'[102] The apparent decline in operative surgery in the 1880s may have been due to the advent of urban hospital-based specialists. It has been observed that some physicians began a trend towards heroic and hopeless intervention on the terminally ill, but Langstaff's record suggests that he was loath to inter-

TABLE 7.4
Langstaff's surgical operations

	1850s (5 years)	1860s (1 year)	1870s (3 years)	1880s (2 years)
Tooth extractions	228	46	128	81
Yearly average	45.6	46	42.7	40.5
Chloroform	0	2	19	20
Other operations	132	56	93	41
Yearly average	26.8	56	31	20.5
Chloroform	0	3	4	2
Reason for surgery				
Abscess	82	36	43	20
Lance gums	17	9	5	3
Tongue-tie	6	1	2	0
Amputation	2	1	10	1
Mastectomy	0	0	2	0
Club-foot	0	1	1	3
Harelip	0	3	0	0
Hernia reduction	0	1	0	1
Repair	0	0	0	1
Tumour or polyp	5	1	5	10
Tracheotomy	0	0	2	0
Hydrocoele	0	2	1	2
Swollen leg or joint	20	0	18	0
Other	0	1	4	0

Source: All entries in Langstaff's daybooks for 1849–54, 1861, 1872–5, 1880–2

vene in such settings: most operations were on the external parts of healthy young people.[103]

Langstaff's surgical instruments were never described in detail. He mentioned, at least once, each of the following: probe, knife, bistoury (several types), throat cannula, catheters, bougie, truss, pessary, forceps (several kinds, including bulldog, tooth, small, and polypus), dislocation apparatus, lip-pins, Pingle's tubing, tonsil scissors, syringes, sutures, ligatures, trochar, tourniquet, and stomach pump. He probably acquired an inhaler in the 1860s, and an estate inventory shows he owned a 'hand atomiser,' an 'aspirator,' and a 'hypodermic syringe' – items that may have been used to induce local or general anaesthesia.[104] The comments that do appear are more or less complaints about the inadequacies of his tools. For example, when he tried to tie a cut radial artery, he wrote, 'I would have done better with a pair of bulldog forceps';[105] in resecting a small tumour, he found the 'tonsil scissors answered better than [a] knife.'[106] Sometimes he modified his equipment: he dipped an enema syringe 'in melted tallow until a coating [was] formed over it so as not to irritate' a patient's piles.[107] Once only he watched a colleague use 'wire galvanism' (electrocautery) to arrest bleeding during surgery.[108]

The most common operation in every decade analysed was dental extraction, apparently Langstaff's only solution for dental problems and a service he performed forty or fifty times every year. Beginning in December 1859, his use of chloroform in dentistry increased until the final decade when it constituted well over half of the anaesthetic administrations. Langstaff employed chloroform in approximately twenty-five per cent of his dental procedures, especially in multiple extractions.

In the early 1860s, dentists N.J. Peck and Dr A. Robinson came to the region. As the itinerant Robinson's long-running newspaper advertisements promised and Langstaff's daybooks confirm, the dentist spent the twenty-fourth day of each month in Richmond Hill, 'thankful for the favours of the past twenty years' and offering his services with the benefit of 'vitalized air.'[109] Langstaff recorded his assistance to Peck and Robinson in multiple extractions; sometimes he administered anaesthetic for several patients in succession.[110] Relations seem to have been cordial; in some surgical cases Langstaff apparently counted on them for help or equipment; they called him for advice when they were ill.[111] Since the doctor was prepared with anaesthetic for the dentists' visits, he seems to have arranged his own elective surgery procedures near the same dates.

Matthew Teefy's family continued to see Langstaff for tooth extractions even after the dentist came to Richmond Hill. The oldest daughter, Clara, in whom Langstaff was beginning to suspect tuberculosis, had difficulties with her teeth and required several extractions. When she was almost twelve years old, he gave her chloroform before pulling two teeth; the process must have been fairly tolerable because during the next ten years she returned several times for dental care under anaesthetic. Teefy's younger children Louise and Armand were also sent to the doctor have their teeth pulled, but as they did not receive chloroform, it is likely he was simply obliging them or their parents by removing already loosened infant teeth.[112]

Amputations were usually done as a clean completion of a serious traumatic laceration or crush injury; Langstaff, therefore would be obliged to do his work in great haste at the site of the accident, be it a barn, a mill, or a field, and often without anaesthesia. Of the twenty-six amputations he performed in forty years of practice, fourteen involved loss of digits or hands, usually the result of saw and axe injuries – the cogs of the 'cutting box' (straw cutter) were particularly dangerous. In addition to causing many other injuries, threshing machines claimed one hand and one foot. Only one amputation (of a thumb and part of a wrist) was ascribed to a firearm.[113] Often the member was completely severed before Langstaff arrived: the fingers and thumb of a child who had placed his hand in a cutting box; the arm of a man who had lain with his limb in the path of a train 'while drunk.' All the doctor could do was dress the stumps.[114] The amputation of entire limbs was mercifully infrequent: Langstaff tended to three severed arms and two legs, all but one the result of violent injury.[115]

On occasion Langstaff amputated for intractable medical conditions such as mortification following frostbite. A man lost nine of his toes in four successive procedures over the two months following a trip from Toronto in a severe March storm.[116] Once Langstaff amputated the extra digit of a child born with two thumbs.[117] An elderly woman lost her leg at the upper third of the thigh after she had suffered with a swollen, painful knee, which had been punctured and drained more than sixteen times during the previous fourteen months. At first he had 'feared' her swelling was 'from disease of the heart,' but he concluded it had 'extended from' a problem in the knee-joint. As his note suggests, the operation occasioned the special attention of interested witnesses: 'Dr L. Langstaff, Dr Armstrong, Wm Cross my student, Ernest Langstaff home from U.C. College and young Neil with Armstrong from Stoufville [sic] present.' Langstaff had some difficulty controlling bleeding with a 'turniquet' [sic]' as 'every time the blood burst from the raw surfaces upon the knee.' Finally he asked an assistant, 'Mr Bliss the waggon maker,' to compress the artery at the groin and moved swiftly to complete his task: 'I screwed [the tourniquet] up very tight very quickly and amputated suddenly in about $^1/_2$ min. by two cuts after the one pierce through the limb. i.e. First pierced limb just below tourniquet apparently passing through its centre, then cut suddenly out towards knee with one stroke of knife making a flap about 8 in. long along the only sound part of limb ... knife so sharp and long it passed through without sawing motion.'[118] In the first post-operative week Langstaff described how the woman developed phantom pain; seventeen months later the stump was inflamed.

The most common non-dental operation in all periods was incision and drainage of abscesses and swellings. This procedure represented sixty per cent or more of operations throughout the forty years of practice. In the pre-antibiotic environment of the mid-nineteenth century, advanced infections were common. Accumulation of pus and organization of an infected wound were recognized components of the healing process, but evacuation was essential to its completion. Failure to do so, fumbled technique, or a premature attempt before the abscess was 'ripe' could lead to death from widespread infection or septicemia.

With a knife and usually without anaesthetic, Langstaff 'lanced' the abscess, drained its contents, and occasionally described the colour, smell, or quality of the pus – since these characteristics were related to prognosis. Unless the wound closed before complete evacuation had taken place, he did not return to see the patient. For example, of the thirty-six such operations performed in 1861, four were repeat incisions on two different patients; of the forty-three done in 1872–5, ten were repeats on five patients.

Particularly common in women were abscesses of the hand or fingers beside the nail (felon), often the result of infection of a small irritation or cut sustained in daily activities. Sometimes inflammation of the face or the ear could progress to an abscess, which had to be drained. Langstaff named 'carbuncle' as the specific type of abscess on many other occasions and twice at least mentioned 'anthrax.'[119] The term 'anthrax' is now reserved for a specific infection spread from animals, but during Langstaff's practice the possibility of infection from animals was under dispute and the word could apply to a wider range of inflammatory lesions, especially 'malignant boil' or gangrenous inflammation.[120]

Most abscesses were located on the surface of the body, but at least twice Langstaff inserted a needle into the chest to treat empyema (pus in the chest).[121] Opening the chest or abdomen was dangerous; it is clear that Langstaff viewed it as a desperate measure, waiting until the 'chest bulged forward' and the diagnosis, together with its dismal prognosis, had become indisputable. He sometimes 'tapped' abdominal fluid, or ascites, with a needle and syringe; only once did he open an abdominal abscess, after which the patient appears to have survived; he recorded draining fluid from an ovarian cyst.[122] He witnessed other cases of internal abscesses and may even have suspected the diagnosis prior to the patient's demise, but he did not operate. One child succumbed after many weeks of illness from an internal abdominal abscess, likely the unrecognized result of a ruptured appendix.[123] Several other patients died of conditions like appendicitis or thoracic and abdominal abscesses, without any attempt having been made to operate on them. A few of these abscesses ruptured spontaneously and drained to the outside or into another body cavity,[124] but some were not diagnosed until death and autopsy. There is no evidence that Langstaff knew his nearby contemporary Abraham Groves, who claimed to have removed the first Canadian appendix in 1883.

Tracheotomy, invented by Pierre-F. Bretonneau in 1826, was used as a life-saving measure for suffocation caused by diphtheria, a major source of paediatric morbidity in the nineteenth century. Following a theoretically simple procedure reserved for emergencies, the operator made an incision in the front of the neck into the trachea through which the child could breathe. As the patient was generally unconscious or close to it, anaesthesia was generally neither necessary nor safe. Langstaff's first attempt at a tracheotomy may have passed unnoticed, obscured by the more commonly written expression 'lanced throat,' since among the many lesions he had incised were abscesses in the mouth, tonsils (quinsy), throat, and neck.

The first surgical management of a case suggestive of childhood diphtheria was seen in May 1853: a tracheotomy was not done, but an abscess was lanced inside the mouth on two separate occasions in one week. The outcome is unclear, but the grim clinical description suggests it is unlikely the child survived; Langstaff did not mention her when he assisted the newly bereaved mother in childbirth two days later.[125] In 1870 one other patient paid two dollars to Langstaff for 'removing tonsils,' but no other tonsillectomy was mentioned.[126]

The four certain attempts Langstaff made at tracheotomy were marked by hesitation and failure. The first took place on 12 March 1866 and may have been encouraged by reports on tracheotomy in his journal literature in the preceding year.[127] The patient was a 'nearly exhausted' young girl with diphtheria, whose blue lips and dark blood were a sinister indication that she was suffocating. Langstaff's trepidation was apparent: 'I attempted to open the larynx above cricoid ... *black* blood [spurted] from *arteries* ... goitre being large, cricoid being deep ... and not having a suitable canula, I desisted rather than run risk.'[128] The girl died.

Two days later Langstaff purchased a 'tracheal trochar & canula' for $4.25;[129] however, he does not seem to have used this new equipment until nearly six years later. This next patient was a boy whom he had followed for a week in his rapid downhill course diagnosed as 'scarlatina.' The child was blue, his pulse 140, respirations 36, and a hard lump had formed beside the larynx so that he could not open his mouth wide enough to put out his tongue. Langstaff 'passed a small trochar & canula into crico-thyroid space, first making puncture of lancet a little more than through skin.' The boy probably died soon after, as he was not mentioned again, even though two days after the surgery Langstaff was tending his mother and his sister, who had contracted the same disease.[130]

One year later Langstaff attempted a third tracheotomy, on a little girl whose 'croup' and 'suffocation' had followed that of her sister. When her difficulty of breathing increased, Langstaff decided to operate, but he 'had to wait till [her father] came home. [I] opened the windpipe and got a quill in and child breathed through it with great force but quill was too long and after withdrawing it to shorten the quill it could not be introduced again properly. From having bad light & there being veins & arteries all around the opening and the child being prostrate & blue & the discharge from the windpipe being exceedingly tenacious, I doubted of the operation succeeding, if ever so successful in itself. I *desisted*.'[131] This child too appears to have died.

The last and possibly only successful tracheotomy that Langstaff did was at the telegraphed request of a colleague in 1877.[132] Perhaps because of his dismal personal experience or because specialists may have appropriated the technique, he does not appear to have used it again, even when confronted with situations that seemed to merit this form of intervention.[133] There is evidence that he doubted both the value of tracheotomy and his own skill in performing it.

Other more simple procedures were fairly common early in the practice, most notably the lancing of gums in teething children and the cutting of the lingual frenulum to release tongue-tie. These operations were quick and the infant patients received neither anaesthetic nor follow-up attention; sometimes, however, Langstaff was obliged to return because what he thought had been irritability due to teething was actually the beginning of a more serious problem. Two-and-a-half-year-old Baldwin Teefy's meningitis had presented in this manner: Langstaff observed a slightly feverish and cranky little boy, noticed molars were erupting, and decided to lance the child's gums since it had seemed to help him earlier; meningitis was evident and teething no longer seemed an adequate diagnosis.[134] Perhaps because he had many similar experiences, there seems to have been a relative as well as an absolute decline in the frequency of procedures for lancing gums and releasing tongue-tie in the last two decades. This decline could also have resulted from heightened awareness of the concepts of infection or an increasingly non-interventionist stance in the profession at large.[135]

Major elective operations seem to have taken place in the patients' homes or, if the weather permitted, outside on the porch or in the yard. In the later years Langstaff indicated that he observed operations in the hospital in Toronto, but he did not organize hospital-based procedures himself and there is no evidence that he operated in his own home. About one year into his practice Langstaff performed his first 'big' elective operation: a cystotomy, or opening of the bladder, on a man with urinary retention whom he had already been following for six weeks. He left a long description.

After many daily visits and one wakeful night with the man, whose 'bladder [was] quite even with the umbilicus,' Langstaff 'opened the bladder above the pubis; drew off about a gallon of urine leaving about a quart, that the canula might retain its position in the bladder. A catheter was rendered inefficient from small clots in the last part of the urine.' No ether was given, but the patient may have been drowsy from his fairly advanced renal failure and the fact that he 'had taken two glasses of wine & some laudanum ... before the operation.' This produced 'an approach to coma – snoring under jaw retracted; easily aroused, but suddenly dropping to sleep again.' Post-operatively, Langstaff found the patient more comfortable, his pulse stronger and slower, but four days later he wrote 'mortuus est.'[136] Despite the death of this patient, Langstaff's practice immediately became busier: and within the month his average daily visits increased from fewer than one and a half to more than four, a rise inviting speculation on the relationship between the young doctor's perceived ability or renown stemming from this surgical case and the increasing public confidence.

No mention was made of any attempt to induce coma in the second 'big' surgical case of Langstaff's career, two years later, and the record suggests that none was made. The young doctor had been following a man for a large 'tumor,' more properly a cyst, abscess, or diverticulum, in the neck. The patient's symptoms were not given, but Langstaff described the swelling, which 'extended rather farther forwards than the larynx; backwards beneath the sternomastoid nearly to the transverse line drawn across the back of the neck. It forced the side & angle of the jaw somewhat up; & was so close upon the clavicle below that the point of the finger would not go readily between them.' The doctor was concerned about eventual difficulties, such as choking, suffocation, and stroke, and consulted his colleague Dr H.H. Wright. The following is twenty-seven-year-old Langstaff's account of their collegial disagreement over the surgery and his confession of errors in judgment and technique:

Dr Wright did not like that we should operate but I urged that we should, that the tumour could not ... be more malleable than it was & consequently inferred that it was not strongly adherent to the surrounding parts & that in dangerous parts, the tumour might be separated by the handle of the scalpel. ... Contrary to our expectations the tumour was strongly adherent to all the parts ... & to the jaw & to the common carotid vessels. In dividing the integuments ... the lips of the wound did not draw asunder & the coverings were literally cut off & at every 2nd or 3rd cut a small artery spirted [sic] out & from the toughness of the tissues all knives appeared dull. When ... the tumour was fully exposed ... [I] opened by accident the sack & out came dirty purulent matter. We tried without avail to tie the opening ... then when the tumour was near empty [I] drew it out rather strongly & was separating it from the carotid artery & vein divided some of the [tissues] causing great pain & next made a slight cut into the internal jugular, but with some difficulty we got the section of the vein tied chiefly through the expertness of Dr Wright.[137]

Langstaff continued with a description of his closure of the four mangled 'flaps' of the rather gaping 'cavity' by 'interrupted sutures' and the dressing of 'lint' dipped in tincture of 'benzoin' and sealed with 'adhesive plaster.' Characteristically, he made a learning experience of this unpleasant adventure and concluded his note with recommendations to himself: 'In removing tumors, have about four times the means or implements for arresting haemorrhage that are though[t] likely to be required. Never feel sure that the elasticity of the skin will allow you to make a small opening or that any of the cellular tissue will yield to the handle of the knife, particularly if the tumor is large or has ever been in an inflammatory state.' Miraculously perhaps, this patient survived and Langstaff busied himself with seven others that same day. During his recovery the man's wife fell seriously ill with tuberculous pneumonia, but five follow-up visits later she was better and the man's surgical wound was healing rapidly too. No first name was given, but the surname was longstanding in Langstaff's practice, a finding that hints at the man's possible longevity.

In the 1860s Langstaff seems to have been more confident: he did more elective procedures on conditions that were not immediately life-threatening, such as congenital deformities and tumours. For these he usually gave anaesthetic. He may have read about the surgical techniques, but there is little indication that he observed doctors other than his professors to learn operative technique, although others liked to watch him. A planned procedure with the use of anaesthesia seems to have been something of a social event. Langstaff relied on a variety of attendants to help with chloroform administration: family members, other doctors, or interested people, like Rob Law and the doctor's old friend and brother-in-law Simon Miller.[138]

Langstaff had learned to make prior arrangements for the post-anaesthetic revival of his patient which could sometimes be quite difficult, especially if a lot of blood had been lost. He relied on a variety of modalities including a 'cold gust of wind' and displayed some creativity in his solutions. For example, in the presence of his physician-brother, another doctor, and his son Ernest, Langstaff used chloroform and 'removed [a] cancer about the size of an egg' from the right side of a woman's head; he 'operated on the back stoop in the rocking chair which is handy to tip back when the patient gets faintish.'[139]

In mid-life Langstaff seems to have become a local expert on the surgical treatment of club-foot, which was a fairly common birth defect (Table 7.5). Beginning in April 1856 he operated more than twenty-five times on thirteen different children for this condition; the boy who was his first patient to receive chloroform suffered from club-foot or a similar problem caused by previous injury.[140] To correct a club-foot, Langstaff partially cut the Achilles tendon to lengthen it and, if necessary, would repeat the surgery several months later. He followed these patients assiduously, measuring, ordering, fitting,

TABLE 7.5
Chronology of some operations in Langstaff's practice, 1850–89

Year	1850–4	1855–9	1860–4	1865–9	1870–4	1875–9	1880–4	1885–9	Total
Mastectomy	1	1	3	7	4	3	0	0	19
Club-foot	0	3	10	8	3	1	3	0	28
Harelip	0	0	3	2	0	2	0	1	8
Tracheotomy	0	0	0	1	2	1	0	0	4
Hernia	0	0	0	0	0	0	1	1	2

Source: Langstaff's daybooks, 1849–89

and repairing the special devices they wore. After one little boy broke his wooden boot for a second time, Langstaff ordered a special leather shoe.[141] Two children seem to have been brought some distance for Langstaff's surgical care, since he indicated that one child was 'stopping on the [Richmond] Hill' and the other was 'kept by Mrs Johnson at York Mills.'[142]

The ongoing contact with these children drew him close to their families. In one example of such interaction, Langstaff first operated on Elizabeth, whom he came to call 'Miss Lizzie,' in May 1864. By the end of three weeks he judged the result to be 'halfway to natural.' He repeated her operation twice in the next five years, saw the girl regularly for traction, splints, braces, and boots, and eventually considered her condition 'improved.' For the next twenty-five years the family always consulted Langstaff for their minor and serious illnesses.[143]

Harelip with and without cleft palate was a disfiguring birth defect that Langstaff treated in six different patients with eight plastic interventions; two children had double harelip and each side was treated separately. From his description it appears that he preferred to close the defect with needles rather than sutures, although in one case he used both.[144] The first correction of harelip was done in May 1861 on a two-year-old boy with a severe form of double harelip and cleft palate that caused the middle portion of the lip to be 'projecting beyond the nose, a round nob with one tooth in it.' Langstaff decided on a two-stage procedure: he 'divided ridge of hard palate & septum nasi within mouth so as to allow the ... [protuberance] to be forced back.' Five months later he administered chloroform and inserted needles in one side, but he blamed himself a week later when one needle ulcerated out before he removed the strapping: 'I should have told them to bring the child out,' he wrote, but observed that the lip 'has knitted well considering the great chasm there was before the operation. Will operate again in about 6 months when the cheek gets accustomed to being brought forward & the lip more to the natural length.'[145]

Langstaff actually mentioned the use of chloroform in only three of these procedures, although it is unlikely he ever attempted such a delicate operation on young children without it. Once, however, he noted that the anaesthetic 'did not take effect.' The attendants 'let' the five month-old baby 'lie in the cradle,' while Langstaff's brother Lewis did the cutting with apparent success: 'Good job very,' said the note.[146] This may have been Lewis's first attempt at a harelip operation; the day before, he had assisted with the same procedure on a different child.

Most harelip patients were young children, but one was a twenty-year-old unmarried woman who had a partial deformity. Langstaff operated in the open air with the assistance of his physician-nephew Elliott and his son Ernest: 'Ernest held her head standing behind her chair as she sat in front of the house in its shadow, Elliott gave the chloroform on her right, I on her left drew down the lip with my left forefinger & thumb & entered the point of the narrow curved bistoury in the nostril & carried the edge gradually through the right edge of cleft.' The note continued with a detailed description of how both edges of the cleft were neatly peeled away with the final turn of the knife towards the cleft to leave a small 'point' or 'teat' on each side. He inserted the upper needle first, then the lower, and 'then points squeeze[d] together without any stitch.' Sealing wax, 'not too much & not in way,' was left on the needles. Typically, this account was sprinkled with axiomatic statements and advice on management: 'The object is to take away all the depressed portions of lip. Left side bled freely ... The side nearest angle of mouth always bleeds ... hold needles by pair of incisor-cutting tooth-forceps close to lips [and] stand in front with little fingers on skin.'[147] Six days later he reported that the young woman's incision had 'knit splendidly.'

Mastectomy was an operation Langstaff had no tendency to avoid. During the forty years of his practice he performed nineteen mastectomies on fourteen different women: two women had the procedure repeated when their tumours grew back;[148] one was operated on four times over the course of three and a half years even though her first operation included removal of the underlying chest muscles, an early 'radical' procedure.[149]

Langstaff's treatment of breast cancer began in 1854, when he made

a 'call by permission' to a patient who had been concealing her aggressive breast tumour, a 'fungus haematodes,' for eighteen months
and treating it with 'quack plaster,' which was 'eating it down' and
causing 'great pain.'[150] He did not operate on her, nor did he see this
fearful patient again, but he probably remembered her dreadful condition as he performed his first mastectomy sometime in the second
half of the same year.

This first mastectomy patient had been nursing at the time and
may have had an abscess, since she survived to give birth to another
baby seven years later; however, the original record of her operation
is among the few documents missing from the daybooks. At the
birth of her older child, Langstaff wrote, '7 years since last [child]
was born, just after, left breast & parts above it amputated ... lacta-
tion was going on at the time & small part of gland was left. Milk ran
out as knife passed through it.'[151] He did not mention whether or not
he had employed anaesthesia, nor did he give the reason for surgery,
although in most other cases he specified 'cancer.'

In the second mastectomy – the first for which there is an original
record – Langstaff was assisted by another doctor, a neighbour, and
a medical student. He 'amputated right breast leaving nothing of the
gland but a little of the capsule at the lower side.' He made no
mention of anaesthesia; yet the following day the woman was 'strong
and cheerful' and two weeks later her wound was 'almost entirely
healed.'[152] An observation that invites speculation as to whether or
not it was used, chloroform was not mentioned until the eighth
mastectomy. This was the third of the four operations on a woman
with persistent 'fungus haematodes.' Despite the use of anaesthetic,
speed and technique were given capital importance:

Dr Geikie, Dr L. Langstaff, Dr Pierson & Mrs Webb came to look on. Gave
her chloroform & removed left breast in less than $3/4$ of a minute. It was as
large as a child's head, globular & a little nodulated, blue in spots & full of
large veins. I stood with my right side opposite her shoulder; placed the left
hand below the tumor, drew it up & placed the edge of the knife below it,
then carried the edge of the knife inwards around the tumor to the place of
beginning with one steady sweep, cutting through the skin & fat too for
about an inch to half an inch deep, then drew the tumor inwards from the
arm pit & a little downwards, cut deep from above & within, downwards &
outwards, raising the outer side of the tumor & cutting more horizontal to
the surface of the pectoralis major muscle a part of which I cut away with

tumor [previously]. I removed it with about six cuts following each other as rapidly as they could be made. The lower part of the pectoral was removed so the heart could be seen beating against the intercostal muscles. About twenty small arteries bled rapidly for a short time, tied only four. The cool north wind blowing into the house helped to stop the haemorrhage & revive her. The wound was about eight inches in diameter. Laid dry linen on it.[153]

Nine months later Langstaff removed a metastatic gland from her armpit, tying off the subscapular artery. There is no other mention of this patient.

Even with anaesthetic Langstaff continued to be concerned about speed. Perhaps to avoid allowing himself to slip into lethargy, he kept in mind the patient in whom the 'chloroform effects went off' half-way through her mastectomy. When he had to repeat her operation sixteen months later, he did not mention using chloroform at all, but he did note that his 'cutting lasted two minutes.'[154] The technique described, a sweeping circular cut and six hexagonally arranged slices parallel to the chest wall, appeared in other cases, as did the restorative 'gust of wind and cold to the face.'[155] The practice left a gaping wound that healed slowly and only rarely by 'first intention' (with the edges approximated and no pus).[156]

The most common complication following mastectomy was bleeding, which could recur as late as two months after surgery. Langstaff was interested in ways of preventing haemorrhage and experimented with different techniques: tying arteries, applying snow and lunar caustic to oozing surfaces, and, in the late 1870s, twisting rather than tying vessels. When one patient bled to faintness after he had twisted the vessels, he wrote, 'I think [vessels] should not be twisted off but twisted and released.' One month later, he declared this patient 'healed.'[157]

In contrast to the doctor's accounts of tracheotomy, optimism pervaded his records on mastectomy. After surgical haemorrhage one woman 'soon rallied' within the hour and another was found sitting up and 'quite jolly' two days later. A patient was first seen in an unfavourable condition, with a 'rapidly growing' and 'stinking' cancer that she had secretly been treating with 'cancer plaster'; less than two weeks after her operation she was said to be 'healing rapidly' despite 'the maggots upon [her] sheets.'[158]

Four of these patients went on to bear children; Langstaff seems to have been constantly aware of the relationship between breast function and pathology. He noted in one case that coexistent pregnancy 'favoured' the healing; unfortunately, the child was stillborn five months later.[159] He observed that a patient's breast which had been 'amputated' seven months previously was swollen two days after her delivery, 'though *none* of the gland was left'; she nursed her child on the opposite side.[160] One woman with left-sided breast cancer reminded the doctor that she had had an abscess on the right, but her children had always 'liked the left one best.'[161]

Langstaff performed no mastectomies in the last eleven years of his practice (Table 7.5). It seems probable that this highly elective procedure was quickly taken over by surgical specialists in the nearby city. The daybooks tend to support this statement. In 1875 he observed Dr Geikie perform a mastectomy at 'the hospital' in Toronto; in 1881 he was in the city again, watching Dr Aikins resect part of a tongue with 'wire galvanism.'[162]

Other tumours appear in the surgical record, through often a lesion Langstaff would call a 'tumor' was not a cancer or even a benign tumour, but simply a swelling or a cyst. Using chloroform, he did remove a 'cancerous tumor' from the knee of a woman and 'she said she did not feel it at all.'[163] With great care and difficulty he resected four large 'fatty' tumours from the back, over the deltoid muscle, and once from the hip, but it seems likely these were benign lipomata.[164] Two of these cases involved family members; it seems that for one Langstaff travelled to Wallaceburg to perform the surgery. Small moles were 'ligated' or occasionally cauterized rather than cut, except he once 'shaved off' a melanotic tumour overlying 'dense tissue' and found this was an *excellent plan.*[165] Langstaff managed the 'cancerous lymphatics' of one elderly man with a fairly extensive axillary dissection. One month later he removed three more glands. The note 'entirely healed,' written four weeks after the second resection, seems poignantly optimistic, since the enlarged nodes were likely malignant.[166]

The difficulties created by this kind of intervention are vividly described in the account of the surgical removal of 'a large cystic tumor' of the vulva, possibly a Bartholin's cyst, in a colleague's patient: 'Dr Hunter gave chloroform & held left knee ... Her husband held her legs and Mrs Craig [held] one knee & the tumor some of the time ... Haemorrhage was profuse part of the time, beside the main trunk of pudic [sic] artery, there were about half a dozen that spun into my face and hair. The spectacles were a great protection to the blood blinding me.'[167]

There were other minor operations: twice Langstaff divided sternomastoid muscles in children with wry neck; on many occasions he punctured legs swollen with 'dropsy'; four times he treated a retracted foreskin or paraphimosis; and he excised wens and nasal polyps, 'a little like pulling out soft guts,' he once wrote.[168] Often he was called upon to remove insects, peas, beans, and choke-cherries from the noses and ears of little children. Sometimes the summons for these mundane tasks came in the small hours of the morning, as it did the night he went out at two o'clock a.m. to relieve a man with an insect in his ear.[169] Inexplicably, in the spring of 1871 he extracted three fish-hooks from three little boys, though he never did so again. Removal of 'motes' (minute foreign bodies, especially 'barley beards') from the eye was common. Needles and pins also required removal, but the community seems to have been sanguine about the urgency: 'been there four years', he wrote of a needle extracted from the abdominal skin of a little girl.[170]

Langstaff lanced swollen testes or hydrocoele at least ten times, but seven of these operations were for a single patient, whom he tended off and on for twenty-four years.[171] He attempted to drain large ovarian cysts in three different patients, in efforts ranging from the simple – 'ran a little yarn into it' – to the ambitious, the removal of nine pints of fluid repeated three times until he could write that the cyst was 'entirely gone.'[172] The declaration was premature, because the patient's abdominal fluid reaccumulated within two months, although she lived for at least two more years.

Hernia was not uncommon; however, until late in Langstaff's practice the only treatment was reduction and support by a truss. Langstaff treated strangulated hernias several times: he gave the patient liberal doses of opium, 'grasped the skin around the tumor & kept up a steady gentle pressure upwards ... & continued pressure for about an hour.' If he was successful, 'the tumor gradually passed & slowly so as to be imperceptible.'[173] Strangulated hernia could be lethal; the doctor was not always successful in his management, even when he used chloroform. Frustrated in his attempts, he was obliged to stand by helplessly, offering only opium, while his patient died a slow, painful death.[174] In 1881 he attempted an unspecified surgical procedure for an inguinal hernia. Once again, however, the description displays his innate conservatism when it came to untried surgery: 'I got into [an] abscess and stopped.'[175]

Finally, in 1883, Langstaff was confronted with the desperate condition of a man who 'had been vomiting faeces for several days, thick as mush and horrible stench,' because of an incarcerated femoral hernia. The ageing doctor, who had been operating less and less in the previous five years, resolved to perform the only herniorraphy in his entire career. His anxiety could only have been heightened by the eminent gathering crowded round the table:

Dr Armstrong gave chloroform; Dr Doherty helped hold flesh; Dr Robinson sponged wound; McLean, high school teacher held arms; his brother watched legs ... First incision by lifting skin and passing knife through fold deep enough to reach as far as I wanted first cut; enlarged the stricture distinctly by finger outside the sac but could not reduce the gut, then used forceps scissors probe & blunt pointed bistoury, but made little progress; *then* used forceps & scissors till I came to gut; then director passed readily down through stricture and hernia knife passed on it through stricture ... but could not possibly be reduced until I separated the adhesion all around the gut by the finger keeping the nail outward from the gut which was almost black & thickened but tough. Sewed up wound closely, net with weak solution of carbolic acid, then pledget of linen wet with comp tinct benzoin, then strapping.

The patient did well post-operatively, but Langstaff had doubts about the nursing care: 'Two hours after operation, he was without a bad symptom altho' not under opium. Laudanum had been left by Dr Tabor, but friends would not give it as their grandmother had been poisoned by it *they thought*.'[176]

Injuries and fractures were a common feature of life in nineteenth-century Ontario; most of Langstaff's surgical activity was devoted to the emergency care of wounds. The change in the frequency of some injuries seems to reflect the increasing mechanization of his society. He also performed a variety of operations, ranging from common tooth extractions to relatively rare elective procedures such as mastectomy and correction of birth defects. Langstaff used chloroform to induce anaesthesia and adopted carbolic acid dressings shortly after they were introduced. In the 1860s and 1870s his operative initiative grew, together with his confidence in anaesthetics and antiseptics, but it declined slightly in the 1880s, possibly owing to the presence of specialist surgeons in the nearby city. There is little evidence to suggest that the increase in operative procedures seen in the middle two decades of his practice was a result of heroic intervention on the terminally ill. Most of the new operations seem to have been for mastectomy and the correction of birth defects, while his operative intervention for emergencies, such as the incision of abscesses, remained relatively stable and may not have been associated with anaesthetic use.

CHAPTER EIGHT

Birthing and Its Problems
in Langstaff's Practice of Obstetrics.

Over the course of the nineteenth century birthing was 'medicalized' – it ceased to be perceived as an entirely natural process and the exclusive domain of midwives or other women attendants and was increasingly viewed as a potentially dangerous, almost disease-like condition amenable to a variety of treatments, involving special instruments and medication that properly belonged in the hands of doctors. Historians have been divided over the question, to whom was the change more beneficial – the birthing women or their male physicians?[1] Those emphasizing the benefits to women refer to the ghastly agonies of an earlier period and contrast them with the decline in perinatal and infant mortality rates, which they attribute to the 'achievements' of the nineteenth century; however, the decline in mortality did not begin until several decades after medical men entered the birthing room.[2] Those emphasizing the greater benefits for doctors cite the apparent rise in perinatal mortality throughout the second half of the nineteenth century, which they attribute to the newer 'interferences' with natural processes; they also cite the loss of women's employment due to an associated decline in midwifery, the 'construction' of female diseases through gender bias, and the monetary gains for physicians from medical midwifery.[3] The issue is complicated.

During the period of Langstaff's training, James Young Simpson recommended the use of chloroform anaesthesia for obstetrical cases, and the role of physicians in the spread of childbed fever was recognized by Oliver Wendell Holmes and Ignaz Semmelweis, who suggested that contagion was spread to birthing women on the hands of examining doctors from other patients and cadavers. In the late 1840s, just as Langstaff completed his training, Semmelweis introduced his successful practice of prophylactic handwashing in chlorinated lime. Antisepsis and anaesthesia were both controversial techniques in obstetrics.

Until the 1880s many physicians resisted the idea that they could spread infection by their interventions. Doctors found it difficult to accept responsibility for the horrible deaths of their patients and were reluctant to abandon the instruments and procedures that seemed to both hasten birth and make it safer. When germ theory replaced older atmospheric or miasmatic theories in the late nineteenth century, a new concept of disease transmission made the ideas of Semmelweis seem more plausible and antiseptic techniques were adopted. Similarly, anaesthesia during childbirth had its detractors, who decried the associated loss of consciousness and questioned the moral rectitude of its use, citing scripture to prove that women were meant to experience pain in labour; however, it also had its advocates, who emphasized the relief of pain but who may have been more interested in providing an 'unresisting body' for their interventions. The potential of a general anaesthetic to harm a foetus, now well known, was not yet an important factor in the anaesthetic debate. Historians have poured much ink over the social reasons for these controversies.[4]

The Langstaff daybooks afford an opportunity to examine how an individual doctor and his women patients reacted to medical midwifery and the controversial new techniques. It is clear that Langstaff viewed himself and was viewed by his society as an appropriate attendant at births. In his entire career he attended the birth of about 4,000 babies, approximately a hundred every year. This estimate is supported by the observation that he attended forty-three twin and two triplet births.[5] During the first five years he was called to an average of fifty confinements per year, but his obstetrical practice peaked in the 1860s and 1870s at close to 110 'confinements' or deliveries a year. There was a slight decline to roughly ninety-five deliveries a year in the 1880s, following, but not as great as, the twenty-two per cent decline in his overall activity between the last two decades (Table 8.1). This absolute (but not relative) drop in obstetrics could have been owing to the presence of other doctors in the community or to the fact that his patient population was ageing with him.

Langstaff's obstetrical practice was not confined to deliveries; he saw women patients in a variety of other situations related to reproduction, including visits after births and for menstrual difficulties, spontaneous abortions or miscarriages, and mastitis or inflammation of the breast. But women consulted him frequently for other problems too. In every decade studied, visits to married women patients filled a larger proportion of Langstaff's activity than would be expected given their numbers in the population (Table 5.3). The extra attention they received compared with male patients, children, and unmarried women seems to be entirely accounted for by birthing and its complications, which grew from roughly seven per cent in the 1850s to fifteen per cent of his practice in the 1860s and stabilized at about twelve per cent thereafter.

Comparison of the Langstaff documents with the census of his region for each decade shows that he was present at an ever-increasing proportion of the births in his region (Table 8.2). By 1860 he was attending at least forty per cent of the births in his immediate area; in the 1870s and 1880s the figure was closer to seventy per cent.[6] Some women called him back for six or more deliveries. This seems to be a relatively early date for physician-attended birth: in her study of birthing in the United States, Judith Leavitt has shown that it was approximately 1900 before fifty per cent of American births were attended by male doctors.[7] Since the deliveries recorded in the local district represented only thirty to fifty-seven per cent of the deliveries Langstaff attended in any given census year, it seems that at least half of his obstetrics patients lived in different census districts more than three miles from his home.[8]

The most likely reason for the doctor's presence at many local births is that the mothers and their attendants desired his help; there is nothing in the record to suggest otherwise and there are many instances where it is clear that the mother, her family, and her attendants were grateful for his presence. In only one case (cited below) did a birthing woman seem to have been less than comfort-

TABLE 8.1
Langstaff's obstetrical practice

	1850s (5 years)	1860s (1 year)	1870s (3 years)	1880s (2 years)
Obstetrical visits	491	507	1,299	646
Percentage of all visits	6.8	14.8	12.4	11.8
Births	241	111	312	156
Yearly average births	48.2	111	104	78
Natural abortions	17	8	14	4
Twins	5	2	8	1
Triplets	0	0	1	0
Stillbirths	8	3	14 (18)*	8
Maternal mortality	4	2	9	4
Fatal haemorrhage	1	0	1	1
Post-partum fever	3	2	8	3
False labour	12	6	3	1
Forceps	6	5	129	55
Ergotamine	5	7	27	22
Chloroform	0	0	1	4

* Fourteen deliveries resulted in stillbirths, including two sets of twins and one set of triplets.

Source: All entries in Langstaff's daybooks for 1849–54, 1861, 1872–5, 1880–2

able with Langstaff's presence, but her own mother and husband were eager for the doctor to stay, and the woman herself claimed that she had not wanted him simply because he had come too soon.[9] Indeed, some pioneer women, like diarist Mary Gapper O'Brien, indicated their desire for a doctor's presence even when one was not available.[10]

The birthing experiences of Mrs Betsy (Clarkson) Teefy, the postmaster's wife, may reflect the growing trust of community women in the doctor's obstetrical skills. The family had been consulting Langstaff since shortly after he set up practice in Richmond Hill: Teefy himself had been to have his chest examined in early 1850 and the older children had been seen for various minor problems. Over her life, Mrs Teefy gave birth to nine children, only six of whom survived infancy. The first two babies were born before Langstaff came to the community; the next four were born between January

TABLE 8.2
Local births in census* and in Langstaff's practice

	1851	1861	1871	1881
Population	5,150	2,581	2,920	2,637
Births in local census	134	98	76	67
Births/1,000 population	26	38	26	25
Census births attended by Langstaff (%)	16 (12)	31 (32)	52 (68)	43 (64)
Births above as % of all births attended by Langstaff in that year	41	30	57	43

* 1851 Districts: Vaughan II, Markham I; 1861 Districts: Vaughan II, Markham III; 1871 Districts: Vaughan II, Markham II; and 1881 Districts: Vaughan II, Markham I, Richmond Hill

1851 and December 1853 without his assistance, although the family was aware that he was available; the last three were born between January 1859 and May 1862 in the presence of the doctor but without his intervention. Perhaps Mrs Teefy had been attended by midwives or another physician during her first six labours; perhaps she had been disturbed by the death of a child immediately after birth in 1853. It does appear that she did not deem the doctor necessary for her labours until she was older and he had already been observed 'in action' for other reasons.[11]

For a short time Langstaff kept a separate record of his obstetrics cases in the back of the little notebook he had used at Guy's Hospital. That similar documents have been found for other doctors, suggests this was a common practice, which may have been designed to create a reference book for future cases.[12] Langstaff remembered and learned from his experiences and applied his knowledge to later deliveries for the same woman or to other patients. For example, when a recently widowed woman gave birth to a daughter, he noted that her 'case resembles that of Mrs Jo Williams about six years ago.'[13] Retrospective analysis confirms the accuracy of Langstaff's recollection concerning both the details and the date. Sometimes the application of a learned experience was immediate. In confusing the position of a baby's head by 180 degrees, he wrote, 'I think I've never met a case placed like this before'; the following day he made special note of his examination and uncertainty over the orientation of another baby's head.[14]

Langstaff rarely indicated if his women patients were pregnant. Retrospective analysis of the records shows that in the first decade twenty per cent of the patients Langstaff attended in childbirth had consulted the doctor while pregnant, but their symptoms usually had nothing to do with pregnancy or its complications (Table 8.3). This figure rose to thrity per cent in the last three decades. The average number of visits to those pregnant patients who were seen was between two and three per patient, but the figure is skewed upwards from a median of approximately two visits by the presence of a single serious case of fever or pneumonia, which accounts for more than twenty visits to one patient in each of the last three decades. Approximately half these women were attended for false or prolonged labour over several days.

Langstaff's understanding of the physiology of pregnancy and the causes of its complications is only sparingly alluded to in the day-books. Extremes of temperature, either hot or cold, were held responsible for complications in pregnancy and labour; it was clear, moreover, that the pregnant woman should avoid psychic or physical stress. In the first week of April 1861, as if he had some fresh interest in the expected duration of pregnancy, he noted the precise time lapsed from the day three of his patients were married to their deliveries; in one case of illegitimacy he recorded the date of 'coitus.'[15] Aside from two other such notations during the next year,[16] these comments were exceptional. Langstaff usually counted dates only to explain possible symptoms, abnormalities, and complications, or to note coincidental ironies. For example, one patient had been 'married for 5 months' and had 'vomited for three,' suggesting pregnancy; another, in labour, had been married six years without having other children; another, 'married last New Year's Day,' gave birth to her first child at 11:15 p.m. on December 31.[17]

Although Langstaff may have been present at a large proportion of the local births, he did not spend much time with a patient during her pregnancy, during her labour, or in the post-partum period. Pregnancy seems to have been considered the normal state for a married woman, as the remarks cited above seem to suggest. One mother who had just delivered her second child had 'not had her turns' after the first, so quickly did she become pregnant again.[18] He seems to

TABLE 8.3
Langstaff's visits to pregnant and post-partum women

	1851 (1 year)	1861 (1 year)	1881 (2 years)
Births	33	111	156
Visits to pregnant women	29	85	137
No. women who received antenatal visits	7	30	55
Average antenatal visits per all birthing mothers	0.2	0.8	0.9
Post-partum visits	59	259	323
Average visits per all birthing mothers	1.8	2.3	2.1

Source: All entries in Langstaff's daybooks for 1851, 1861, 1882–3

have had some sympathy for the ravages of repeated childbearing. He noted as he attended Mrs Peter Rupert for her '15th acouchment [sic]' that the thirty-nine-year-old woman was 'still fat, plump, and fair.'[19] Reports made during the week-long pneumonia of Mrs Jeremiah Nelson included incidental references to her pregnancy: 'false pains' and 'threatened' with labour. When after much pain and difficulty in breathing she died, presumably taking her baby with her, Langstaff wrote that he 'was glad she was out of her sufferings.'[20] The following day he 'opened the chest' to determine the cause and extent of her disease, but no further mention of the infant was made. It cannot be determined how many of his other patients were pregnant when they died.

All indicators suggest that Langstaff usually arrived an hour or less before the baby was born; if it was longer, he recorded the length of time he 'staid [sic]' or had been 'detained,' ranging from one hour to two days. If the mother could be left, he might return up to a dozen times in a single day.[21] In the last decade of his practice he seemed more inclined to tarry with birthing patients having 'tedious,' 'hard,' or 'slow and deceitful' labour. For two cases in the last year he spent more than forty-eight hours at the bedside; once he 'wanted to leave but she wouldn't let me.'[22]

Usually it was the expectant father who brought the summons, or if a messenger or telegraph was used, the doctor was often met by the father along the way. On a few occasions the man would find the doctor absent and would follow him to another patient's home. In darkness or very cold weather Langstaff seems to have been grateful for company on his journey, since he recorded the fact in his book.[23] For roughly one case in every six the summons came so late that Langstaff missed the delivery altogether, but in about half of these he arrived before the birth of the placenta. In a few of the late cases it seems that the family had been planning to do without the doctor until a frightening symptom caused them to change their minds, a situation that has been observed elsewhere.[24] Sometimes it appears the call had nothing to do with the birth itself and was a response to complications that arose post-partum, such as retained placenta or severe afterpains.

Delay was not for lack of haste. Several times the doctor described the speed at which he travelled to the labouring mother in the company of the father: 'we went out in 34 minutes over 7 miles,' but the baby was born 'just as I got into the house.'[25] Francis Button managed to return with the doctor to his labouring wife just one hour and fifteen minutes from the time he had set out on his eight-mile round trip; when sent for help during her next delivery two years later, he found the doctor on his rounds and hurriedly helped him saddle his horse, leaving the gig behind.[26] At 3 o'clock one morning Langstaff lost patience with a particularly anxious father who roused him because his wife had miscarried and was faint from loss of blood: 'he rang the bell about six times hard as he could ring it, worse than ever rung before. In hurrying lest he should ring again, I knocked over our best lamp and spilled coal oil on the floor.' Langstaff's seemingly disgruntled state persisted two days later, when he blamed the wife for the loss of her infant because she had taken 'too much senna contrary to orders. Its action brought on expulsion of contents of uterus and haemorrhage.'[27]

Scant remarks throughout the records reveal the importance and continued presence of women attendants, though not surprisingly their names and exact duties are rarely described and the word 'midwife' is never mentioned. Since there was no organized midwifery movement in Ontario, as there was in Quebec, physicians may not have been threatened by the activities of female attendants.[28] In a few thousand deliveries Langstaff bothered to comment on women attendants only fourteen times; these people observed the progress of labour, followed (or failed to follow) his orders, changed the sheets, adjusted the bed, and generally kept vigil. More than tolerated, it seems likely from these records that the women were expected to be present and often decided when to call for the doctor. In one case he and the midwives were summoned simultaneously, since the child was born before 'I or any of the women got there.'[29]

The patient's mother was often among the attendants and would make important decisions. For example, when a woman's bleeding slowed and, after days of watching, she finally fell asleep, 'her mother blew out the candle and all went to bed.'[30] This supports the observations of others, who have suggested that women dominated the confinement as long as it remained a home-based event whether or not a male physician was called.[31]

Although Langstaff tried to leave quickly, sometimes he had to wait to be of assistance. He did so in the case of the woman who was ambivalent about his presence in conflict with her own mother. Langstaff wrote about how he arrived at 11 o'clock p.m. and found as follows:

Her pains have gone off and she says she is sorry she sent for me. Took a teaspoonful of laudanum an hour ago ... as everything she takes goes right through her and has done (for weeks I believe). Pulse 140 and she looks very anaemic. I lay down for an hour but slept until $1^1/_2$ A.M. ... got up when I heard her coughing and went into her room where her husband was also fast asleep; all the house had gone to bed; fire out; just a lamp burning in her room. She said I had better not go yet as she had some little pains beginning again. I went outdoors & back to the lounge again and covered up as it was very cold. In about an hour, say half past two, I awoke & heard her straining hard on the floor in her room in a sitting posture ... she thought it would be born right away. I called her husband in from the kitchen to help lift her into the bed. She said she was still loose ... heavy constant labour was continuous; no fire on yet. She would not allow me to assist or hardly touch her. I found the cranium in the os externum and would have used forceps if she would have let me. After about ten or fifteen minutes [3 a.m.] child born almost asphyxiated but recovered well, a stout boy. I told her she had been in labour two days ... she gave a knowing look but said nothing in contradiction. Pulse still rapid, respiration laboured, uterus contracted tolerably but I hurried to get some ergot which with a tablespoon of brandy & three spoonfuls of milk I got down her. She got weaker and weaker, said she was dying, twitching of face set in & she died at 4:10 A.M. I kept a cold wet towel often changed to uterus which was quite hard much of time. No flow externally. On passing finger up vagina along cord placenta not reached. I felt also in bed & on withdrawing not a stain of blood. Husband stood at foot of bed and saw no blood on my finger or hand, this was about ten minutes before she was entirely gone. I waited about an hour until Mrs Sam Lyons her mother was brought and explained the circumstances to her. She said she was there yesterday and told her she was in labour but her daughter did not want her to stay.[32]

Most indicators suggest that the attendants welcomed the doctor's presence and that he appreciated theirs, but relations were sometimes strained. Of the fourteen obstetrical cases in which Langstaff specifically bothered to mention the women attendants, more than a third indicate criticism or disagreement. For example, Mrs Devlin was blamed for giving a parturient mother a teaspoon of hot liniment in water, causing the pulse to rise to 140; Mrs Henricks, together with 'Mrs B,' was criticized for giving 'brandy punch by her own will' when there was 'no need.'[33] The doctor seemed to be most critical in the first decade of his practice: a Mrs Miller was blamed for not evacuating the bladder of one labouring mother; when a 'child nearly bled to death' a 'woman' was held responsible for 'not having tied the naval string tight enough.'[34] Langstaff wrote that he was summoned at 3 a.m. one cold night in 1858 to an arrested labour after the 'hand was discovered down ... and the pains became weak (perhaps from the fright of the old women).' He brought down the baby's knee and accomplished 'expulsion in about ten minutes ... the child living.'[35]

Sometimes, as in the last-mentioned case, the doctor seems to have been quite proud of his ability to intervene successfully or content to have company during the delivery. Thus, when the hips of a birthing mother 'cracked' as the foetal head passed through the bony pelvis, 'a woman sitting nearby perceived it';[36] when premature twins were born, 'an RC woman gave them a private baptism.'[37] Once the efforts of the doctor and his labouring patient were musically 'accompanied' by 'Elder Hawkins troop singing on the Hill at the same time.'[38] In the last decade of his practice there were no critical remarks made of women attendants. For at least one patient, 'blue and faintish' from haemorrhage, the 'woman' worked as a partner, 'pressing externally [on the aorta] and applying cold water freely' while the doctor raised the foot of the bed and extracted the retained placenta manually.[39]

A prospective analysis shows that at least one post-partum visit was the rule in approximately sixty per cent of all cases; at this time the doctor would often collect his fee. Attendance in the post-partum period was quite variable and, like most of his other activity, depended entirely on the patient's condition and a summons. A very sick patient could be seen more than thirty times. For the three-year period beginning February 1872, more than five post-partum visits was a poor prognostic sign, since these frequently seen mothers died in nearly forty per cent of cases.

The newborn baby also was a concern for the doctor. At almost every confinement Langstaff noted whether or not a son or a daughter had been born, the presentation, and the time of birth; however, if the infant was crying 'lustily' and breathing well, his attentions to it seem to have been less important than his care for the mother. He did record the gestational age in cases of prematurity. Only rarely did he note the child's weight, usually if the baby was exceptionally large. For example, he had already delivered twins weighing 8.5 and 9.5 pounds and a singleton weighing 11.5 pounds before he delivered Mrs Young of an 11-pound daughter – 'the fattest ever seen.'[40] One remark hints at a mistrust of the accuracy of scales. Mrs Sam Mager's baby girl became the 'largest [he] ever saw,' weighing 13.5 pounds, but, wrote Langstaff, 'I think [it] was heavier.'[41]

In several instances congenital abnormalities were recorded involving the feet, fingers, face, and spinal cord. There was one baby with imperforate anus and another with a condition suggestive of a blocked oesophagus, atresia or fistula; both appear to have died within a few days.[42] In only one family did the abnormalities appear to recur: two children born to Mrs James Shaw had supernumerary thumbs.[43] On three occasions in 1868–9, Langstaff surgically tapped the backs of children with spina bifida.[44] Cleft palate and harelip seem to have been common in his surgical practice, but if he noted these abnormalities at birth he did not record them. Two children died soon after birth with cyanotic heart disease, 'morbus caeruleus.'[45] Once he saw evidence of trophoblastic disease, in the form of 'hydatids,' which he 'washed away' by 'flooding' the uterus with carbolic acid through a large gum catheter.[46]

Anencephaly was the most common of the congenital abnormalities in the daybooks. It occurred in nine births over the forty-year period.[47] Here, especially, Langstaff seems to have learned from his own experience how to predict the deformity. In 1861 he wrote of a woman, 'married eight months today but abdomen as large as at ninth month ... a quantity of water discharging during most of the labour ... two pailfuls at least. ... the large mouth & hand of the

monster first felt, head & face & neck like a toad with a large bloody
tumor on one side of neck.'[48] In two subsequent cases of anencephaly
he also noted the large quantity of water. In 1865 he observed a
woman's 'uterus [to be] on the stretch'; when a great quantity of
water gushed out following rupture of the membranes, he 'told them
that the child would most likely be dead & deformed & it was.' He
then wrote, 'Deformity is generally attended with a great quantity of
liquor amnii.' Fourteen months later he attended the same patient in
the delivery of a normal healthy girl.[49] Even the knowledge that one
such tragedy did not always lead to another served him in his practice. Three weeks after Mrs Fred Gaby gave birth to an 'acephalous'
baby, the doctor was called to reassure her because 'she thought that
she had been poisoned.'[50]

Perhaps the most impressive of Langstaff's abilities, in the eyes of
the attendants, was his use of artificial respiration to save apparently
stillborn children. He used the 'Biblical' method (blowing into the
mouth) at least eight times in his forty-year practice.[51] Sometimes he
explored other methods: 'raising the ribs by the fingers under their
margins increased the frequency of the child's breathing after it had
been resuscitated by blowing into the mouth & keeping the trachea
gently back so as to keep the oesophagus closed.'[52]

The first such attempt at artificial respiration was in 1853, for a
baby delivered from an unfavourable position:

Mrs Young of a son 3³/₄ P.M. sent for about 1¹/₂ P.M. Husband said pains had
been on but an hour but on arrival found os fully dilated & she had had
some pain all night but she had been accustomed to somewhat similar & did
not mind it. The waters broke while she was sitting in the chair waiting for
the bed to be prepared [she] was immediately given opium and while she
lay on her left side, [I] used r[ight] hand felt hands first; then the side of the
thorax wh[ich] first appeared to be the head but I could distinguish the ribs;
then felt the knee; then the foot & brought it down as it wedged against the
back of uterus; a gentle pain & it came to within the vulva, another not
strong & it came out of the vulva; another & the body was expelled as far as
the navel. The cord I felt beating *weakly* & only about 30 in the minute: I
protected it from the pressure of the perineum. After a time another pain
expelled it to the shoulders (the other foot had come down previous to the
expulsion of the nates & with a crack & I thought the thigh bone must be
broken but was agreeably mistaken). The next pain expelled the shoulders
and the head (I drew gently at each pain). All beating of the cord [ceased] &

as far as I could perceive of the heart; but by taking fresh breath frequently
and blowing into the mouth & repeatedly following it with pressure upon
the epigastrium & chest while the child was in warm water; the child sighed
and after a time came to, but did not become strong enough to cry. *Putting
the finger into the fauces produced no effect.*[53]

It is not clear how long this child may have survived. Sometimes
Langstaff observed that resuscitated babies were 'quite limpsy' long
after they began to breathe.

Some babies were revived more readily, like a child with 'no pulse
when born ... but one puff of breath into the mouth caused it to draw
a breath.'[54] The long-term outcome in successfully resuscitated infants may have been ominous, especially for one baby who was 'stillborn $1^1/_2$ hr before it breathed.' Langstaff 'held its nose & breathed
gently into mouth & compressed chest alternately. [Two hours later]
it breathed about twice a minute.' He recommended the family 'roll
it occasionally from one side to the other & tickle it gently by gentle
friction.'[55] A common feature in these records of artificial resuscita-
tion is the frequent use of the word 'gentle.'

Infant death, before, at, or shortly after birth, was the most common cause of death in all age groups in every decade studied. Some
of the deaths took place days or weeks before delivery; Langstaff
was able to estimate how long before by the presence or absence of
peeling foetal skin or decomposition. He relied on the mother's history and attributed death in utero to 'false [labour] pains,' a 'rough
ride,' and a 'fright' sustained two months earlier.[56] Several mothers
had repeated stillbirths, most more or less premature. One bore nine
children, of whom the last six were healthy girls born in Canada, but
the first three were 'boys all dead and born in the old country.'[57] In at
least two cases Langstaff noticed that the child had a large liver,
suggesting what is now called blood group incompatability.[58]

Many of those babies pronounced dead at delivery or shortly after
were destroyed by the birth itself. An abnormal presentation, such as
a breech, a prolapsed cord, or strangulation by the cord around the
neck, could result in loss of the foetus. Sometimes these children
were injured by the doctor's use of forceps to terminate prolonged
labour in the case of a narrow pelvis and a large child.[59] In such cases
the mother might have died, too, without abrupt delivery. At least
three times, once for prolonged labour and twice when twins presented in interlock, the baby was deliberately destroyed by

'embryotomy,' evacuating the contents of the foetal brain with a perforator and removing the pieces of its dismembered body with a hook.[60] The incidence of this procedure seems to have been equivalent to that in other practices: two of Langstaff's contemporaries each faced this gruesome task four times.[61]

Birthing is a potentially lethal event. In nineteenth-century Ontario perinatal mortality was very high; the most common causes were haemorrhage and infection (puerperal sepsis).[62] Langstaff was well aware of the complications and viewed the reason for his presence at a delivery to be the detection, prevention, and treatment of these life-threatening situations. Obstetrical causes of death ranked third or fourth in the list of all causes of death in every decade studied and were the most common cause of death for all adults. The majority of women who died succumbed to infection, but a few in every group bled heavily and died of exsanguination, usually within a few hours of delivery. Langstaff's maternal mortality rate seems to peak in the third decade at 29 per 1,000 (Table 8.1).

Suffering in labour was also greatly feared; patients looked to the doctor for rapid delivery in order to reduce the duration of pain as well as to minimize blood loss. Sometimes a patient would labour for three days or more before the doctor was called. Rupturing the membranes was the simplest solution Langstaff could use, but it had usually happened naturally or had been done for him by one of the other attendants before he arrived. In the first year of his practice he helped to deliver a 'crossbirth' child by rupturing the membranes and bringing down a foot (podalic version):

Mrs J. Stewart, of a son, Friday 11³/₄ P.M. On my arrival the os uteri was fully dilated and the membranes not ruptured ... I introduced my left hand which had reached partly into the uterus when something suddenly ... caused the mother to start as if the head [moved] from the right iliac region towards the fundus ... I felt the hands and feet above the symphesis [sic]. I took the left foot by the ankle between my fingers & ruptured the membranes between the nails of my forefinger & thumb, when the water pushed out & the foot came readily down & out of the vagina. The breach [sic] very soon entered the vagina & the cramps which she had been subject to in previous labours now commenced; the pains were powerful very soon expelled the breach & abdomen. The pains now became extremely powerful & the cord ceased to pulsat [sic]. I extricated the arms, & the pains being excessive frightened the attendants to almost shriek like the mother. I passed my finger up & into the mouth wh[ich] was as much as I could reach, depressed the chin as much as possible, the head & the placenta were soon *shot* at once *through* the pelvis & from the os externum.[63]

Reports of this happy outcome told by the 'shrieking' attendants no doubt enhanced the young doctor's midwifery business.

In order to hasten or terminate delivery Langstaff came to rely increasingly on obstetrical forceps, spoon-shaped instruments designed to grasp the foetal head and facilitate its passage through the birth canal. Although there is some controversy over whether or not forceps were used in Roman antiquity, these instruments were invented (or re-invented) in the seventeenth century and brought into obstetrical practice in the eighteenth century. There is some evidence that their use in the nineteenth century was a matter of medical controversy, especially in the later decades, but Langstaff appears to have had few doubts about their use.[64]

It is not known when or how Langstaff learned to use forceps. He first used them in his own practice in 1851, but he employed them only six times in the 1849–54 period (Table 8.1). In the first decade he indicated difficulty, 'as usual,' in applying the blades because of their orientation: not quite forward or backward enough or 'not pointed sufficiently toward the umbilicus.'[65] He once wrote that he applied forceps while his patient was lying on her right side, but the usual posture he preferred birthing women to adopt was not indicated.[66]

Langstaff slowly became adept in the use of forceps, noting cases in which they had been 'easily applied,' or 'adjusted very nicely and all did well.'[67] From these experiences, he observed that they are 'easiest to apply just before the head reaches the perineum.'[68] He began to test various models. In 1863 he bought a pair of used forceps at the sale of a dead colleague and noted that they 'worked well'; two years later he referred to the efficiency of 'Rigby's forceps' in a delivery that 'did not last two minutes.'[69] Later he began to use the instruments to change the presentation of the foetal head to a more suitable position when it 'did not seem disposed to change of itself,' or because it would not be born or turn without them.[70] In urgent situations that required rapid termination of labour, such as haemorrhage, he sometimes applied the forceps 'above the [pelvic] brim' or 'before the os was $1/2$ dilated.'[71]

Reflecting confidence in his new skill, Langstaff's use of forceps increased from 4.5 per cent of deliveries in the 1860s to 41.7 per cent in the 1870s; in other words, two babies in every five born in the later practice came into the world with the help of instruments. This is a high rate of forceps use: for example, Langstaff's contemporary Horatio Burritt used the instruments in only 5.6 per cent of the births he attended; other Canadian practioners employed them with varying frequency ranging between two and forty per cent of births.[72] Since Langstaff's colleague Burritt did sixteen embryotomies as opposed to Langstaff's three, it is tempting to suggest that the relatively higher rate of 'successful' delivery in Langstaff's practice may have been due to his use of forceps and at the expense of the health or long-term survival of the infants he delivered. In other words, the overall survival of infants in Langstaff's practice may not have been any better than in Burritt's when embryotomies are included.

Langstaff did record many instances of evident success with forceps, when babies were born after difficult labours, 'with the greatest of ease,' in 'less than fifteen minutes,' using only 'gentle traction.'[73] If he happened to be without his instruments, he noted unnecessary bleeding and 'delay' for up to five hours 'for want of forceps.'[74] He may have been interested in delivering himself as well as his patient from her confinement, but the patient came first. Recording the case of a thirty-three-year-old mother who lay swollen in prolonged labour of twins, he wrote, 'She asked if there were lightening bugs all around and said there was fire all around, her body & limbs next moment stretched out & began to quiver, face dark & whole body began to twitch, I ran for forceps in my gig ten rods away, applied them and delivered as fast as possible.'[75]

Even in the later period the doctor sometimes met with difficulty or failure in applying the forceps.[76] The instruments were dangerous for both mother and baby. They could cause severe lacerations of the birth canal, introduce infection, and destroy or severely damage the child. Langstaff seems to have been careful to avoid these complications, but he did record consulting on several of his colleagues' patients who had been more brutally managed.[77]

Langstaff may have been cautious to avoid injury to the mother and seems to have recognized and almost accepted the damage the instruments could do to the child, but it is impossible to determine what proportion of the stillbirths in his practice were the result of intervention. Forceps offered a way to save at least one of two persons otherwise condemned to death. One baby, too large to pass through a narrow birth canal without a 'strong pull' on forceps, was born with a 'jerk'; others were 'palsied,' or 'nearly gone,' or died the next day.[78] Once only he recorded a skull 'fracture of both parietal bones ... only the left dinged in but badly so.' He tried to save this baby, whose chin prior to delivery had been impacted from a transverse lie, by placing dry cups over the indentation on the side of the baby's head; the outcome was not recorded.[79] In a case of a child stillborn with forceps, he seemed to exonerate the instruments while recognizing their risk, 'I think it had been dead since before I was called.'[80]

In the final decade, perhaps because of an increasing awareness of the dangers of maternal infection and foetal damage, Langstaff used forceps in 33.9 per cent of deliveries, slightly less often than in the previous years and with apparent decline between the two years studied (from 36.6 per cent to 30.3 per cent between 1882 and 1883). Indeed, his colleagues were increasingly cautious about the associated dangers, but in the context of his record it is difficult to characterize Langstaff's frequent recourse to instruments as 'abuse.'[81] His diction suggests some hesitation even when the indications are clear: 'I had to insist on applying forceps,' he wrote concerning a woman who developed pallor due to bleeding during a labour that failed to progress.[82] He justified their use by claiming that they 'had to be applied before [a child] could be turned.' Once he indicated using forceps at a patient's request.[83] Like the two-day birth attendance in his final year, the decline in forceps use may reflect a greater willingness to wait in a mature physician.

Langstaff's confident proficiency in the use of forceps, his concern for his patient's modesty and well-being,[84] and his discomfort in a professionally delicate situation are bound together and amply reflected in this 1863 case history that merits citation in full:

Whealon Mrs of a [blank – sex of child not recorded] Forceps used, 2nd pos, left hand and the cord down.
Sent for ¹/₄ to 6 A.M. Whealon came himself with [Dr] Hostetter's chesnut [sic] horse & cutter, said that I could ride with him. H[ostetter] had sent him for [Dr] Duncomb but that he came for me, was coming for me in the first place, but met H on the road. I rode my own horse & passing him Hostetter's horse balked. On arriving at the house, the children were all crying. H was examining the presentation & after a little invited me to examine it. The chord [sic] & left hand were down along the side of the head. After waiting a while I recommended the use of the forceps as the pulse was weak & the

breathing was panting. I offered to operate with my own forceps but he produced a pair of crow bars & held them along side of mine said they would take up less room; the woman having been placed partly across the bed he without asking my permission sat down by the bed threw the clothes completely off (the woman lying on her back) began introducing his instruments. After labouring for some time he got them introduced but could not lock them he therefore drew without locking them when they slipped off he seemed to think the head was born (I had partly covered her again). He repeated this operation several times, then tried using one of them as a vectis; the long crow bar handle gave him great power particularly as there was a hook at the end but this slipped off also & when I objected to the use of those huge crows any more, he was then for grabing [sic] my instruments which lay on the table behind him, but I objected somewhat as they were of a peculiar make and one not used to using them might fail. (Mrs Doyle the only woman present had motioned to me while he was working at this barbarous practice that I should take his place.) I consented as he coaxed & looked imploringly he asked which I introduced first. I said, 'sometimes one & sometimes the other.' He had a fair trial with mine & failed also & was about to take his own again when I thought it my duty to object, said I would try mine & if I failed we could use the perforator. I had her brought close to the edge of the bed with a foot on each side of me upon a chair. Told him to put something more under her shoulders when [he] grasped the end of all the blankets & was putting them under her but I secured one & covered her from the waist down & applied the instruments with the greatest ease & had the head nearly extracted before he had time to run round the bed to see how I applied them. He however peeked under the clothes just as the head was delivered to his great disappointment. I had just time to tie the chord once when he ran with the scissors & clipped it off. The child was dead however. He went to work to bandage her & seemed determined to make her shout a few times more as his hard knuckles seemed to hurt her abdomen. I cleaned my instruments & at once left. I was in the kitchen some of the time while he was operating & remarked to the husband that it was customary for the physician attending to operate.[85]

There was no other mention of this patient.

In Langstaff's time Caesarean section could save a child, but it usually resulted in the death of the mother and was reserved for those instances when the mother was already dead or dying. Langstaff never performed a Caesarean section operation. His reluctance to jeopardize the mother's life to save a child was shared and endorsed by most other practitioners, including his Ontario contemporary Horatio Burritt, who did sixteen 'embryotomies,' all without anaesthesia, to destroy the foetus and save the mother in cases of protracted labour.[86] In situations involving the death of a woman in labour or late pregnancy, Langstaff's decision against the operation may have been reinforced by his recollection of the difficulties experienced by his brother Miles, whose wife had died in childbirth, leaving him to father three children and a newborn. In Quebec, however, from at least 1830 some support for Caesarean operation hinged on the possiblity of baptizing the child; similarly, destruction of the foetus to save the life of the mother was frowned upon by the Roman Catholic clergy.[87] The difference, if any, between the incidence of Caesarean section in Quebec and Ontario practices is unknown.

Haemorrhage at delivery occurred fairly frequently. Langstaff knew it was caused by a malpositioned or retained placenta, abortion, and surgical tears, all of which he was prepared to correct. Over the entire forty years, nine women bled to death of the thirty-nine who appear to have died of birthing complications. Twice he blamed haemorrhage on warmth or 'the heat of the house' from 'baking on a hot day';[88] several times he recognized that some women were 'disposed' to this problem at every delivery.[89] Sometimes he saw menorrhagia, or bleeding as a complication of normal menstruation, and he managed this as he would a post-partum haemorrhage. Pallor, fainting, and loss of pulse were danger signs even if haemorrhage was not apparent; he was alert also for a characteristic 'sickly smell' of 'flooding.' Although he did not measure arterial blood pressure, he noticed whether the 'system' or the veins were 'full' or not.[90]

The presentation of a haemorrhage could be dramatic, as Langstaff himself described: 'I was sitting by the bed holding the pulse (not fearing much of anything) when I perceived it intermit a beat. I sprang to loosen bandage when she said she was faint.' The resultant 'immense flood' could produce loss of consciousness and blueness of the face and hands within minutes.[91]

Removal of the placenta was the first step in such a situation. Sometimes this was difficult if the mouth of the uterus had contracted first. Once, because there was flooding and the placenta was 'adherent' and 'would not separate,' he extracted it manually, 'clawing with two fingers' as quickly as possible.[92] This patient later developed fever. On another occasion when an 'adherent placenta tore apart,' he introduced his arm to the elbow and 'peeled' the remainder off, 'causing great pains,' but, he added, for 'only about minute.'[93] He was summoned to a case of retained placenta by his anxious brother Dr Lewis Langstaff, 'who met me at the gate,' but he let Lewis perform the operation while he gave instructions.[94]

In his last decade Langstaff rarely removed the placenta manually. Perhaps he had become aware of his own role in puerperal sepsis or sceptical of the value of intervention; indeed, one of his colleagues confessed to a change in practice after making the discovery that manipulation favoured bleeding.[95] As for the decline in forceps use, it could also be that in his later years he had simply become more patient. Sometimes, if there was no haemorrhage, he would wait till the following day.[96]

To stop bleeding, after the placenta had been delivered Langstaff 'applied child to breast,'[97] as he knew the suckling of the baby could help reduce bleeding by causing contraction of the uterus: 'pains all over when the child nurses' was once a reason for his being summoned.[98] He also regularly used tampons and tents in the vagina, sometimes dipped in alum, lead acetate, tea, or another 'astringent.' Sometimes he raised the foot of the bed and put pressure on the abdominal aorta to reduce the blood supply to the haemorrhage. In winter, he hoisted the window and applied snow or ice water to the abdomen and vagina. These measures were always adopted in great haste and had to be sustained for hours, but he had confidence in their value. Thus, when Mrs Ed Saunderson flooded for the second time after a delivery, he 'staid [sic] about four hours' and 'saved life perhaps by pressing the aorta for about 2 hours.'[99] Similarly, Langstaff 'staid' an entire day with Mrs D. Eyer, Jr, who was 'nearly gone' from flooding and had 'bid adieu to her children,' when, subsequent to his applying dressings and raising the bed, she 'rallied' and survived.[100] He recorded seeing very few lacerations, but once he sutured the ruptured perineum of a woman who had delivered unattended five days before; four days later he noted that the 'hole in which the suture lies [was] larger considerably than the ligature.'[101]

Ergotamine, a drug derived from the 'rust' parasite of rye wheat, is a specific remedy for perinatal haemorrhage. It acts by provoking contraction of the blood vessels and of the uterus. Its general effects had been known for centuries, since consumption of bread made with contaminated flour produced a dangerous illness called St Anthony's Fire. It may have been used by midwives as a folk remedy, but it was brought into obstetrical orthodoxy in 1807 by John

Stearns, who claimed to have learned of its use by 'an ignorant Scotch woman.'[102] Enthusiasts for ergot emerged in Quebec as early as 1826.[103]

Langstaff used ergot only once or twice a year (2 per cent of cases) in the 1850s, but this figure increased to 8 per cent and 8.7 per cent of cases in the middle decades and 14 per cent in the 1880s (Table 8.1). At first he employed it only 'at the end of labour,' but he was impressed with how it quickly and efficiently dealt with slow, ineffective labour and post-partum haemorrhage.[104] In the early 1860s he became increasingly comfortable with its use prior to delivery for women known to be bleeders or already bleeding. Doctors were aware that it might have a harmful effect on the baby, partly because the uterine contractions could delay birth. Langstaff was careful to observe the newborn and seems to have conducted an ad hoc 'clinical trial' in his own practice. Thus, after 'early' and 'moderate' administration, newborns were noted to be 'lively notwithstanding the ergot'; once, when he 'gave ergot pretty freely' before delivery, it 'did not affect child's hart [sic].'[105]

With time Langstaff seems to have become more cautious: he indicated that ergot was given only 'towards the last,' or 'as instruments applied,' or not 'till after the placenta,' or 'after flooding began.'[106] Several times in the later years he specifically mentioned when no ergot had been given at all,[107] but in at least one of these instances it was to absolve himself of iatrogenic responsibility for a contracted uterine os and retained placenta, a complication that might have been caused by the drug had it been given.[108] An exception to this was his management of a case of placenta praevia, during which he steadily kept his fingers between the placenta and the baby's head, giving ergot throughout the delivery until the happy outcome.[109]

Sometimes patients flooded though 'all precautions' including ergot were taken.[110] Despite these treatment failures and his later caution, his confidence in the drug was unshaken. When confronted with a haemorrhage he would 'send for' ergot if he had none with him;[111] in 1882 he watched as one patient 'flooded to death in about 2½ hours in spite of the cold douche and compressing aorta; I had no ergot with me.'[112] If Langstaff did attempt a blood transfusion – as his son maintained he had – it seems that it would have been in precisely this setting.[113]

For a six-month period in 1869 Langstaff adopted an unusual form of treatment for menorrhagia, or increased menstrual bleeding: uterine cautery. He introduced a caustic agent such as silver nitrate through a gum catheter directly into the uterus. Several of the seven women treated in this manner received the cautery more than once.[114] The method was abandoned as abruptly as it appeared.[115] Cautery or irrigation of the uterus with cold or astringent solutions to induce contraction had been recommended for many years for uterine inflammation or bleeding,[116] but this particular method seems to have been inspired by the work of Joseph Lister. Langstaff's adoption of the new technique came a little more than one year after the virtues of carbolic acid were first discussed in the *Canada Medical Journal* and just as William Canniff published articles on its relationship to germ theory and its properties in toothache and skin disease. Langstaff abandoned the uterine carbolic wash a few months before a report by T.G. Roddick of poisoning by carbolic acid and one year *before* a Canadian article appeared to describe the uterine application.[117] It appears that for this single therapeutic modality his practice preceded advocacy in the Canadian medical literature.

Rapid delivery seems to have been Langstaff's preferred method of relieving pain, but sometimes the pains were 'hard,' 'severe,' or persistent. In these cases he would give a medication, usually opium. His inclination to do this increased over his final three decades, to a peak of approximately twenty-five per cent of obstetrical patients. Nevertheless, in all periods he used medications far less often for perinatal women than he did for the population at large (Table 8.4). An interesting feature of his prescribing practice was the fact that in the majority of situations in which a medication was given he had arrived too late for the delivery. No information allows the observer to choose between several plausible hypotheses: prescription of a drug may have made him feel as though he had done *something* to justify his authority or his fee when he had failed in his main purpose; or perhaps the summons came late in some labours *because of* inordinate pain in the second or third stage, making his ability to offer analgesia the prime reason for his presence.

Anaesthetics were introduced into obstetrical practice in the late 1840s, just as Langstaff completed his training at Guy's Hospital, where he first witnessed their effects. Although he had employed ether and chloroform in the 1850s and early 1860s as medical analgesics and surgical anaesthetics for cases that included post-partum complications, he did not use an anaesthetic for a delivery until 1865. The first patient to enjoy the oblivion of chloroform was his wife,

TABLE 8.4
Medication at deliveries and Langstaff's time of arrival

	1850s (5 years)	1860s (1 year)	1870s (3 years)	1880s (2 years)
Total deliveries	241	111	312	156
No. given medicine	7	10	53	28
On time for delivery	214	82	269	133
% given medicine	2.8	7.3	11.5	10.5
Too late for delivery	27	29	43	23
% given medicine	3.7	13.7	51.2	60.8

Source: All entries in Langstaff's daybooks for 1849–54, 1861, 1872–5, 1880–2

Mary Ann, as she laboured for the sixth of her eleven babies.[118] She did not receive the anaesthetic again, however, and Langstaff used it only sparingly for obstetrical cases: just one (0.3 per cent) delivery in the 1870s and four (2 per cent) in the 1880s. Thus, his frequent use of forceps seems to have been quite independent of anaesthesia, although historians have found that anaesthesia and instrumentation went 'hand in hand.'[119] There were no reports of ill effects on mothers or children in the daybooks.

Between 1858 and 1863 a few Canadian deaths were attributed to anaesthetics, including one in Toronto.[120] The drug's danger for the foetus was suspected though unproven. The aforementioned Burritt used chloroform even less often than did Langstaff: only twice for deliveries and apparently never for his sixteen embryotomies. Burritt's hesitation may have derived from his first delivery with the anaesthetic, which he suspected had caused the child's death.[121]

From Langstaff's earlier experience he knew that manipulation of the womb and its contents could result in severe pain. He noted that when a colleague had removed the 'placenta in [a patient's] other two confinements by grasping with hand [he had caused] more suffering than all other [aspects of birth] together.'[122] For at least one less affluent patient, Langstaff used chloroform to ease this management of a dangerously complicated labour. He had already attended Mrs Charlie Morrison at least three times over the previous decade for stillbirths, one of which involved the loss of triplets. He arrived at 5 a.m. to find the 'shoulder presenting [and the] hand hanging out. Waters gone off five hours, child compressed, uterus hard.' Version or turning the baby from within was the method of choice for delivery. He administered opium and then 'chloroform so as to keep the patient only partially conscious. Os not fully dilated but sufficient to admit the hand, which passed up very slowly & easily, as the pains would relax a little, till the finger reached the bend of the knee, on catching point of middle finger into back of knee joint & drawing down, child [a living daughter] came away entirely in 2 seconds with the greatest ease. Placenta soon followed.'[123]

According to published fee schedules, use of chloroform could double the cost of attendance during delivery, from five to ten dollars.[124] This may be why its infrequent use seems to have favoured women in comfortable circumstances. Among the birthing women to whom Langstaff administered chloroform were the wife of the newspaper printer, the wife of a minister, and both his own wives.[125] Professional courtesy extended to the families of clergymen as well as doctors; thus, of this group only the printer would have received a bill. These were, however, the women of the community most likely to know about the drug and most able to insist upon its use. Judith Leavitt has shown that increased medicalization of birth was sometimes endorsed and encouraged by women.[126]

Toxaemia of pregnancy, or eclampsia, was a condition that Langstaff did see from time to time, in the form of generalized swelling, protein in the urine (which he demonstrated),[127] and convulsions. One woman died of it while in labour of a full-term baby, as Langstaff and two colleagues stood helplessly by.[128] Some cases of convulsions in the perinatal setting may actually have been due to infection rather than eclampsia, but the doctor did not distinguish between them. He seemed to be aware that certain drugs favoured seizures, and blamed one father for having given laudanum, though 'he said [just] a drop,' for a persistently crying newborn who had 'convulsions repeatedly since.'[129]

Langstaff managed 'fits' with fever therapy, such as bleeding and cold to the head, and in the late 1860s he added bromides, a treatment he found to be very effective. One new mother was 'first rate' a day after her seizure, during which she had emitted a 'low plaintive cry.'[130] Several times he seems to have been similarly impressed with how quickly patients could recover following seizures: one woman was 'uncommonly well' the next day; another, whose fit he had related to delayed menses, 'looked only a little wild' immediately after a convulsion and was later found 'doing her ironing.'[131]

Langstaff seems to have been able to recognize the clinical setting that favoured seizures, and was anxious to prevent them. For example, a mother was delivered of a daughter and left in a 'cheerful' condition with a 'healthy flush.' During this labour he had observed that the 'colour came and left her face suddenly several times ... also a sudden dark blush came over her whole face like a shadow dark and sudden' and she had 'pain in top of her head.' Later the doctor wrote, 'I was out round the barn when [her husband] came suddenly to the door, "she is in a fit." (I had told them she was threatened with fits).' Langstaff rushed to her side, showered her head, bled her 'freely,' and gave antimony potassium tartrate and bromide. When he came to attend this patient and others in later confinements, he used bromide before delivery to 'ward off convulsions,' as he had used cold to the head in the past.[132]

The most common cause of perinatal morbidity and mortality in every decade studied was the infection called childbed fever. Less abrupt than haemorrhage, the infection usually took two or three days to develop and was characterized by fever, rapid pulse, persistent swelling and tenderness of the abdomen and uterus, skin changes, absence of breast milk, and, in severe cases, kidney failure, confusion, loss of consciousness, and seizures. Women who died usually did so within two days to two weeks of delivery; some developed chronic illness that waxed and waned until death up to four months later.[133]

The most compelling evidence that the disease was spread on the hands of examiners is the apparent rise in maternal deaths during the later half of the nineteenth century in a manner that parallels the rise in physician-attended birth.[134] It is not difficult to find cases that may have been infected by Langstaff, who visited women with childbed fever and children with apparent streptococcal infection on the same days as he attended other birthing women who later developed fever.[135] He used forceps with great frequency; it is known that childbed fever occurs more commonly in situations involving manual or instrumental intervention. For instance, a young woman bled profusely following her confinement, to which Langstaff was summoned three hours late when the placenta would not come and the 'cord had been pulled until it had begun to give way.' He introduced his hand and extracted the placenta, and observed the uterus contract and the bleeding stop, but ten days later the patient lay feverish and 'sinking' with a 'death rattle' in her throat.[136]

The mortality rate in Langstaff's practice rose in the third decade to be among the highest reported for his century; however, statistics on maternal mortality have been notoriously difficult to gather with precision and their interpretation is 'tricky.'[137] The nine puerperal deaths out of 312 deliveries translates into a high mortality rate of 29 per 1,000, but these numbers are quite small; as will be shown below, it would be wrong to conclude they reflect the entire practice. However, it is reasonable to ask if the high mortality rate in Langstaff's practice had anything to do with his frequent use of forceps. To answer this question, many factors must be considered.

First, some years saw several puerperal deaths, others, none, although Langstaff's forceps rate rose to high levels and remained constant. The most significant factor that could explain the variability in maternal mortality is the effect of concomitant epidemics of erysipelas, scarlatina, and sore throat, caused by bacteria that can also cause childbed fever. Families lived in houses that were small, crowded, and poorly ventilated, especially in winter. Mothers could be infected by exposure to their sick children as well as by the examinations of their doctor, who tended them all; several instances of childbirth immediately after attendance on sick children were mentioned in chapters 5 and 7. Childbed fever occurred more commonly in years with a high incidence of these streptococcal infections and diarrhoea, a correlation lending support to the observation that outbreaks could be related to the appearance of particularly virulent strains of bacteria.[138] For example, in the worst such season, the winter of 1871–2, nine children died of scarlatina and four women succumbed to puerperal fever between the end of February and early April. These four maternal deaths also contributed to the gloomy statistics for 1872–5, but in the next twenty-seven months only one such death occurred. Langstaff indicated that at least three women who died had been sick before they went into labour; in at least one other case a newborn acquired erysipelas before the mother developed a fever from which she eventually recovered.[139]

Second, Langstaff became a popular consultant for midwives and younger, less experienced clinicians, who summoned him when they encountered a difficult case. This factor might tend to make the death rate falsely high: if his maternal mortality rate is to be expressed as a function of birth rate, it should include all other mothers delivered by the people, midwives or doctors, who had consulted Langstaff. Of the nine women who died of childbirth in the years between 1872 and 1875, only one had not been seen by Langstaff during labour.

This problem is more evident in a consideration of maternal deaths over the entire forty years: of the thirty-nine women identified as having died of post-partum complications, sixteen did not see Langstaff until some time after giving birth, when they were already sick; thirteen of these women delivered by midwives or other doctors died of fever, three of bleeding. Seven of nine women who died in the 1850s do not appear to have been attended by a physician at their deliveries.

Third, Langstaff's use of forceps seems if anything to have been somewhat lower among women who eventually died than among his other patients. Of the nine women who died in 1872–5, only two were delivered by forceps, both were haemorrhaging before he applied the instruments, and one died within minutes of delivery; one other woman bled to death and the remaining six died of fever – but he had not used forceps at their deliveries. Of the thirty-nine women found to have died of childbirth complications over the forty years of practice, only eight were delivered by forceps, but one of these had been seen by another doctor (whose efforts had caused a laceration). The forceps rate among the twenty-three women attended in labour by Langstaff and who eventually died is therefore 30 per cent, which is lower than the frequency of use in his later practice. Of the seven women he delivered by forceps, three quickly bled to death, but it is entirely possible that the remaining four who died of puerperal fever may have developed their infection from the doctor's instruments. Nevertheless, Langstaff's tools cannot be held accountable for thirty-one other deaths of puerperal fever in women who had been delivered neither by forceps nor by him.

Finally, if doubts can be raised about the actual maternal mortality rate in this practice, I believe doubts can also be raised about figures based on sources that include obstetrical casebooks. Maternal deaths have been defined as occurring within the 'puerperum' or the three to six weeks following birth.[140] However, this arbitrary time-limit can falsely skew the death rate down; I did not use a cut-off date in analysing Langstaff's practice. If a mother contracted her illness at or immediately after birth, I counted her death as puerperal even when it occurred up to four months later. The advantage of a daybook over an obstetrical notebook is that the daybook permits the identification of such cases that might not have appeared in an obstetrical record, not because of deliberate attempts to falsify but because of the nature of the document: doctors may have followed a time-limited definition of puerperal illness; or they may have come truly to believe that a woman's prolonged illness could have had nothing to do with a labour that took place months before; or they may have intended the obstetrical notebook to serve only as a guide to future interventions at the birth itself. In other words, mortality rates based on obstetrical casebooks may be suspected of being falsely low. As I said at the beginning of this chapter, the issue is complicated.

Langstaff used the word 'metritis' (inflammation of the uterus), but it is not always clear if he distinguished between various localized and potential causes of childbed fever; there seems to be some overlap between his recognition of this condition and that of mastitis (inflammation of the breast), another type of postnatal fever. From the earliest days of his practice, Langstaff washed his instruments and used wine, known to have mild antiseptic properties, as a vaginal douche. There is no evidence, however, that he understood his own role in the transmission of this disease until perhaps late in his practice, when he often mentioned the use of carbolic acid and once the changing of his clothes prior to a delivery.[141] The figures are too small to allow statements about the impact such procedures may have had on mortality in his practice.

Despite his potential responsibility for causing fever, Langstaff treated the women so afflicted with great care, visiting them daily, sometimes three or four times a day, until they recovered or died. The measures taken to treat childbed fever were almost the same as those used for other fevers: cold to the head, warmth to the feet, venesection, cupping, broths, and opium if needed for pain. Tartar emetic was used less often. Langstaff saw one patient, who lived four miles from his home, thirty-four times in the six weeks between her confinement and her death.[142] More than half of those who developed fever recovered. He made remarks that indicated his hope for recovery: for example, he described how a woman who had been extremely ill with fever, diarrhoea, and skin abscesses since the birth of her daughter five weeks before lay in a 'stupid sleep ... a dreamy state with her eyes wide open ... at the same time losing their lustre, but the lustre returns in a twinkling on speaking to her & she says, "I am not sleepy."' In spite of this hopeful sign, she died two days later.[143]

Mastitis, which Langstaff called 'gathered breast,' was fairly common. When it 'threatened' he used topical remedies, poultices, breast pumps, 'false nipples' (nipple shields?), and analgesics.[144] One woman was reportedly 'applying a weasel skin' to her 'threatening' breast, but exactly how was not stated.[145] If an abscess formed, as happened in one to two per cent of all mothers delivered from the 1850s to the 1870s, he incised it. One such case drained 'about a quart' of purulent fluid; only once did he record using an anaesthetic for the procedure.[146] There seems to have been a general decline in the absolute frequency of this complication, from approximately two or three times a year in the 1850s and 1860s to once in the 1870s. Although two women developed mastitis, no cases of breast abscess were seen in the 1880s. This may have been the result of improved aseptic technique, but again the figures are too small for definite statements to be made.

While feverish, many women developed psychiatric symptoms. It is impossible to separate these secondary causes of mental disturbances from the condition known as post-partum psychosis (see chapter 6). The content of his patients' delusions interested him. He recorded how one mother, whom he had not attended in her labour two weeks earlier, spoke nonsense, pinched her breasts, bit her fingers until they bled, and made attempts to bite those around her: 'she said, "I am not going to get well anyhow" [and] she fancies the baby smells bad and wants it buried.' Langstaff showered her head, offered opium, brandy, camphor, and chloroform, and sat with her until she fell asleep; she died the following day.[147] Another, who was 'obstinate about taking anything but [could] be humoured to do so,' complained that her doctor was 'always teasing,'[148] and another, whose 'reason was gone' and who had been seen by the doctor 'a dozen times in one day,' thought she had been 'a long time ill.'[149] Several women in delirium, even those who had not been confined, had 'fancies' concerning birthing or 'seeing [their] children when not present.'[150] Once only, Langstaff specifically indicated a diagnosis of 'puerperal mania' in a woman who 'persist[ed] that she is going to die.'[151] He took these presentiments of death very seriously; in his experience they often came true.[152]

There appears to have been no specific treatment for post-partum women with psychic symptoms. The doctor would prescribe 'anything that agrees,' but it is clear, from his detailed knowledge of their fantasies, that he listened to their ramblings and was not above doing seemingly futile things to please them. Ageing and ailing himself from the illness that would claim his life only months later, he sat and 'talked a little' to a young mother feverish and confused five days after the birth of her first baby. At first she thought she was in

Aurora, but when the doctor questioned her, she reasoned that the door and the wallpaper were like her own. Her 'mind wanders,' he wrote, and she 'fancies things,' but 'she is very *good natured*' [Langstaff's emphasis] .. She wanted me to take hold of the point of her tongue. I did so and she became calm at once and relapsed into a stupor.'[153] She died five hours later.

Approximately one per cent (thirty-nine) of all birthing mothers in Langstaff's practice were unmarried; three gave birth to two or more illegitimate babies, as much as twelve years apart. In Langstaff's record these women are identified as 'Miss' and the name of their own parent, usually but not always their father. Some appear to have held a nebulous marital status, since Langstaff would designate a woman as a dependant of an unrelated man, possibly her employer, possibly the child's father.[154] Illegitimacy occurred at a constant rate; Langstaff's contemporary Dr Burritt recognized it with the same one per cent frequency. Furthermore, there does not appear to be any difference in the number of visits or the nature of his treatment between married and unmarried women.[155] The doctor's language suggests he may not have been particularly sympathetic: words like 'another bastard' and 'grandbastard' appear occasionally, but the words may have seemed less disparaging then than they do now.

Attention was paid to paternity, not simply for settling the doctor's bill, but also for support of mother and child. In this matter the mother's word or that of her family appears to have been accepted. Thus, the hired man at Burns's mill came forward to pay for the delivery of an unnamed woman working there; 'old Fox' was identified as the progenitor of another child; 'young Warren at whose father's house she has been living' was similarly named; and the uncles of an illegitimate child claimed that 'Snider the late Dutch preacher is the father of it.'[156] One dark young woman, a few days prior to her delivery of a blond child 'begot up West,' was 'dropped' by Francis Button at the door of a home, where, perhaps because paternity was implied, the reception was less than warm. 'The boys are mad,' wrote Langstaff.[157] Privacy for unmarried mothers in the lower social class was non-existent. The newspaper reported information about paternity supposedly 'confided' to the doctor, but the daybooks tend to refute the accuracy of such stories.[158]

A significant proportion of these women appear to have been in service as domestics. This might have been because of the pregnancy, but it is possible they became pregnant through the sexual exploitation that came with service employment.[159] They often had their babies in the home of a neighbour rather than at their parents' house. Thus, Susannah Doner gave birth in the home of Adam Sturm, just as his family came down with severe scarlet fever. The Sturm children seem to have recovered, but their father died. Miss Doner developed post-partum fever and after more than twenty visits from Langstaff she died too.[160] Langstaff had attended Susannah's family for many years; he indicated that her mother nursed her through part of her last illness, even though she lay in another's home. Six months later, for some unexplained reason, possibly compassion, guilt, or paternal duty, a man paid the doctor thirty dollars for his attendance 'on the late Susannah Doner.'[161]

Most of the unmarried mothers had uncomplicated deliveries not requiring extra attention; however, two cases late in Langstaff's career show that he could be indignant when he thought that they had been maltreated. In the first he was summoned by telegraph to attend an unwed mother on her third post-partum day; she lay dying of 'metritis' due to a 'severe laceration through anus & lower part of rectum' made 'by Dr Hammil' and his use of forceps.[162] In the second he visited a young woman who had given birth twelve days before and still had an enlarged uterus; he wrote, 'Dr Knill has been there & "gone on terribly, will give Dr Langstaff to understand that he knows as much as Dr Langstaff." He hoisted the window & gave her cold & now she is going to have a gathered breast.'[163]

The long-term problems of repeated childbearing seem to have occupied Langstaff but little: twice he prescribed pessaries for uterine prolapse,[164] and he kept a newspaper advertisement for an effective uterine support in his daybook. Fertility rates declined in the second half of the nineteenth century; it seems women sought to control their reproductive functions.[165] There is no indication, however, that Langstaff gave advice for birth control. It is possible he may have advised prolonged breast-feeding, a traditional method that had received medical endorsement in Britain in the first third of the nineteenth century.[166] Nevertheless, he may have witnessed failures of this method, attributing a stillbirth to a 'ten-mile rough ride' the mother had taken 'while nursing a three year old in the bottom of a sleigh.'[167] In this context 'breast-feeding' seems the most likely meaning of the word 'nursing.'

How long mothers chose to nurse their children cannot be determined from this medical record, but most did nurse, since a 'wet nurse' was not specifically mentioned until 1888.[168] Langstaff noted that the child in question was still nursing at three years, as if this were late; he recorded that one baby had been weaned at three months, as if this were unusually early.

The difficulties facing a single mother in Victorian Ontario guaranteed that a few would either attempt to terminate the pregnancy, or failing that, commit infanticide; however, there were strict penalties. Ontario law, based on the British law of 1803 amended in 1828, 1831, and 1861, defined induced abortion as a statutory offence, made third parties responsible for aiding and abetting, and eliminated any distinction between early and late abortion. By 1861, women who attempted to induce their own miscarriages were felons.[169]

Langstaff did not perform abortions. When he was called either to help save or help evacuate the 'ovum' and contents of the uterus, most of these miscarriages appear to have occurred spontaneously. Thus, a fifteen-year-old girl who had 'never menstruated' was seen for severe pain and an abdominal 'tumor just like a $4^1/_2$ month uterus,' which 'disappeared' after a flow of 'bloody water'; married women also presented in similar circumstances.[170] Some spontaneous abortions occurred in clusters, especially during times of epidemic diarrhoea, suggesting an infectious cause.[171] Langstaff usually estimated the age of the foetus and occasionally noted when the child could be seen 'transparently' through intact membranes.[172]

Sometimes a traumatic cause for abortion was named, but one woman, who 'fell against a washtub' and miscarried, appears to have had two other abortions for unnamed reasons.[173] A few abortions were complicated by profuse bleeding and fever, symptoms suggesting but not confirming that the abortions may have been induced. The number of spontaneous abortions in the daybooks appears to decline with time: Langstaff recorded miscarriages in 8.3 per cent, 6.2 per cent, 4.5 per cent, and 2.6 per cent of his obstetrics cases in the 1850s, 1860s, 1870s, and 1880s respectively (see Table 8.1). Belying the presence of a large abortion industry, however, the figures in all decades studied are considerably lower than would be predicted simply using the natural incidence of spontaneous abortion (one in six). This discrepancy suggests that women who miscarried consulted the doctor rarely and with decreasing frequency throughout the second half of the nineteenth century.[174] Even less often did Langstaff directly indicate that he suspected illegal activities on the part of community women and medical colleagues.

Abortionists operated in the Toronto region, but they did not come to attention unless a death occurred; several regular practitioners were accused of having done abortions when pregnant women died in suspicious circumstances, but the actual frequency of these apparently common cases is not known.[175] Langstaff was involved in two cases of illegal abortion; both implicated the same physician. In March 1868 Langstaff was summoned to his own patient, nineteen-year-old Sabra Wright, daughter of William Wright. She lay severely ill with fever in the Queen Street office of Dr Moses Hilton Williams, a licensed physician newly graduated from Toronto's Victoria University.[176] Langstaff had known the girl since she was a child; she had recently been coming to see him for dental problems and headache.[177] The scenario is reminiscent of the deathbed confession, often used in American courts to implicate abortionists.[178] Very weak and capable only of a whisper, Sabra told Langstaff that Williams had 'used an instrument' that produced pain. Her countenance was very pale, her lips white, nose sharpened, eyes sunken, and her tender, hard abdomen signalled peritonitis.

Sabra was too sick to be moved back to Richmond Hill. Langstaff asked his old friend W.T. Aikins to continue her care, but Aikins refused because Williams 'was an abortionist.'[179] She died shortly after and the authorities prepared for an inquest. Langstaff wrote to Aikins expressing his fears that the family would testify against him and saying Williams's brother-in-law had been 'out here feeling the people.'[180] He was worried that Sabra's cousin and employer, Elizabeth Ann Harrington, would confirm that the girl had been in chronic ill health, but he hoped that Elizabeth's father, Amos Wright, who was also Sabra's uncle and the former Reform member of parliament, would testify against his own daughter. The doctor could not be assured of Wright's support, since Amos was locked in an ongoing court battle with Langstaff's brother John.[181]

An autopsy and inquest were held, both of which Langstaff attended. He was kept in the witness box for two hours. The court accused Williams of having performed an abortion, but he denied the charge, claiming Miss Wright had come to him in desperation after months of medical mismanagement by Langstaff. The autopsy revealed trauma to the cervical os, but since the prior pregnancy could not be proven, the case was dismissed.[182] Langstaff was clearly uncertain about the fact of pregnancy, but he did refer to Williams as an 'abortionist' in his records.[183]

Langstaff's suspicions regarding Williams had already been raised at their meeting, just a few months before the death of Sabra Wright, when he had been called to see Mrs Martha Basingtwaite (or Besingtwait), vomiting and febrile, following her miscarriage in the fourth month of pregnancy. She had been to Toronto to see Williams and had been given some unidentified medicine 'before she aborted,' but, Langstaff later testified, 'he did not tell me what he gave her then.' Mrs Basingtwaite and her sister, Miss Hunter, 'were impera-tive on me that I was not to stop the labour.' During the next month Williams came to Richmond Hill at least twice to see Mrs Basingtwaite. Langstaff had trouble with her compliance: he wrote, 'I am thinking of discontinuing as they don't go according to orders.' Perhaps the patient was concerned that Langstaff's discovery of her actions would bring about prosecution. She died after four weeks of severe illness.[184]

The Richmond Hill newspaper had followed both stories and openly linked the case of Sabra Wright to that of 'Mrs Basingtwaite who died here a few weeks ago.' It reported that Sabra's lover, 'Jim,' had displayed total disregard for her plight, telling her in a letter that 'it was a pity she had not committed suicide four months ago.' There is no doubt,' the editors continued, 'but Dr Langstaff could a tale un-fold in this case that would raise a storm, but as it would not bring the dead to life, we presume the Doctor prefers to observe his usual reticence.'[185]

One month after the inquest on Sabra Wright, another inquest was finally called to investigate Mrs Basingtwaite's death of six months earlier. John Palmer, the local hotel keeper, came forward with an incriminating letter from Williams that 'embrace[d] sundry glaring offers of money if Mr Palmer could procure evidence to prosecute some one for defamation of his character.' The jury decided that Basingtwaite had died 'in consequence of having procured an abor-tion' with the help of her sister, Miss Maria Hunter.

Warrants were issued for the arrest of Williams, of the sister as 'aider and abettor,' and of the husband 'as accessory after the fact.' But Williams had 'left for parts unknown before the constable had time to arrest him.'[186] This experience does not seem to have left a permanent mark on Williams's career. Fifteen years later an adver-tisement in the *Globe* announced that he was proprietor of the 'On-tario Pulmonary Institute' on Jarvis Street.[187]

Infanticide was also known. In mid-nineteenth century England and the United States a significant proportion of coroner's inquests were held upon the bodies of newborn children.[188] Prosecution of this crime increased in nineteenth-century Britain, but beginning in the 1850s there was a parallel trend to more lenient punishment for the financially disabled and 'ruined maid.'[189] Infanticide was differentiated from murder and given a lesser penalty, partly to enhance the possibility of conviction.[190] Sometimes it was easier to prosecute the mother for concealment of birth than for murdering her child. The frequency of infanticide in nineteenth-century Ontario is uncertain, but the many newspaper reports suggest it was not uncommon; studies show that there were dozens of coroner's inquests in the second half of the century.[191] Like their British counterparts, Ontario doctors and courts also seem to have been relatively lenient, often recommending clemency and thereby provoking the *Globe* to suggest, in 1870, that 'surely juries are becoming merciful to a fault.'[192] An editorial in a Canadian medical journal attacked an American coroner for having decided a baby had died of asphyxia, without having the well-to-do unmarried mother charged with murder.[193]

Langstaff seems to have been vigilant for the crime, but his opinions regarding prosecution and punishment are not known. On being summoned to attend an unmarried woman, he 'removed the placenta' but was too late to deliver the child, 'supposed to be George Stephenson's.'; 'I know by the shape of the head,' he wrote, that it was 'born before I arrived and nearly smothered in the vessel.'[194] He may have suspected foul play also in a few of the stillbirths he arrived too late to deliver. His diligence in examining the state of the body to determine the approximate date of death (i.e., *prior* to delivery) may have served to prevent such charges.

Langstaff was involved in two trials held for suspected infanticide. Ann Brophy, an unmarried servant in the home of Peter Rupert, was charged with concealment of birth. Mrs Rupert told the jury that she had had no reason to suspect that Brophy was 'about to be confined,' but she found her servant in the privy 'one hour after she had excused herself.' Mrs Rupert and her daughter helped Ann Brophy back into the house, where Mrs Rupert made an 'examination' that 'satisfied her that she had given birth to a child.' Her husband went to look for the baby near the privy and, noticing broken snow behind the fence, found the body. Mrs Rupert said that Ann Brophy had claimed to have been 'insensible' and unaware of her actions, and added that the girl 'would have died in about half an hour had I not found her.' Langstaff, who had attended 'plump and fair' Mrs Rupert in some of her seventeen deliveries and one apparently spontaneous abortion, was called to an inquest. The case proceeded to trial in Toronto, where he gave evidence before a grand jury, but no record of his testimony has been kept. If the doctor favoured conviction, his statement was not convincing: after 'a powerful and feeling appeal' by Brophy's counsellor, the jury brought in a verdict of not guilty.[195]

From testimony in this and the abortion cases, it seems that males in authority adopted the role of inquisitors. Their doing so may have been partly to shelter themselves from being named accessory to the crime. In the Basingtwaite case the Methodist pastor John Bredin testified that he had asked the patient's mother 'whether [her daughter] had been confined or not,' because he had been 'credibly informed there was a premature birth,' but was told 'nothing of the kind was the matter with her.' When the mother later apologized for having misinformed him owing to her own ignorance, he expressed his 'surprise to Miss Hunter [the patient's sister], who was sitting close by, that she should allow her mother to misinform me by telling an untruth [to which], she replied "you did not ask me the question."' It was neither stated nor questioned why such information should be the privilege of the minister not yet a father himself.[196] Similarly, Peter Basingtwaite took pains to show he had 'never' called for Dr Williams' but had 'fetched' Dr Langstaff instead. He reported that Langstaff had asked if there had been any 'foul play' and had warned that the miscarriage 'might cause some trouble or mischief.'[197]

Given the legal situation, it was in the best interests of a husband, a doctor, or even a preacher to distance himself from any possible association with an abortion, natural or induced. Solidarity among women, married or not, may have kept most abortions from the attention of men. In such a climate the relatively small and declining proportion of natural abortions or miscarriages attended by Langstaff may reflect mistrust of males and anticipation of the interrogation women might receive should they miscarry.

If there was female solidarity, Langstaff's second infanticide case suggests that it was not universal. Furthermore, it shows that the doctor spoke out on a patient's behalf when she stood accused by her peers. Thirteen years after the Brophy case, Langstaff gave medical evidence on behalf of Fanny Williams, a thirty-eight-year-old widow accused of infanticide. He had attended the birth and assisted the delivery with forceps, but he thought the child was one month premature, 'from appearance of the nails.' It died thirty hours later having had several seizures. The press reported that the coroner, Dr Reid, received a 'communication that the child had met with foul play.' On the morning of the inquest Langstaff visited Mrs Williams, already under arrest, and he gave her some medication. The paper quoted him as saying, in her defence, that he 'thought the child was one of eight months' and that he 'did not think it would live'; perhaps he was aware of some damage caused by his use of forceps. The charges had been made by 'some neighbour women' who had also been present at the delivery and others who claimed to have heard Mrs Williams speak of her plans to destroy the baby, before its birth, by taking drugs and/or throwing herself down stairs to induce premature labour. Five women who testified to that effect convinced the jury. In spite of Langstaff's testimony and that of three other doctors who had agreed with him, Fanny Williams went to jail. The York Herald's commentary on the 'disreputable affair' made it clear that the press sympathized with the verdict and with the jurymen, who had to endure the 'hisses of an impatient and indignant little crowd' who believed that 'the whole affair was an uncalled for aggravation of the misfortune and disgrace that she had brought upon herself.'[198] Three months later Langstaff went to Toronto on Mrs Williams's behalf and her case was dismissed.[199]

The Langstaffs were no strangers to tragedies of birthing. The doctor and his wife often shared the painful conditions that plagued their neighbours; their experiences reiterate a common pattern. Langstaff delivered all but one of his first wife's eleven children, all four of his second wife's children, and most of the ten babies born to the wives of his brother John and his brother-in-law Henry Miller, Jr.

Langstaff's first born, Lucy Dorothea, died at nine months of age, at quarter past one in the morning of 24 September 1857.[200] He did not identify the cause, although there were several cases of diarrhoea and sore throat in the community at the time. Two years later, a boy, named Wickliffe Ogden, was born. Langstaff seems to have been looking forward to the new child and may even have discussed the event with his patients, as two months earlier he wrote 'Wickliff Langstaff' in the margins of his daybook after a visit to a woman patient who had perhaps suggested the name.[201] When Wickliffe was almost two, another baby was born, but it was a month premature and died three days later; Langstaff recorded the birth, but not the death. One year later there was another little girl, Lizette, but before she was a year old Wickliffe had died, at three years nine months; six months later Lizette died too, just after her first birthday.

The following month on a Saturday at noon, Mary Ann gave birth to another baby boy, but her labour 'pains [were] slow and weak.' Langstaff wrote that he gave 'ergot in small doses gradually increased ... forceps used after the head was noticed several times after intervals of some minutes to give sudden spasmodic twitches. It came down and turned into 1st position by slight force – forceps removed to be applied as in 1st pos[ition] but it was found difficult, head having gone back & turned into its old position [4th]. F[orceps] withdrawn & applied as at first & completed [delivery] easily, but chord down & flaccid, pulseless, but the child rallied.'[202] These remarks hint vaguely at the scene as the two so recently bereaved parents watched their baby struggle for ninety minutes before it died. The doctor saw nine other patients that day and did one other delivery. And so the Langstaffs buried their fifth child.

Sometime in the following few months, the couple adopted Ernest Franklin, who, though he was just a bit younger, was said to resemble blond, blue-eyed Wickliffe. Ernest's birth date is known, but his biological parents cannot be identified.[203] At Mary Ann's next confinement Langstaff administered chloroform – apparently for the first time at any delivery – and all seemed to go well, but little Herbert died six months later. In the next seven years Mary Ann had five more children, three of whom, Mary Lillian (Lily), Rolph Lewis, and Louisa Eleanor (Nelly), grew to be adults. Lily and Rolph lived to be more than one hundred years old. The Langstaffs' last baby, named James Dick for the long-time Presbyterian minister, died at ten days of age. Mary Ann's last confinement, was the only one Langstaff did not attend. He was off visiting patients in Markham that day, his absence suggesting that the birth may have been unexpectedly abrupt or premature.

Both Langstaff's wives spent a large proportion of their married years either pregnant or nursing. Since eight of Mary Ann's babies died in infancy, the time she gave to nursing was short relative to the time she spent pregnant. Following the birth of children who survived longer than six months, Mary Ann Langstaff conceived an average of twelve months after delivery, a calculation strongly supporting the notion that she nursed her babies for about a year. This figure is skewed upward by the final interval of twenty-three months between the birth of Nelly and that of the last baby; the suggestion is that Mary Ann may have nursed the older children for approximately six months and adopted prolonged nursing only at the end of her childbearing. Langstaff's second wife, Louisa, would spend three of her seven years of married life in a state of pregnancy (see chapter 9).[204]

In June 1879, six years after the birth of her eleventh baby, Mary Ann fell desperately ill during a heavy menstrual period – a time in which Langstaff and his contemporaries thought women were particularly vulnerable.[205] The reasons for their attitude may have been rooted in other beliefs, but it is significant that Langstaff's comments about menstrual vulnerability were the expression of fears of infection rather than injunctions against physical activity; moreover, all but one were written after antiseptic principles had been accepted.[206] He seems to have viewed the menstruating womb, like the post-partum uterus, as an open wound at risk of infection.

Indeed, Mary Ann's febrile condition was not unlike post-partum fever. Her son, Rolph, ten years old at the time, recalled her craving for strawberries and his own frantic search in the garden to please and perhaps cure his ailing mother. After just a few days she 'passed away having made peace with God at 10 min to 12 noon,' on 21 June 1879. The daybooks do not really describe her illness, but in brief comments Langstaff revealed his understanding of germ theory, curiously intermingled with miasmatic principles, and his sympathy for Ontario's nascent public health agenda. He attributed her death to 'menorrhagia then typhoid fever from slaughter house & pig pen stench on Matthew McNair's premises.'

On the day of her funeral he wrote, 'Interment of the remains of late Mary Ann Miller, beloved wife of James Langstaff ["MD" was added later]. Sermon by Revd Isaac Campbell to a large concourse of people, even the stairs seated, all could not get in. The pulpit ornamented with flowers, pew draped in mourning. A beautiful chant sung, fine sermon, short appropriate eulogium.'[207] The local paper said that she had been 'highly respected and admired by all,' her 'circle of friends was the very largest,' and many followed 'her remains ... to their resting place.'[208]

But that was not the end of the case. Langstaff had twice been sued by McNair over matters pertaining to real estate. Now feeling much maligned, he waged a campaign, through the authorities and the press, against the intransigent neighbour who refused to 'clean up.' Three years later, the doctor was still brooding over his loss and what he perceived to have been its cause: he wrote again, 'Mrs Mary

Ann Langstaff passed away from earth to heaven this day three years at 10 m to 12 noon calmly & peacefully. Death caused by slaughter-house stench during a period of menorrhagia.'[209]

❧

Obstetrics made up roughly ten per cent of Langstaff's practice, with a rise in his middle career and a slight decline at the end. It appears that birthing mothers and women attendants were willing to have his help; by 1871 he was delivering half the babies born in his census district. Over his career Langstaff increasingly used forceps to assist delivery and ergotamine to control bleeding, but there was a small relative decline in forceps use in the last decade of his life. On rare occasions from 1865, he gave anaesthetic to his patients, usually edu-cated women of means, and he generally seems to have avoided giving any medicine in the birth period. After 1867 carbolic acid figured in his obstetrical record.

Perinatal mortality rates in Langstaff's practice appear to have been high in comparison with others available for his era. The elevated mortality may have been related to his use of instruments, but other factors have been identified to explain them, including concomitant epidemics of scarlet fever and his consultation practice. In cases of puerperal fever Langstaff made repeated visits, his notes of which display concern for his patients. He did not perform abortions, but twice he testified in coroner's cases concerning abortion and once he spoke in defence of a woman patient accused of infanticide. The declining number of miscarriages in his record suggests that there was a certain reluctance on the part of his community to invite the doctor to attend, since his visit might raise suspicions for all con-cerned of deliberate interference with pregnancy.

Langstaff used his techniques of intervention, including forceps and anaesthesia, on members of his own family. He attributed the death of his first wife to infection contracted during a period of heavy menstrual flow. His anger over a neighbour's perceived re-sponsibility for her death and his conviction about germ theory prob-ably led him to take a more active role in politics and public health, the topics of the next chapter.

CHAPTER NINE

Therapy through Social Action:

Lawyers, Politics, and Public Health

The last two decades of the nineteenth century saw increasing agitation for sanitary reform and public health throughout the western world; Ontario was no exception.[1] In 1882 Robert Koch's proof that tuberculosis was caused by a bacterium added to the growing evidence for the germ theory of disease, recently endorsed by the work of Louis Pasteur and Joseph Lister, and gave a final 'scientific' boost to the sanitary movement that had originated in older theories of noxious airs (or miasmata). In the past, sanitarians have been portrayed as opponents of the more 'scientific' theory of micro-organisms, but Nancy Tomes has recently argued that the sanitary reform movement 'paved the way for the rapid acceptance of the germ theory.'[2] Although medical professionals may not have understood the germ theory, they did become supporters of government intervention to control risks to the public well-being; the leadership taken by physicians in the public health movement may have helped their efforts to gain greater control over the management of their profession.[3]

The Langstaff record affords an opportunity to observe when and how an individual physician and his community reacted to the legislative and social changes brought about by the public health move-

ment. The gathering of statistics, an essential part of the early movement, placed demands on both municipal officials and physicians
because it required meticulous reporting and agreement on a repro-
ducible classification of disease. By the time Ontario had enacted
laws to make these impositions, Langstaff had long been ready to
cooperate and was a strong supporter of tightened legislation for
public safety in matters pertaining not only to hygiene, but also to
the risk of accidental and violent injury. It seems that he viewed his
commitment to public health as an extension of his medical therapeutics. Some of the evidence for these statements is taken from his
ongoing contact with the law.

Possibly more than his late twentieth-century Ontario counterparts,
Langstaff had frequent contact with lawyers and judicial processes,
as the inquests into abortion and infanticide discussed in the previous chapter may already have implied. In his forty-year career he
was involved in a total of seventy-one different legal cases, involving
roughly 120 court appearances, which necessitated many additional
trips to Toronto (and elsewhere) for preparatory meetings with lawyers (Table 9.1). Slightly more than half (thirty-eight) of the seventy-
one cases were civil suits or arbitrations in which he was plaintiff,
witness, or defendant. He also appeared before a judge to settle the
expropriation of his property for the widening of a Toronto street.

Coroner's inquests made up nearly half (thirty-three) of the seventy-one cases in which Langstaff appeared; in half of these he gave
autopsy evidence. The majority were handled in the immediate vicinity. Inquests in his practice seem to decline in the 1880s whereas
other cases increased, perhaps because the coroner preferred to hear
the opinions of specialists or younger, 'more scientific' physicians
(Table 9.2). Accidental death and suicide, usually attributed to 'temporary insanity,' were the most common reasons for an inquest. Some
accidents were related to lack of safety standards for farming implements and the dangers of travel over the York roads. 'Foul play' was
often suspected, especially in the case of a homeless man found with
his skull smashed and another whose body was exhumed four months
after death because of rumours that he had been poisoned.[4] The
more usual verdict, however, was death by natural causes, which
was cited in at least five cases and possibly also some cases with
outcomes that are now unknown. Information on inquests is derived
mostly from newspapers; then, as now, the press was more interested in gore and sin than in disease.

TABLE 9.1
Legal cases in Langstaff's practice, 1849–89

	Civil cases		Coroner's inquests	
	Witness	21	Reason: Accident	8
	Plaintiff	10	Suicide	6
	Arbitration	4	Unknown	6
	Defendant	2	Natural	5
	Unknown	1	Murder	3
			Infanticide	2
			Septic abortion	2
			Exposure	1
Total cases		38		33
Court appearances		56		63*
Trips to Toronto		63		12

* Includes 5 trials
Source: Langstaff's daybooks, 1849–89; newspapers: *Globe, York Herald, Liberal*

TABLE 9.2
Civil and coroner's cases in Langstaff's practice (by decade)

	Civil cases	Coroner's inquests	Total
1850s	8	5	13
1860s	13	10	23
1870s	5	17	22
1880s	12	1	13
Total	38	33	71

Source: Langstaff's daybooks, 1849–89; newspapers: *Globe, York Herald, Liberal*

Murder was not unheard of in the Richmond Hill area, although most chroniclers, possibly reflecting the ideas prevalent in their own time, tell only about the famous case of Captain Kinnear.[5] Two of at least three murders from Langstaff's sphere went to trial: Susan Heatherington and Mary Ann Moore were both beaten to death by their husbands, and Langstaff had performed their autopsies. Matthew Teefy was the foreman of the coroner's jury in the Moore case. In correcting errors in the newspaper reports, he told how the jury had not given a verdict of 'manslaughter,' as had been said, but had found that the woman 'came to her death from inflammation of the bowels caused by violent blows and kicks inflicted by her husband.'

The inference of course was murder or manslaughter, but Teefy pointed out that a coroner's jury could not give that verdict. Recognizing the now-familiar pattern of chronic abuse, he claimed that Mrs Moore, a 'quiet sober industrious woman of strict temperate habits,' had suffered much horrid treatment from her husband but had 'tried to keep her secret to herself.'[6]

In both murder trials the doctor's testimony supported the verdict of guilty, but despite the jury's opinion and much to the disgust of the local papers, the husbands were convicted of the lesser crime of manslaughter and given light sentences. Langstaff was called to give medical care to both men, one in prison and the other after he tried unsuccessfully to commit suicide by slitting his throat. The doctor's notes suggest that he may have felt himself to be in a dilemma: attendance on wife-beaters was distasteful, but in all his years of practice he never refused a request for care. Perhaps taking advantage of the situation, or more to register his annoyance, he charged the exceptionally high fee of four pounds, ten shillings (eighteen dollars) for medical attendance on Heatherington in the penitentiary.[7] Experience with violent deaths reinforced the doctor's temperance sympathies: alcohol was a factor in both murders and in at least three other accidental deaths.

Serving as a witness and performing autopsies at the coroner's request could be lucrative, since the York County treasurer was supposed to pay between four and fourteen dollars for each case, depending on the time involved and the distance travelled. In recording these accounts Langstaff jokingly inscribed his debtor as 'Queen, The' or 'Our Sovereign Lady etc.' Reimbursement could take two years or more; the delays increased in the late 1860s and early 1870s, to become a matter for discussion in both Quebec and Ontario medical journals.[8] In 1876 Langstaff was paid for two autopsies: for the first, he had waited thirty months; for the second, twelve years.[9] The situation eventually improved and he was usually paid within two months.

More important, perhaps, from the perspective of changing medical practice was the ever-present threat of prosecution for malpractice. Unfortunately, there are few histories of medical malpractice in North America, but not for any lack of material: much can be found in newspapers as opposed to medical journals.[10] Malpractice trials are thought to have been 'rare' in Ontario until after 1890, but the possibility of malpractice lay behind several inquests into accidental deaths and abortions held in Toronto, including the case of Sabra Wright (see chapter 8).[11] When new drugs were introduced, doctors and pharmacists were said to confuse them with poison or be ignorant of the correct dose. The Toronto inquests of 1855 involving Langstaff's associates Aikins, Rolph, Philbrick, and a medical student, made this painfully obvious: the doctors were accused of having killed their patients with inappropriate doses of morphine.[12] Langstaff may have been present at these widely publicized inquests: he owned a pamphlet describing them and his friend Abraham Law had served in one as a juror.

In 1871 a chilling death brought this type of problem even closer to Richmond Hill, when a man was accidentally poisoned with the strychnine he had kept for killing rats by confusing it with morphine powders Dr Hostetter had given him for back pain. Langstaff and Hostetter performed the autopsy together; for once the rivals seem to have agreed completely.[13] In 1879 Langstaff's colleagues determined that a Markham man had died of an 'accidental' overdose of the morphine and chloral hydrate he had been given by Dr Pingle for 'dyspepsia.'[14] Five years later Dr F.R. Armstrong published a warning about a pharmacist who had mistaken aconite for brandy; ironically, this was just eight weeks before Armstrong's own demise related to drugs and alcohol (see chapter 2).[15]

Other contacts with lawyers came with the doctor's duties as executor of relatives' wills and in efforts to collect debts. It appears that estate affairs could be difficult to arrange. When Langstaff assumed the care of his dead sister's children, Susannah and Henry Burkitt, he made five trips to Toronto before he was able to register the documents properly: once he came on the appointed date, but the papers were not ready; twice he had all the papers and witnesses with him, but the judge failed to appear.[16]

Langstaff sued for non-payment of medical bills and twice appeared as a witness for other doctors against recalcitrant patients or their estates.[17] Similarly, he served as a witness for two insurance companies against clients who had been patients of other doctors.[18] Contingency fees were not legal, but the daybooks show that bonuses were part of informal practice: Langstaff wrote that he would give his lawyer '$3 for pleading my case; if in my favour, $2 more.'[19] Under duress, patients would settle out of court by paying an amount they deemed appropriate, usually much less than the doctor had charged. Langstaff seems to have turned the same practice on members of the legal profession. In 1883, as a board member of the Ontario Industrial Loan and Investment Company, deadlocked for two months over how to settle a lawyer's account for $1,600, he moved that they 'pay $1,200 instead.'[20]

Twice only, the doctor was a defendant in a trial; both times, he felt he had been gravely wronged; both times, he had to face Matthew McNair, the same man whose 'foul' slaughterhouse Langstaff would later blame for his wife's death. In neither case had there been any question of his medical judgment. First he was charged with having sold a property that the witnesses, including McNair, 'made out was covered with logs and thistles'; he appears to have lost.[21] Later he was accused, again by McNair, of allowing water to flow onto the latter's property. The suit, which caused Langstaff to make seven trips to Toronto, was reduced to an argument over the boundary between two lots. Twenty-five people made statements; the doctor gave $1.50 to each witness who appeared on his behalf. He wrote that McNair had set 'the example of some pretty strong false swearing.' When the court found for the doctor, he recorded the judge's 'severe rebuke' and his words 'I never gave a verdict with greater satisfaction.'[22] The press agreed that the suit had been a frivolous waste of public funds worth many times more than the cost of the land in question.[23] 'False swearing' was intolerable to Langstaff. In another case he attended as a witness, he claimed, 'three of them made up a false oath,' and observed that it was 'hard to prove that a thing has not been seen or heard.' Six weeks later he seems to have derived some vicarious pleasure from reading that a 'court suit in Washington brought fraudulent action' and was 'thrown out.'[24]

The interface between law and medicine probably also had an effect on Langstaff's record-keeping and on his opinions about social practices. The diligent maintenance of the daybooks, to which he referred in court, the increasing indications of precisely when he told a patient to stop treatment, and the notation of disagreements with colleagues may have been a response to the perceived threat of lurking lawyers. His convictions about the need to control alcohol and to improve roads, his anger at the unsanitary and unscrupulous practices of McNair, and perhaps a certain sense of professional vulnerability may have helped confirm his decision to try lawmaking as a means of coping with lawbreaking.

Six months after the death of his wife Mary Ann, Langstaff was elected reeve of Richmond Hill by a margin of two votes.[25] The doctor's sympathies for the Reform party were more than apparent to his community. Reeve was not his first public office: he had thrice served as a grammar school trustee, had been a Vaughan township councillor for three consecutive years, and a village councillor for one, and, indulging his pet peeve, had put in two years as a commissioner of roads. Later he would convince the authorities to allow him to conduct experiments on road maintenance.[26]

Perhaps typifying other Ontario communities, Richmond Hill took a dim view of partisan politics in municipal affairs and was even more wary of medical men who mixed health care and politics. The *York Herald* criticized an unnamed doctor of Langstaff's political stripe who had warned a patient of the opposite persuasion that going out to vote would be bad for his health.[27] Seemingly unintimidated by public disapproval, doctors on both ends of the political spectrum were conspicuously open about their sympathies. Grand examples were set by Langstaff's teacher Dr John Rolph and by Dr Charles Tupper, a 'Father of Confederation,' who served more than a dozen years in Sir John A. Macdonald's Conservative cabinet before he became prime minister in 1896. Several of Langstaff's colleagues, including Drs Hostetter, Lynd, Reid, Strange, and Widdifield, had entered the fray, running for provincial or federal seats.[28] Some chose the Conservative party, but Rolph's former students seemed to have embraced his Reform (Liberal) politics, just as Langstaff had done. George Brown, founding editor of the Toronto *Globe* and another Father of Confederation, had given front-page coverage to a petition encouraging him to run for office, bearing the names of medical Reformers, including Drs W.T. Aikins, H.H. Wright, and Walter B. Geikie.[29]

It was an exciting time to be an Ontario Liberal. The party held provincial power in the later part of Langstaff's career, first under the leadership of Edward Blake (provincial premier from 1871 to 1872 and leader of the federal opposition from 1880 to 1887) and then under Oliver Mowat (premier from 1872 to 1896). The policies of the Mowat government, especially with respect to social and agricultural reforms and public health and welfare, reflected the concerns of James Langstaff; it is possible that the mature practitioner did not find it a coincidence that he enjoyed prosperity during Mowat's term.[30] On the federal level, Alexander Mackenzie had wrested the reins of government from Sir John A. Macdonald in 1873, but only for a single term. For a committed Liberal there was always work to do.

Political activities of all types seem to have interested the doctor. He dropped in on Tory events when Sir John A. Macdonald was the featured guest,[31] and he intently watched crises, like the 'great Finian [sic] excitement' of 1866.[32] On 1 July 1867, the day of the Confederation of Canada, he was visiting patients; however, he attended political meetings in the weeks just before and after that important day. Until 1888 the franchise belonged only to men who owned land; Langstaff's Toronto properties therefore gave him the right to cast his ballot in the city. He recorded voting in at least six West Toronto elections, always for Reformers, who did not always win.[33] He attended nomination meetings in the city and in both East and West York,[34] and he was seen at Reform conventions,[35] picnics,[36] and banquets,[37] where his presence and sparse comments were sometimes documented by the press. The doctor helped the campaign of a medical colleague running on the Reform ticket, by driving him up and down the second concession of the township and into Thornhill to canvass votes.[38] When he needed a lawyer, he engaged the former rebel and temperance advocate Charles Durand.[39]

On other occasions Langstaff went to hear Reform leaders, such as Blake, Mowat, Mackenzie, and Brown.[40] It is not certain if Langstaff was in nearby Aurora to hear Blake, famous for his 'able' and rousing delivery, give his oft-cited 1874 speech, in which he promised 'nothing in advance of popular opinion.'[41] He *was* present, however, in the July heat of 1879, when a crowd of two thousand gave the former premier a 'storm of applause' for an address that lasted two and a half hours; the tired doctor thought the speech had gone on longer.[42]

Despite their many successes, the Reformers were not always united. Langstaff and Matthew Teefy both had differences with the influential George Brown. At a nomination meeting in Weston, Brown named the doctor as one of the ringleaders of a 'bogus' delegation of suspect allegiance who had 'excluded true Reformers.' Langstaff's version was different. Believing Brown had no business in the rural meeting in the first place, and possibly chuckling over the outcome, he wrote that there had been 'two delegations from Vaughan ... Brown thrown out.'[43] Postmaster Teefy had no sympathy for old rebels, blaming his father's 1838 death on fatigue from his winter service as a volunteer 'defending Canada from invasion ... after W.L. Mackenzie was defeated,' but he seems to have supported Reform with some reservations. As an Irish Catholic, Teefy complained that he had been

'insulted' by Brown's decision not to support separate school education, a gesture that brought mollifying letters from other local Reformers.[44] Years later, party solidarity won out, and the doctor and
the postmaster both seem to have forgiven or forgotten the insults.
After Brown died a lingering death from an infected wound caused
by an assassin's bullet, Langstaff paid the considerable sum of four
dollars to buy his portrait; a picture of Brown 'dedicated to the Reformers of Canada West' can be found in the Teefy papers.[45]

As a township councillor from 1864 to 1866, the doctor was involved in the administration of public welfare, which depended on
the ad hoc generosity of municipalities;[46] he often moved that money
be given to the support of destitute persons. The same paupers were
recommended to financial aid month after month and council usually responded. In addition, Langstaff took a visible stand on the
issues that had always provoked his ire: the deplorable availability
of drink and the equally deplorable state of the York roads. He had
tried to limit alcohol by his motion for local prohibition and with his
support for raising the fee for a tavern licence. Poor road maintenance not only hampered his house calls, but also increased his
workload with the anxiety, frostbite, and accidents of the 'travelling
public.' He made certain that the township discharged its monetary
debts to hospitals and to those who had been injured on its roads
and bridges. Only once did he refuse to support a claim: the horse,
he decided, had been lost through its owner's neglect.

In 1878 Langstaff served a one-year term as councillor for the village of Richmond Hill (incorporated in 1873). In the weeks leading
up to that election, there had been complaints about the infamous
York roads and the do-nothing Conservative council that had been
acclaimed year after year.[47] Letters to the editor, signed by 'Onlooker,'
lamented the bad roads in medical terms: 'no wonder there is many
a sickness even death as the consequence.'[48] The protests, which the
doctor may or may not have penned but with which he openly sympathized, seem to have had the desired effect. A new council was
elected; Langstaff was proud to have tied for the most votes with
Abraham Law, another Reformer, who had already served as the
first reeve.[49] The village business, like that of the township, involved
deliberations on money for paupers, sidewalks, and a device to scrape
the roads.[50] The greatest achievement of this council, however, was
its impact on the local press.

Whether Richmond Hill liked it or not, its municipal affairs were deeply tainted with partisan politics; supporting and perpetuating the situation was the biased reporting of the town's only paper, the *York Herald*. The new, Reform-dominated council of 1878 came under immediate attack by the Conservative editor, who took every opportunity to disgrace the disorganized and incompetent 'Grit menagerie,' unable even to muster pay for the Patterson village marching band.[51] Two months after its election the *Herald* issued a snide report on a meeting about establishing a new paper, held by the 'Grits of the village,' including James Langstaff and Abraham Law.[52] The threat soon materialized and the first issue of the Richmond Hill *Liberal* rolled off the press that summer. The *Herald* fled to Bradford under a new banner proclaiming it 'a Conservative Journal,' but six months later it was back providing alternative coverage of all village events to the delight of its Tory constituency and present-day historians.

The *Liberal* outlived the *Herald*, but its early years were plagued with difficulties, not all due to partisan politics and none more vexing than the 'blaze' in 1883. The Toronto *Telegram* claimed that a hostile crowd had deliberately set fire to the *Liberal* office and taunted its charismatic editor, Sturgeon Stewart, by burning his effigy together with that of a certain 'grass widow,' with whom, it was said, he had been 'too intimately associated.' The indignant town council registered a formal protest to the *Telegram* at the insult of the 'false assertions' and the 'unfounded slander against the inhabitants of this village.' It is not known whether the councillors were angered by the unwelcome publicity or by its lack of veracity.[53] Over the years Langstaff gave medical attention to all the editors of both papers and their families; in his records, however, there are no clues to the mysterious cause of the *Liberal* 'blaze.'

Given the doctor's evident commitment to politics, his stature in the community, and his experience as a councillor, it seems only natural that he would run for reeve. Other events in the preceding months may have influenced the timing of his bid. He had helped fight a huge fire that had destroyed valuable properties and threatened a large portion of the town, making the acquisition of a better fire engine a top priority.[54] Three months after his wife's death he had been robbed of seventy dollars by a thief who had entered his home while he and his motherless dependants were asleep.[55] He was still deeply concerned about the management of the York roads and had been at the massive indignation meeting held in October 1879.[56] In fact, a letter about the mismanagement of the roads, bearing his signature, had been published in the *Globe*. In it he used an analogy to 'false swearing' in the law to point out that the road was getting thinner: 'any who deny this will be like the lawyer who undertook to prove the prisoner innocent – only two witnesses had seen him steal, but the lawyer could bring thirty to prove that they did not see him steal.' The same letter was reprinted in his home town, with unfortunate timing, as it appeared on the same page as his wife's obituary.[57]

Important as these issues were, I think the main reason Langstaff decided to run for reeve was his belief that Mary Ann had died of the emanations from McNair's slaughterhouse. In this period of rising agitation on sanitary reform, the town had been laconically demanding action on the public nuisances in many yards in a 'state calculated to breed fever'; the paper kept reminding its readers that 'a dollar spent on cleanliness may save a doctor's bill, and perhaps lives.'[58] Rhetoric about the apparent increase in typhoid and other diseases of 'filth' was common. Local outbreaks received press coverage; particular attention was paid to the death of John McBride, a former Richmond Hill high school headmaster, who had turned to the study of medicine and had allegedly contracted typhoid while attending patients in the Toronto hospital.[59] As a physician and a Reformer, Langstaff could do no better for the cause of public health than set out to clean up his town. It lends support to the observations of those who have found that the sanitarian movement was a positive influence on the acceptance of germ theory, and is perhaps significant in itself, that his commitment to this issue predated the discovery of the tuberculosis germ and the formation of a permanent Provincial Board of Health.[60] While there is no evidence that Langstaff refused to accept the tenets of germ theory, he appears never to have used the words 'germ' or 'bacteria' in any of his writings, as if they were related but secondary to his primary goal of public hygiene.

For a widowed country doctor, being reeve was not an easy task. Langstaff's nephew Elliott had joined him in practice, but inexorable medical duties caused the reeve to miss nine of the twenty-two meetings held during his year-long term. Sometimes the council met without him, but two meetings had to be rescheduled for lack of a quorum; Teefy's thinly veiled annoyance can be read between the lines of his minutes. A decision was taken on the new fire engine and Langstaff watched the county council endorse a plan to build a House of Refuge for indigents, a house of industry that promised to offer comfort for an amount less than the combined municipalities were already spending on relief.[61] He also had the cathartic opportunity to address the entire York County council on the state of the roads. The superintendent had submitted a report claiming that the roads were in 'excellent condition,' but Langstaff spoke of the futility and expense of the system of snow removal and of scraping, which removed the high rounded surface and hampered drainage. He recommended that county councillors assist the superintendent in his assessment. Backed by an impressive petition bearing the signatures of 800 ratepayers, he said 'he did not expect these resolutions to be carried – he did not much care whether they were or not – (laughter), but the agitation of the question would make itself felt at the next election.'[62] The *Globe* reported that his long address 'was listened to with great attention.'[63]

Langstaff's tenure as reeve was marred by two incidents, one frivolous and the other deadly, and both destined to erode respect and block his hefty agenda. The former event became known as the battle of the 'Pound-keeper and the Reeve.' The doctor's young son, Rolph, had been driving two cows to pasture when one of the animals wandered into an orchard. The boy chased after the stray, while pound-keeper Richard Jordan, who had been hiding in the bushes nearby, pounced on the other hapless bovine left meandering down Yonge Street. The reeve demanded return of his cow, denying charges that it had been 'running at large'; the pound-keeper refused. The reeve sued, the pound-keeper resigned, and the case dragged on for months. Langstaff claimed that his quarrel was not with the law, but with Jordan, who had been accused of excessive diligence in the past, although he had yet to be convicted of wrongdoing.[64] The press had a heyday with the shenanigans: 'To beef or not to beef,' the *York Herald* quipped, and it accused the rival *Liberal* of trying to protect its indefensible 'patron.'[65] The court threw out the case on a technicality and charged a fine and costs to the reeve; Jordan was reinstated. Such was the nature of this small world that the pound-keeper summoned the doctor for medical care in the years that followed, and, apparently without rancour, Langstaff went.[66]

The other incident was far more sinister: smallpox. On 2 February 1880 Langstaff visited the Horner household and recognized the dreaded variola rash. He 'vaccinated the whole family,' imposed a quarantine, returned home, changed all his clothes, and went out to attend a delivery.[67] Smallpox was often fatal; those who survived could be left disfigured or blind. In Ontario the disease was endemic and exacted a constant low level of mortality, but the years 1879 and

1880 were exceptionally difficult.[68] The newspaper reported that Langstaff 'refuses to attend [the sick], but will give them all the medicines they require, if they procure a nurse from the hospital. The doctor takes this course in the interests of his other patients.'[69] The daybook entries confirm that he did not go back to the Horner house.

Prior to this outbreak Langstaff seems to have done vaccinations in an ad hoc fashion at a declining rate amounting to less than ten per cent of the birth rate in the practice. But in February 1880, vaccinations were all the rage in Richmond Hill; droves of people came forward in groups of ten or more. The disease spread from the Horner family to several others, until thirty people were afflicted and five died.[70] Panic reigned: one man was attended simply 'for fear of smallpox.'[71]

Two weeks into the epidemic Langstaff came to the disastrous realization that despite his precautions, he was harbouring the scourge in his own home: his physician nephew was 'bad with variola.'[72] Elliott, the second son of Langstaff's brother John, had only just completed his studies at the University of Toronto. Moreover, it was Langstaff who had attended the birth of Elliott and all his brothers and sisters and Langstaff who had failed to vaccinate them. The *York Herald* quoted the reeve as saying that his nephew had chickenpox not smallpox, but even if the doctor did tell this supposedly reassuring lie, no one was fooled.[73] Elliott's name figured in the published lists of victims; the pretence of isolation to prevent the spread of contagion had to be abandoned. Langstaff continued to live at home and tend other patients.

After being 'shut up over five weeks' in Langstaff's house, Elliott went home to his family for another month of convalescence; the relieved father had the recovery announced in the paper.[74] Fear subsided and vaccinations waned to resume their low background level, until five years later, when word of the 1885 Montreal epidemic reached Richmond Hill, provoking new hysteria and another flurry of vaccinations and special meetings, which Langstaff attended.[75]

The rules for such situations were far from clear. Responsibility for the 1890 fiasco did not rest with the doctor alone, nor did it belong, as the press believed, to the 'negligent community.'[76] An anonymous doctor, believing that physicians could spread the disease, had recommended that only one medical man be assigned the task of caring for all the sick.[77] Some people refused vaccination, compulsory measures were controversial, materials needed were not always available or reliable, and a system of checks and reminders was non-existent.[78] A few years later the Ontario Public Health Act of 1884 specified smallpox control by notification, isolation, quarantine, and terminal fumigation and recommended 'systematic and compulsory performance of vaccination' in the event of an epidemic; regular vaccination was to be promoted through education and persuasion.[79] The new rules may have increased the tendency of medical professionals and society to blame the victim: in 1885 an official visiting the region claimed that 'people nowadays who get smallpox thoroughly deserve it.'[80]

The little epidemic of 1880 demonstrated that even when a means of prevention was somewhat understood, the health of the public required more than a quick fix and a dedicated reeve. Langstaff was committed to organized public health, but when his frustrating year as reeve expired, he did not seek re-election; nor did he run for office again, although rumours circulated that he would.[81] He did remain a supporter of the right of the government to intervene in the interests of public health.

In the mid-1880s the public health movement became a greater preoccupation of the Ontario government. Some physicians agreed with this stance, including prominent leaders in the Canadian Medical Association; a committed few championed the cause.[82] Dr Edward Playter, a Liberal, who had practised at Richmond Hill in 1873 and whose family had been among Langstaff's patients, began to make public health his specialty. He had founded the *Sanitary Journal* in 1874 and for years had been encouraging his colleagues to see that prevention, though unfamiliar, was far better than treatment: 'medical science,' he said, 'appears to have been built up so to speak on the wrong side of disease.'[83]

Public health had been in the hands of random and capricious local boards of health, but it became a permanent provincial responsibility in 1882; standards were set and inspections arranged. Although questions have been raised a century later as to the real value of these measures,[84] Langstaff assimilated the concepts providing new justifications for his old beliefs. For example, he had seen privies as a dangerous source of morbidity (especially harmful to the urinary organs) owing to the necessary exposure to 'cold,' but he came to regard outdoor facilities as the cause of infectious fever.[85] Rather than run for office, Langstaff may have determined to exercise his influence through this new bureaucracy. In the fall of 1882 he sent a letter to the Vaughan council warning that 'the health and lives of the inhabitants of the village are endangered by the filthy state of certain premises.'[86]

The provincial board of health became increasingly active in 1883; its secretary, Dr Peter Bryce, began insisting on medical reporting of infectious disease, a systematic classification of disease, and regular reports on the state of municipalities and their incipient local boards of health. As clerk of the village Teefy received these circulars and dutifully read them at council meetings. His response to Bryce's questionnaire sent 30 May 1883 gives a vivid description of the town.

In Richmond Hill slop water was 'thrown about the yards in most cases,' and vegetable waste was 'fed to pigs and cattle.' A 'little stagnant water in a ditch' was about to be drained by order of the village council, but there were no rules governing the disposal of human excreta. 'Each householder [could] do as they please' in dealing with human waste, but privy pits were the most common; no bylaws governed their use, but none were closer than twenty-five feet to wells providing drinking water. In the previous twelve months there had been two cases each of scarlet fever and diphtheria and one of typhoid, but no cases of smallpox, measles, or whooping cough. When asked how the diseases were propagated, Teefy wisely wrote '[I] cannot say'; possibly trying to deflect blame, however, he volunteered that the children with diphtheria 'came here from Toronto' and that the case of typhoid might be related to 'filthy premises.' In response to the question of 'nuisances, such as neglected slaughterhouses,' he alluded to McNair: 'There is a certain premises [sic] in the village where caracases [sic] are boiled for the fat – occasionally.' Teefy was 'not aware of any' disease transmitted by privies, garbage disposal, or contaminated wells; as to whether or not he thought cases of disease might have been reduced by 'proper precaution,' he again replied, '[I] cannot say.'[87]

Teefy also had to acknowledge that the municipality had yet to appoint a local board of health and that children were not required to have a medical certificate in order to enter school. Perhaps lack of action on these issues may explain why he seems to have ignored another request for information sent fifteen months later, although both he and Langstaff kept reminding council of its duty. The town finally appointed a local board of health and Dr William J. Wilson its first medical officer of health in 1884.[88]

In the fall of 1883 Richmond Hill had its first visit from Dr William Oldright, chairman of the Ontario Board of Health. He came to investigate a 'complaint of certain nuisances calculated to be injurious to the health of the inhabitants.' Exactly who had complained was not revealed, but McNair's slaughterhouse was one of the problems. A special meeting of the village council was held; Teefy's minutes show 'Doctor James Langstaff' in bold 'Hancock-sized' script, listed at the head of eleven concerned villagers, including one other physician.[89] Oldright heard the grievances and followed up one month later with a letter demanding to know what had been done. Since nothing had been done, the frantic council formed a committee to examine the by-laws relating to nuisances.[90]

A year later, 'Senex' and 'Citizen,' authors of letters to the *Liberal*, complained of the stalwart inaction of the village council and were explicit in their criticism of the 'blood-boiling' and 'bone-boiling' stench of McNair's premises, offensive to the 'olfactory organs' and the 'orbits of vision.'[91] Once again the anatomical references suggest a medical author. Seven years after Mary Ann's death and despite repeated inspections and warnings, the intransigent slaughterhouse still caused distress.[92]

During this time Langstaff continued to wage epistolary warfare on the York roads. The reactions his letters provoked suggest that some citizens did not like the activist doctor. Beginning in 1879 he convinced authorities to let him and four other men experiment on the management of a five-mile section of Yonge Street, but he was annoyed when the practices he had proven to be effective were not adopted.[93] Thinly disguised as 'Observer,' he wrote four letters on the subject in the winter of 1885–6, offering detailed suggestions as to the proper management, which if implemented, he said, 'would be a great luxury to the travelling community after pounding over the rough York Roads for so many years.'[94] His recommendations were the same as they had always been: 'I would say, stone your road early in spring, – where hollowing, fill the centre, – where crowning, fill the ruts, – where gravel can be got, use a little to bind the surface, – and do away with all hoeing, raking, and picking, and tinkering.'[95] He cited his successful experiments of 1881 and 1882 that had demonstrated the virtue of this frugal method: 'There has been great improvement in the York Roads ever since 1880, when I was in the County Council and made the superintendent fill the ruts in the spring ... Before then there used to be indignation meetings on account of the bad state of Yonge Street. Perhaps the superintendent [does not] remember them.' He criticized the managers for having bungled an experiment in 1884 by filling the ruts with mud instead of stone.

Rebuttals were published: first from the superintendent, then from Reeve Pugsley. Langstaff drafted a lengthy and irate reply to the superintendent, which he did not send, and composed a more sanguine letter, which was published: 'Now, if I assert one thing and he the opposite, his friends will believe him and my friends will believe me, but this will not be any benefit to the travelling community.'[96] Reeve Pugsley, exasperated with the onslaught, referred to 'Observer' by his real name for the few villagers who had not guessed his identity and sarcastically pointed out what he considered to be grave inconsistencies in the doctor's critique. Blaming the failed 1884 experiment on Langstaff's own inadequate surveillance, he adopted a high moral tone, saying 'he is not a person of so much superior intelligence to any one else, that he can afford to speak with so much assurance, or to treat the opinions of others with so much pomposity and discourtesy.'[97] How many others sympathized with Pugsley's assessment of the doctor's behaviour is unknown; the letters stopped.

The doctor's compositional skills may have been given to public and partisan ends, but his most famous service to the Reform party was as a physician. It came during a low point in his career, during his widowhood some eighteen months after his humiliating term as reeve. In June 1882 the Honourable Alexander Mackenzie, campaigning for a federal seat, came to Richmond Hill for a Reform meeting, but the Conservative candidate, N.C. Wallace, put in a surprise appearance that turned the Liberal get-together into a public debate. The Tory, who was a more effective speaker, tried to dominate the meeting, but Mackenzie managed to hold forth in a quiet and dignified manner; later that night he collapsed.[98] Langstaff, who as usual had been present at the Reform rally, rushed to tend the stricken candidate.

Illness was all too familiar to Mackenzie. Two years previously his fragile health had caused him to resign as Liberal leader in favour of Blake; his speaking voice had been permanently weakened.[99] For this new attack of 'inflammation of the bowels,' a prominent doctor in Toronto was summoned, but when the city man heard that the former prime minister was in the care of an ardent Reformer and that the 'politically correct' doctor was Langstaff, he said no other physician could do better.[100] Mackenzie stayed at the home of Benjamin McDonald in Markham, 'a white house prettily situated on a green knoll ... immediately opposite ... a substantial white brick Tunker church.' The Toronto papers gave hour-by-hour reports on his condition. Hoping to claim the seat by default, the Tories circulated a 'foundationless' rumour that the former prime minister had died.[101]

Langstaff sprang into action. Daily, sometimes several times a day, he telegraphed Toronto with confident news of Mackenzie's progress and supplied details testifying to the honourable gentleman's continued strength and wit. The *Globe* quoted the doctor's politically barbed medical report: 'There are certain indications that the inflammation is gone. There is an abundant perspiration all over the body. The pulse is 83 and falling. The tongue has now a healthy appearance. The tongue was, however, at the commencement of his illness remarkable. Mr Mackenzie says the Tories have made the same remark with reference to that member.'[102] Langstaff added that he expected a speedy recovery, the patient's 'temperate habits availing him well.'

Langstaff's prognostications made front-page headlines for days.[103] Mackenzie lay ill for three weeks, during which time Langstaff made twenty-one visits, staying up to six hours at his patient's side. He did not neglect the rest of his practice, and tended between four and eighteen other people each day.[104] There is no evidence in the daybooks that Mackenzie was mute or had suffered a left-sided stroke; Langstaff spoke only of weakness, abdominal pain, and drowsiness from the prescribed opium. That is not to refute the claim of Mackenzie's biographer, that he had had a stroke: possibly Langstaff dared not write that dreadful diagnosis in a place where it might be read by political enemies.[105]

The election took place on 20 June, while Mackenzie was abed, but he won his seat with a majority of two hundred. The statesman's health was never completely restored. Nearly three months later he wrote to his daughter that 'some remnant of the disease [is still] clinging to me ... but when I take rest enough I can get over it.'[106] Friends gave a generous sum of money to send him to a European spa. For a long time the Richmond Hill papers took a special interest in Mackenzie,[107] but the political barb was never too far away. When the politician considered a rest cure at Banff Springs, the Conservative *Herald* made a wicked allusion to his physical condition, saying, 'it is whispered around here that the Honorable Alexander Mackenzie is going to resign.'[108] Nevertheless, Mackenzie, who never lost an election, ran at least one other campaign (his last) from his sickbed and served in the Commons until his death.[109] He outlived the doctor by three years.

On the day of Mackenzie's rally, several of Richmond Hill's most prominent women had been seated on the platform, among them the high school teacher Eleanor Frances Louisa Palmer. In 1882 the municipal franchise was extended to widows and spinsters in Ontario, but Canadian women could not vote in federal elections and married women could not vote at all, although their political views were thought to influence those of their husbands. Some women who, like Louisa Palmer, wanted the right to vote in all elections became involved in public affairs; because women traditionally supported temperance, allies were found for women's suffrage among men who viewed alcohol as a public enemy. It was not unusual, then, that a few influential ladies graced the Richmond Hill stage on that June day in 1882.[110]

Louisa was the most educated woman in the village, but she came from a humble home – the oldest child of eight in the family of her Ontario-born parents, Jeremiah W. Palmer and his wife, Mary Ann, Presbyterians of Scottish and English descent. They lived in a modest house, on a quarter-acre plot with an orchard and a garden, in the little village of Brooklin, Whitby township, about thirty miles from Richmond Hill. Jeremiah had started out as a shoemaker, but he turned to teaching, perhaps because there was too much competition from the two shoemakers next door. Teaching was not lucrative; by the time Louisa had finished school her father had become the Whitby bailiff. Most of the Palmer children went on to professional studies: the first three, all girls, became schoolteachers, two of the four sons studied law, and one studied medicine.[111]

Louisa had matriculated in the University of Toronto. At that time, with very rare exceptions matriculation was the highest academic goal open to Canadian women.[112] She had achieved honours in mathematics as well as in languages and literature. In 1878, after a period as preceptress at the Ontario Ladies' College in Whitby, Louisa was offered the position of assistant teacher at the Richmond Hill high school, with the respectable salary of $500 per year.[113] The only other academic position in the school was that of the headmaster, whose salary was raised to $1,000 per year in 1878.[114] First Thomas Carscadden and then William McBride occupied the headmaster's position while Louisa worked there. Together these teachers put the village high school on the pedagogic map: by 1880 it was ranked fourth in the province, its students won awards, and popular opinion gave credit to the principal and Miss Palmer.[115] After three years of glorious achievement and just a few weeks after Mackenzie had been saved for Reform and country, Louisa resigned her hard-earned job to marry Dr Langstaff.[116]

Palmer tradition holds that she refused the doctor's first proposal, because she felt obliged to contribute to her brothers' professional studies. Langstaff offered to pay for their education if she would change her mind, and he kept his promise.[117] On 28 September 1882 Langstaff wrote, 'in Whitby married about 5 pm.' He had seen few patients in the preceding week, but had managed to attend a delivery the night before the ceremony. In addition to the wedding preparations, a reason for his apparent inactivity may have been the final illness and death of his long-time colleague Dr John N. Reid. Langstaff was a pallbearer at the funeral five days before his marriage. The wedding took place at the Palmer home; the Presbyterian minister Robert Rogers, of Collingwood, officiated.[118]

According to the paper the couple took a tour of the 'northern lakes,' but Langstaff was back at work six days later. On the evening of their return the newlyweds were serenaded by the town band. 'The doctor being a very bashful man, as everybody knows, did not put in an appearance, but did the honourable thing by sending out a bran [sic] new five dollar bill, which was thankfully accepted by the band.'[119] That night a comet hung in the sky. Perhaps the townsfolk viewed it as a good omen, because it was 'not a little two-for-a-penny comet, but a grand and magnificent looking fellow with a tail many millions of miles long.'[120]

The groom was twenty-six years older than his bride, but at thirty-one she may have been judged lucky to have found a man. How long the new couple had known each other and how they met are not known. Perhaps Langstaff had noticed the teacher when he attended illness in the house where she had been a boarder.[121] It is also possible that they had met before Louisa came to Richmond Hill, since he had made medical visits to her village and to Whitby, where he attended the wife of the Reverend J. Eakins, who 'with a child in her arms [had been] knocked down by passing waggons';[122] summoned urgently to a place far beyond his usual sphere, Langstaff had taken along his wife, who nursed the dying woman.[123] Either because of the much publicized Eakins case or because she too had been active in the church, it is probable that the teacher had also known Mary Ann Langstaff, whose death came eight months after her appointment to the high school; it is certain that Louisa knew the Langstaff children, some of whom she taught.

As the new couple shared concerns about education, religion, and drink, they may have met at temperance gatherings or through the many Presbyterian 'socials' held to collect money for a new church. Langstaff was a member of the building society and had given generously to the project. Fund-raising garden parties, with 'raspberries and ice cream in abundance,' had been held at the widowed doctor's home, his lawn being 'very good [for] an entertainment of this kind.'[124] His marriage to Louisa Palmer and the encouragement he gave to his daughters imply that, unlike some of his colleagues, he approved of higher education for females; indeed, since there was no secret about Louisa's opinion on votes for women, the temperance-minded doctor may have supported this issue too. Canadian women physicians have long been recognized for their activism on the question of women's suffrage, but the attitudes of their male colleagues have yet to be studied thoroughly; indeed, biological arguments against the enfranchisement of women seem to have been abandoned long before.[125]

However much Louisa Palmer and James Langstaff might have agreed politically and philosophically, there is some evidence that the early years of their union were not easy. Was this owing to waning of support on the part of the doctor for his wife's political involvement, or was it simply because of the children's apparently negative reaction to their new stepmother? Langstaff's daughter Lily had entered high school at eleven years of age and was near the top of her class, having completed her fourth promotion (grades 7 and 8) in less than six months.[126] She was headed for a teaching career too; her brilliance and enthusiasm would not have escaped the notice of Louisa, who instructed her for two and a half years. The younger two, Rolph and Nelly, were fond of sport, especially riding and skating, and winter masquerades.[127] At the time of the wedding they were both still in public school, where, perhaps because of serious problems with staffing and crowding, Rolph had been having difficulties.[128] Just before his father married Louisa, Rolph had failed his high school entrance examination, a document Louisa had probably been responsible for grading.[129] The adolescent's opinion of his father's choice may have been unenthusiastic and, after three years of relative independence, his sisters may have sympathized. According to one source, Lily and Nelly temporarily left home to stay with relatives after the marriage.[130]

One year after Louisa entered their home, Rolph was rejected from the high school entrance examinations a second time and his younger sister, Nelly, moved ahead of him; a few weeks later, however, the boy was given special consideration by the inspector because of the unreasonable troubles in the public school.[131] Their stepmother may have used her influence or her skills to help them: Nelly soared from the middle of her class to first place and Rolph's grades improved.

Louisa would have had less contact with Langstaff's eldest, his twenty-one-year-old adopted son, Ernest, who had always attracted considerable attention as an erudite young man about town. It is clear that Langstaff wanted Ernest to become a doctor and take over the practice: he had sent him off to a private collegiate in Guelph,[132] then to Upper Canada College, and on to medical school.[133] Ernest helped in the office and had been present at several of his father's big operations. In the 1881 census twenty-year-old Ernest was called a 'doctor'; the following year Langstaff named him as a partner in his practice announcement. The lad seems to have been bored with the whole idea: doodling in the account books in a transparently veiled code (English minus the vowels), he wrote: 'Smthng t d. gttng trd f dng nthng'[134] Ernest was far more interested in the accounts than in the patients; he collected rents as well as medical bills. He scorned his father's ability to handle money matters: when Langstaff indicated that Mrs Wood had settled her debt, Ernest wrote beside the entry, 'What Mrs Wood'; when the father noted he had done a small business task, the son jotted, 'Did you?'[135]

Perhaps disappointing his father, Ernest eventually stopped the pursuit of medicine and, like Louisa, began teaching, first in Guelph, then in both Richmond Hill schools.[136] He was seen and heard singing at parties, founded a cricket club, and was given to small pranks; his travels to Chicago and to 'the land of the Shamrock so green' occasioned comment in the press.[137] After a time at the University of Toronto, where he majored in natural science, Ernest found his niche as a broker and money-lender. As befit his new status, he became secretary-treasurer to the local Masonic Lodge.[138] Perhaps out of a feeling of guilt he continued to help his father with the medical accounts.

Ernest participated in debates of the Richmond Hill Literary Society, where topical issues were discussed with passion: when it was resolved that 'Married life is more conducive to happiness than single life,' he argued for the negative.[139] Conceived as entertainment, the debates serve as a barometer of the attitudes Louisa or any other ambitious young woman encountered in a late nineteenth-century Ontario town. Scientific and professional subjects were popular. Thus, the Literary Society approved the arguments that 'Vegetarianism is more conducive to health';[140] that 'Doctors are more useful to society than lawyers';[141] and that 'The six days of Creation are geological periods and not literal days of twenty-four hours.' Two Protestant ministers argued for the affirmative in the last-mentioned debate and were declared victorious by the high school headmaster. Debates involving politics were more heated.[142] Dr Armstrong argued successfully for the negative when considering 'Is Politics of more value than science?'[143] In 1878 the Society endorsed the idea that 'Universal [full manhood] suffrage would be preferable to the Dominion of Canada,'[144] but the following week it rejected the resolution that 'Women should be allowed the franchise.'[145] Things were changing, however, and five years later, only six months after Louisa's marriage, a similar topic was chosen: 'It is for the benefit of society that women should have an equal chance with men in the pursuits of life.' The Reverend Mr Campbell, who was the judge, thought that the negative side had won, but he left the deciding to the audience, who chose the affirmative.[146]

If Louisa found it difficult to give up her teaching, she may have derived some consoling pleasure in watching the antics created by her departure. The parsimonious school board refused to raise her old salary and failed to pay the last quarter of the amount owing her until three months after her resignation; even then, it was given not to her but to her new husband.[147] Some members of the school board were not content to offer the job to a woman, but male candidates with dependants found the salary too low. Caught between misogyny and 'miser-y,' they faced their dilemma: hire a woman as assistant teacher or raise the pay; the better-paid job of principal was open only to men. No fewer than nine different replacements came and went over the following year. The problems persisted; five years later a vexed member of the school board complained that a teacher 'could not be found for less than $600 unless it might be a female.'[148]

Almost as soon as Langstaff married Louisa, changes began to take place in his work and in his home. The number of visits he made fell dramatically from an average of ten a day in 1882 to six in the following year. In fairly rapid succession Louisa had four babies, James Miles, Jr, Clara, Milton, and Homer. Langstaff always attended her deliveries; although he did not use forceps, he gave her chloroform three times and ergot twice. To cope with the growing family, Louisa planned major renovations to the house her husband had built thirty-five years before. Eight open hearths were replaced by seven stoves to reduce the threat of fire, and attention was given to decoration. The 'exceptionally fine and tasty job' was considered 'very ornamental and convenient' and featured 'large corniches' in five rooms, 'fancy caps and trusses,' and a 'hall arch ... with a panelled ceiling and enriched with Maple Leaves.'[149]

The renovations may have taxed the new marriage. Family tradition holds that the whistling of the man who carved the elegant bannister nearly drove the doctor to distraction. The younger children sometimes got in the way, even in the office, and the otherwise immaculate medical daybooks were scribbled on and ripped. Clearly irritated by the intrusion, Langstaff wrote on a blemished page: 'Milton tore this.'[150] Louisa acquired fine china, including a set of demi-tasse cups. To tease his upwardly mobile wife, Langstaff tied a long string to one of the tiny cups so that it could be retrieved should he accidentally swallow it. When he once turned to young Rolph and asked, 'What am I going to do with her?' the hopeful lad suggested, 'Shoot her.'[151]

More evidence of domestic stress can be found in difficulties with hired help. A servant was an essential part of any middle-class household; during the twenty years from 1860 to 1880 there had been nine different women, who stayed usually for a year or two each. The family had enjoyed the comfort and support of their servant, Maggie Wood, who lived in the house over the entire period of Langstaff's widowhood. The reader wonders if it had been awkward for the bereaved doctor to effect the purchases of dresses and shoes for his daughters, items which made an exceptional appearance in his account book after the death of Mary Ann.[152] Maggie Wood may have

helped with the buying and sewing of clothes and likely prepared all
the meals. Six weeks after the Palmer-Langstaff wedding, she left.
There followed a steady stream of servants, none of whom stayed
long: eleven different girls in the next seven years. Perhaps the increased turnover was a feature of the changing economy, since women
could find better-paying and more interesting work elsewhere. Perhaps it was a feature of the new order: Mrs Dr Langstaff may have
been hard to please or hard to take.

Louisa's improvement schemes extended well beyond the walls of
her home. She wrote letters on public health complaints and joined
her husband in his assault on McNair's slaughterhouse.[153] She set out
to cultivate the town with charitable parties and concerts; the building plans of the Presbyterian church became a priority. For a 'social'
held on the famous lawn, together with the inevitable raspberries
and ice cream, she arranged to have the garden 'illuminated with
Chinese lanterns' that blended 'harmoniously with the dark foliage.'
The 'Presbyterian ladies, who know so well how to supply,' collected
thirty dollars.[154] Unlike the grand plan of Edward Blake, Louisa's
agenda may have moved a little ahead of popular opinion in her
community: after one of her concerts the York Herald felt constrained
to chasten 'the behaviour of some persons' who, while listening to
the classical music, had managed to knock down two lamps from the
church chandelier. Fortunately, the paper added, there was no fire.[155]

Louisa's greatest energies were given to temperance; in this she
virtually took over from her husband. She was unanimously chosen
to preside at the founding meeting of the Richmond Hill chapter of
the Women's Christian Temperance Union (WCTU) one year after it
became a national organization.[156] The WCTU was dedicated to prohibition, but it was also shaped by antagonism to certain aspects of
'masculine culture that seemed to threaten female piety and religios-
ity';[157] the most controversial of its tenets was the endorsement of
women's suffrage, which had been brewing for several years before
it was formalized in 1891. It has been observed that, within the WCTU,
women were able to use what have been portrayed as 'restrictive
concepts' to extend their power.[158]

Louisa Langstaff served the local WCTU as its first vice-president.[159]
No doubt she endorsed the plea for temperance education in the
schools,[160] but it is not known what stance she adopted when the
movement began asking doctors to stop prescribing liquor as medi-

cine. Given the liberal use of alcohol in the therapeutic practice of her generally sympathetic husband, it was bound to be awkward one way or the other. When the WCTU held its annual convention in Napanee, chaired by its well-known national president, Letitia Youmans, Louisa composed a report for the 'indebted' *York Herald*. She described the sessions in detail, beginning with devotional exercises and progressing through local briefs to demands for action from various bureaucrats. The minister of marine and fisheries, who for some inexplicable reason had been sent instead of the minister of education, gave a complimentary address to the 'immense crowd'; however, he 'implied that the country was not yet ready for prohibition.' Louisa reported that Mrs Youmans 'followed and in a few earnest, forcible words ... dispelled the idea of the country not being ready for prohibition. She censured the government for dilly-dallying with the Scott Act. She wished that the Boys of Canada could be as well protected as the fish.'[161]

The village acknowledged the interest of the doctor's wife in the temperance movement; moreover, her pedagogical background placed her in a leadership role. She was asked to judge entries submitted for an essay contest on the 'Evils of Intemperance.' Louisa chose the composition of thirteen-year-old Helena Wiley, no doubt a relative of Richmond Hill's own Mrs G. Wiley, public school teacher and officer of the WCTU national executive. The precocious Miss Wiley had pretty well covered the territory with her many arguments: the dangerous effects of alcohol on the family; the medical effects on the body and mind; the 'financial facts'; legal statistics; and biblical quotations. She received ten dollars in gold.[162] Louisa's concern for children and temperance led her to invite the sixty members of the 'Band of Hope' to a party on the much trampled but still 'beautiful lawn.' The children sang their 'favourite' song, 'Boys and Girls of Temperance Are We,' before a question-and-answer session on the properties of alcohol, followed by a tug-of-war and other games. 'The evening was very pleasantly spent by all,' the *Liberal* said, 'and the little party broke up by singing the National Anthem and giving *three* cheers for Mrs Langstaff and *one* for the Queen.'[163]

These activities may have benefited the temperance movement and the church, but it seems the doctor soon developed cash flow problems, which became another source of marital strife. Not all can be attributed to Louisa's activities: he may well have discovered that he had an incurable illness as early as 1885, and some monetary difficulties were related to grim legal situations affecting three nephews. Alva Langstaff, son of the deceased Lewis, lost an arbitration.[164] Edwin Langstaff, youngest son of John, Jr, now farming the old homestead, was hauled up on kidnapping charges for having pursued and captured a young orphan runaway who had been his hired hand.[165] Worst of all, Langstaff's ward, Henry Burkitt, became estranged from his wife and two-year-old son for an undisclosed transgression that landed him in the Don Jail. Langstaff made at least twelve trips to Toronto to consult with Burkitt's lawyers, arrange bail, 'hunt up' witnesses, and generally mediate in the problem until a five-dollars-a-month settlement was reached with his wife.[166] Henry moved back into Langstaff's home. The doctor was not poor, but cash was needed and he held a giant auction and 'Credit Sale' to liquidate livestock and implements at the end of February 1885; sales of real estate followed.[167]

The only direct evidence that the new marriage may have been less than perfect was the relatively ungenerous distribution of properties in Langstaff's will written on 12 February 1885, two weeks before the credit sale and around the time of Louisa's second confinement. Witnessed by his nephews Garibaldi Langstaff and Henry Burkitt, this document provided Ernest with the handsome sum of $10,000 for three more years at college, while the Toronto properties were to be divided unequally between Louisa and his two daughters by Mary Ann. The entire value of property destined for Louisa (and all her children) was equal to that bequeathed to the oldest daughter alone. Rolph would inherit the practice, the family home, the farms, and everything else, except lots in Wallaceburg and Chatham left to Langstaff's brother Miles and his nephew James.[168]

It seems that the marital strife, if it had ever existed, did abate. Perhaps owing to the pressures of her own growing family, Louisa's church and WCTU engagements were less visible in the later 1880s. Lily left home, having successfully completed normal school, and began teaching, first in Brampton and then in Goderich. She married Francis McConaghy, who was the son of the town shoemaker and a medical student classmate of her brother Rolph; however, she and her husband seem to have eloped or at least kept their marriage a secret, as there is no mention of the event in the daybooks or the papers.[169] This independent action may have caused Langstaff to draw closer to his second family.

Some relief from the pressures of work may have come from help provided by Louisa's young brother, Jerry, who was indebted to his brother-in-law as a patient. Langstaff had twice raced to Whitby and there spent several days caring for and 'saving' the young man, who had fallen seriously ill of rheumatic fever during his medical studies.[170] After completing his degree in 1887, Jerry joined Langstaff for his first year of practice, as the nephews Elliott and Garibaldi Langstaff had done before, and he assumed a large part of the work. Shortly after his arrival Dr and Mrs Langstaff were able to take a trip to Chicago, the mid-western states, and southwestern Ontario. Unaccustomed to leaving his patients for so long, the doctor was quoted as saying he intended to stay away 'only a short time.'[171] Jerry Palmer moved on to other work in June 1888, whereupon the ailing Langstaff was left to manage alone.

The family had continued to grow and Louisa obviously required more to sustain her family in the event of her husband's death. On 30 November 1887 Langstaff revised his will to make greater provision for his wife and her children. He must have realized he could not live as long as his father had done; just as he expected his patients to look after their affairs in illness, he seems to have been prompted by a change in his own condition: for three days around this date he saw no patients at all. Minor indispositions over his career had briefly caused him to curtail his activities accordingly, but in 1888–9 the daybooks display the effects of chronic illness. The total number of visits made in the final year amounts to half of his usual average, but the visits declined steadily over the last six months. He seems to have been more willing to stay for prolonged periods tending individual cases – probably a function of his own inability to travel.

On 22 October 1888 Langstaff wrote, 'I was sick almost all day – pain in top of head and sick at stomach,' but he went out to attend three people. The headaches came more frequently and he began to notice swelling of his hands and face, symptoms suggesting that his Bright's disease may already have produced a severe rise in his blood pressure.[172] He stayed indoors, but patients came to his house for attention. On 25 April 1889 he wrote, 'Dr Geikie came out to see me today.' Geikie may have recommended total rest, because Langstaff saw no patients for the rest of April or the entire month of May, during which he experienced the ominous symptoms of 'chills and numbness for two hours.'[173] When he went back to work in June, his handwriting was shaky. One of the last cases he attended was the birth of a baby girl, an unaided face presentation, two months premature. The next day both mother and child were 'doing well.'[174]

Rolph was now in his third year of medical school; when classes closed for the summer, he began to see patients on his father's behalf. The community was aware of the doctor's illness and, flattering his long-standing interest in husbandry, invited him to serve as a judge of poultry at the Markham fair.[175] The account books reveal an unprecedented medical income as patients came to settle old debts. Langstaff saw his last patient on 9 July. A month later, at 7:15 a.m. on 5 August, while sitting in the kitchen with three-year-old Milton on his knee, the doctor suddenly collapsed and died. This and the impression of a big black beard and striking blue eyes were the only memories the child retained of his father.[176]

Langstaff was laid in his casket with a great floral pillow bearing the words 'Our Father.' He was said to look 'peaceful ... like a man who had done his duty and died.' The *Liberal* performed its 'painful' task and said: 'though he was ill for several weeks few thought his busy life would terminate so suddenly.' The funeral was conducted by ministers of three Protestant denominations, with a sermon based on the text 'Ye are God's building' (Corinthians 3:10) and the hymn, 'Work for the Night Is Coming.' The pallbearers were physicians, some of them Rolphian Liberals whom Langstaff had known since his youth: Aikins, Bethune, Hillary, Orr, Rutherford, and Wright. The doctor was eulogized in prose, scripture, and verse; the family was consoled by a massive gathering of neighbours, who filled the church to overflowing and assembled on the surrounding lawn. In spite of the unpopularity of the doctor's political attitudes, the perceived value of his other contributions seems to have grown. 'For forty years,' the Tory *Herald* stated, 'he has gone in and out amongst the people of this village ... and his presence will be missed at the bedside of very many sick ones who had every confidence in his ability to aid and help them in their troubles.' Aiming its remarks at the 153 families in debt to the estate, the *Liberal* reported that the 'large congregation comprehended [the minister's] full meaning when he said [Langstaff] was a physician for the poor as well as for the rich.'[177] The doctor was buried in the Presbyterian cemetery, in the grove chosen by his uncle, Squire Miles, near the new church he had helped to construct.

Rolph Langstaff still had two years of study before he would qualify as a physician; therefore, his cousin Dr Garibaldi Langstaff returned to the Richmond Hill practice in which he had first exercised his skills five years before. Rolph, and Langstaff's long-time friend and former brother-in-law Simon Miller, were named executors of the doctor's estate. They set about arranging probate and collecting the $2,500 owed by the 153 families in outstanding accounts.

Legal matters were brought to a standstill when Louisa entered a caveat against the grant of probate, because the will of 1887 had been lost and the executors were using the less generous will of 1885.[178] Since she could not produce the latest will, she was obliged to withdraw the caveat; accordingly, probate was granted to settle the estate according to the provisions of the 1885 will. The collectors had a difficult task, as some patients claimed they had already paid and produced receipts. Others 'claimed they had not consulted the doctor' or 'could not be found' or had 'gone to Manitoba' or 'had died'; their debts were pronounced 'no good.'[179] These duties kept the executors busy for the rest of the summer and into the fall.

The following year Louisa tried to ameliorate her circumstances through the courts; she may have had some success, since the sawmill was sold shortly after.[180] The census of 1891 lists Rolph, Nelly, their cousin Garibaldi, and a servant as occupying the large ten-room family home, while Louisa, her four children, and Henry Burkitt moved into a smaller, one-storey, seven-room dwelling in Richmond Hill.[181] Finally, sometime in 1892, nearly three years after Langstaff's death, Louisa found the 1887 will and sued. She was joined by Ernest and his new family. Rolph argued that his father's widow 'was bound by the former judgement,' that the second will had been 'procured by undue influence,'[182] and that when Langstaff 'executed it, he was not of testamentary capacity.' The court decided in Louisa's favour and assessed costs against Rolph for having 'alleged undue influence.' This success inspired Henry Burkitt to enter his own action against the estate as an excluded trustee.[183] Court battles and legal wrangling between Louisa and Rolph dragged on for years.[184]

The terms of the second will meant that Rolph was obliged to sell the family home in order to provide capital to consolidate Louisa's position. The distress of the situation was alleviated by David Boyle, long-time neighbour and friend, who bought the house for $2,770 in December 1892 and sold it back to Rolph for the same price three years later. Louisa moved to Toronto, where she lived until her death in 1934. Her son, James Miles, Jr, graduated in law with high honours from the University of Toronto, but was killed in action at Vimy in 1917; his 'War Sonnet' and other poems were published after his death.[185] Louisa's beautiful and musically gifted daughter, Clara, also died tragically, of consumption in her early twenties. Louisa's seven grandchildren were the progeny of Milton and Homer, who became successful businessmen and died at ages eighty-seven and sixty-nine respectively.

Of Mary Ann's children, Nelly became a nurse and like her brother Ernest moved to the United States. He cannot be traced, but she died unmarried in California at age seventy-seven. Lily and Dr Francis McConaghy had five children. Widowed at age thirty-four, Lily returned to teaching in her home town in order to provide for her young family; she lived to be 102 years old.

When Matthew Teefy died in 1911 at the age of eighty-nine, he was Canada's oldest and longest-serving postmaster. The six Teefy children who survived infancy also enjoyed long lives. John became a clergyman and died at sixty-three, perhaps still bearing the scar of the deep wound Langstaff had treated under his chin. Baldwin, who as a child had survived both meningitis and a fall from a hayloft, lived to seventy-eight. Armand, who had suffered both scarlatina and a severe case of unexplained fever, first became a teacher and then entered law practice in Chicago. Clara, in whom Langstaff had suspected early tuberculosis and whose teeth he had removed under chloroform, married an Orillia lawyer and lived to eighty-three. Louise, who had been to Langstaff for extraction of her baby teeth, remained single for many years and at the age of forty-seven read a paper to the Ontario Historical Society about the history of Yonge Street, in which she spoke of rebels and the murder of Captain Kinnear, but did not mention her father or her doctor. Five years later she married and went to live in Alberta, until her death at age seventy-four. Teefy's youngest, Mary Alice, the child whose febrile misery had so baffled Langstaff on 3 October 1864, died unmarried in 1949 at the age of eighty-seven.[186]

Langstaff's practice did not die with him; it continued in the same house without a break for the next fifty years, and possibly Teefys still figured among the clientele. Rolph took over from his cousin Garibaldi in 1891, having completed his degree and a year of special training in Edinburgh. He married medical student Lillian Carroll in

1903, two years before she became one of the University of Toronto's earliest women medical graduates. Like his father, Rolph was interested in public health and education. From 1894 to 1911 he ran a private hospital in his house, where he performed Richmond Hill's first operation for appendicitis. He was a charter member of the Toronto Academy of Medicine and often, after a long day's work, cycled the fifteen miles into the city and back to attend the meetings. Rolph served on the school board and as medical officer of health, playing a role in the further sanitation and pasteurization of milk in his community. As a young man he brought the first bicycle and the first automobile to the village; in his one hundredth year he watched the television images of men walking on the moon. Besides running her own busy practice, his wife Lillian was a founder of the Horticultural Society.[187] Together they raised two children and tended the population of Richmond Hill, until their retirement in the late 1930s. The practice passed to their son, James Rolph Langstaff, who witnessed the antibiotic revolution and brought these miracle drugs to the descendants of his grandfather's patients. He retired in 1975 but still resides in the house built by his grandfather in 1849. A wing of the new York Central Hospital was named in honour of the Langstaff family and its contribution to the community. I understand there are a number of medical daybooks extant from the later Langstaff practices ... but all that is another story.

Langstaff practised throughout a period of intense provincial activity in public health. His interest in these issues arose from personal and political convictions that predated Koch's discovery of the tubercle bacillus and the formation of a permanant provincial board of health. It is clear that his concept of public health extended beyond the realm of sanitary reform to the prevention of accidental and deliberate forms of violent injury through improved roads and control of alcohol, but his precise stance on the germ theory remains unknown. His frequent contact with legal proceedings, especially the numerous coroner's inquests into unexplained deaths, served to strengthen these long-held beliefs; while the circumstances surrounding his first wife's death and his deep personal animosity for a neighbour prompted his endorsement of the public health movement. At several times in his career Langstaff was elected to political office, and in 1880 he served as reeve of his village; however, his actions during a smallpox epidemic, his open support of one political party, and other minor incidents show that he was not a universally popular municipal leader. His marriage to the well-educated high school teacher Louisa Palmer who was a strong believer in women's suffrage, hints that, unlike other physicians, he may have sympathized with the women's cause; however, evidence of strain in their marriage invites speculation that its root may have been philosophical as much as personal. Nevertheless, the doctor and his second wife were united on the need for temperance, improved education, and sanitary reform, for which they campaigned tirelessly during the last years of his life.

Conclusion

For forty years in a century of important change, James Miles Langstaff practised in a semi-rural setting, usually alone, with few vacations, and without having attended a medical conference; nevertheless, he was far from isolated and kept abreast of innovation. The science of his early training seems to have stayed with him like an intellectual touchstone and was present in his references to anatomy and physiology in the explanation of symptoms. Examples include his observations on the incongruously deeper breathing of a person recovering from pneumonia, the relationship between function and healing in women with breast cancer, and the mechanism of action in bleeding therapy. Comments in Langstaff's daybooks about novelties range from the enthusiastic to the cautious and even the sceptical; yet, with more or less alacrity, he embraced the innovations adopted by large groups of his contemporaries. An examination of the dates and potential reasons for the innovations suggests several sources of information: encounters with medical students, consultation with other doctors, journal subscriptions, and contact with the legal profession. His numerous personal experiences with illness and death may have contributed to the growing scepticism observable in his later career, especially with respect to certain drug therapies.

The delay between an original discovery and Langstaff's implementation of the innovation in question was variable; the length of the delay seems to have been directly related to the perceived invasiveness of the technique (Table 4.5). For example, the doctor was relatively slow to adopt the dramatically invasive techniques of tracheotomy and general anaesthesia, whereas he quickly included carbolic acid in his management of wounds. The delay between a discovery and its recognition in the Canadian medical periodicals was generally longer than the time that elapsed between the Canadian début and Langstaff's own implementation, which usually took place shortly after publication in the journals he read. His acceptance of a technique was sometimes prompted by oral communication with colleagues: for example, he first used a thermometer during a consultation; on rare occasions, such as the few times he used carbolic acid to irrigate the uterus, he employed an innovation before it appears to have been reported in his literature.

When being up-to-date involved the abandoning of traditional remedies, like bloodletting, calomel, and tartar emetic, Langstaff displayed a greater resistance to change than when it involved adopting something new, but the actual frequency of these treatments in other individual practices is unknown. Restraint may simply be a feature of human nature that is increasingly pronounced with age, but the decline observed during the 1880s in his use of some techniques, especially elective operations, tends to imply that the advent of specialist surgeons may have slowed or halted surgical innovation in his practice. In his later years Langstaff seems to have turned his attention from changes in medicine to political and social reform; however, his actions even in this realm were medical in that they were inextricably linked to his vision of the need to prevent disease and injury. He was especially concerned with education, alcohol, and the state of the county roads and seems to have tolerated if not wholeheartedly endorsed the concept of women's suffrage. The doctor's willingness to support legislative intervention predated the formal adoption of the public health movement in Ontario.

Many questions remain unanswered and others have arisen. Was Langstaff typical of his colleagues in his province, his country, and his century? Did all nineteenth-century medical practitioners accept innovations? Were they equally and persistently inquisitive about the physiological basis for the symptoms they observed? If so, did they share Langstaff's means of continuing education, his hesitation about invasive procedures, and his reluctance to drop old methods in favour of the new? Is it possible that so-called external factors, such as folk attitudes or patients' gender, influenced the preservation of ancient techniques like cupping and leeching? How often did the average family doctor use the instruments Langstaff owned, such as the urinometer, the thermometer, and the microscope? To what extent did the regular physical examinations of healthy subjects, required first by insurance companies and later by employers and schools, influence the use of instruments? Did insurance company reports encourage medicalizing shifts in vocabulary exemplified by the conversion of 'natural' to 'normal'?

Langstaff studied in Canada and England. He was a life-long Liberal, participated in politics, was eager to cooperate with the public health movement, yet was relatively inactive when it came to medical politics or the so-called professionalization of his discipline. It would be interesting to know more about his teacher John Rolph, and whether all his students shared his convictions. Can any difference be detected in the public health or professional commitments of his colleagues who were American-trained or Tory-leaning? Is it possible that other country doctors, like Langstaff, did not often vote in the medical council elections? To what extent, if at all, did rural practitioners feel threatened by perceived incursions on their right to monopolize health care?

Langstaff did most of his work in patients' homes within a ten-mile radius of his own house; although he received payment on only half the debts owing him, he was prosperous and enjoyed diverse sources of income. Future studies based on the extant account records of other physicians could compare practice patterns, amounts, and sources of medical income; combined with census records, such studies would allow more attention to be given to the relative wealth of patients and their willingness to pay. Three of Langstaff's dependents were adopted and he encountered adopted children in other households, but very little is known about the frequency of adoption and the role of physicians in arranging and providing for orphaned children. Habit, geography, moral obligation, and politics were the ties that bound a patient to a certain physician in Richmond Hill, ties that could be broken by disgust or desperation; if the daybooks of two doctors from a single community were extant, it might be possible to explore further the factors determining patient allegiance.

Other community studies might elucidate whether or not the patterns of sickness and injury seen in Langstaff's Richmond Hill are representative of nineteenth-century Ontario. Respiratory and intestinal infections were common and exacted a high death-toll among infants and children; however, tuberculosis, often cited as the single most common cause of death in the period, especially among women, was relatively less apparent and seems to have afflicted men more often than women. Is this finding an artefact of patient consultation or of the doctor's personal reluctance to name the disease, or does it indicate some fundamental difference in the patterns of disease between nineteenth-century Ontario and elsewhere?

Serious injuries were common in the Richmond Hill area; much of Langstaff's surgical care was given to the treatment of wounds. Studies on the epidemiology of trauma in nineteenth-century society would serve to contextualize the accidents seen in his practice that appear to have been related to the advent of industrial machines and the hazards of travel. Langstaff seems to have been comfortable with elective surgical operations such as toothpulling, mastectomy, and the repair of club-foot or harelip, but he avoided procedures that required opening of the thorax or abdomen. Were other country doctors equally bold about external operations and equally shy about internal procedures? When did surgical specialists have an impact on their work? Did they view the loss of opportunities to operate with resentment or relief?

Langstaff was attending more than half the births in his district by the early 1870s, a surprisingly early date for physician-attended birth. Comparison with other obstetrical practices shows that his contained an extraordinarily high rate of forceps use, a high maternal mortality rate, a relatively low rate of anaesthesia, and no cases of Caesarean section. The high mortality rate may have been related to his frequent use of instruments, but it also coincided with outbreaks of similar bacterial infection in children. Furthermore, the grim statistics from this practice may result from the relative 'honesty' of a medical daybook, which provides the opportunity to follow a new mother indefinitely for weeks and months after her delivery, unlike the notebooks dedicated solely to obstetrical case histories that other practitioners kept. In other words, owing to discrepancies in the sources, maternal mortality rates for other practices may be falsely low. Although it is not entirely clear if all instances of surgical and obstetrical anaesthesia were recorded, the low use of chloroform anaesthesia in this practice in conjunction with the high rate of obstetrical intervention challenges some statements concerning the reasons for medical use of anaesthesia at delivery; moreover, the few women who did receive anaesthetic were well-off and educated, in a position to ask for and pay for the additional service. Clarification of the patterns of medical attendance at births in various geographic locations and analysis of sources of information about maternal mortality would be welcome. Similarly, a study of the incidence of Caesarean birth and embryotomy in Quebec or other Roman Catholic communities would help explore the possibility that religious and social factors influenced the choice for the mother's life over that of the child.

Further research might tell us if Langstaff's early and eager involvement with the public health movement was representative of his profession and if medical men, like medical women, supported women's suffrage. If physicians did share his dedication, were they also partisan? Would they have agreed that the definition of prevention should be extended beyond hygiene to alcohol control, road management, and possibly also the enfranchisement of women? How many other doctors became reeves, mayors, or other elected officials? Were they similarly resented by their patient-citizens or frustrated by the difficulties of social activism? Were doctors' wives given to support temperance and suffrage?

Many questions about Langstaff defy the scrutiny of a historian and her computer and will never be answered. Was the strife in the second marriage a product of Louisa's having overstepped the traditional role expected of her? Did it exist at all, or was it a myth fabricated by stepchildren who resented their father's choice? And what if anything does it have to do with the dispute over the doctor's will? Did he enter politics out of grief, medical duty, partisan rivalry, or simple egotism? Is the increasing scepticism perceived in the late practice simply a figment of my late twentieth-century imagination? Or does disillusionment with the therapeutic power of medicine really explain the apparent decline in his more vigorous forms of intervention? How much did maturity and personal experience contribute? Did Langstaff ever realize at the end of his career that some of his early remedies had come to be poisons and that his heavy use of forceps may have killed many infants and some new mothers?

On one point, however, the record is absolutely clear: Langstaff cared for all his patients, was sensitive to their pain, and tried always to help or at least to do no harm.

Appendix A
A Note on Method

The Langstaff daybooks and account books cover the forty-year period between 1849 and 1889 and are separated into two groups (see List of Manuscript Sources). Every doctor-patient encounter in four sections of the Langstaff daybooks was entered into a data-base file (using Claris Filemaker II for an Apple Macintosh Plus computer). The information on each encounter was sorted into records containing fields for date, time of day, name, age, sex, occupation, address, diagnosis, nature of problem, medication and other therapy, house call or office visit, fee, and other details. A single file was created for all visits in each of the four periods analysed: May 1849 to June 1854; January to December 1861; February 1872 to February 1875; January 1882 to December 1883. These years were selected to represent each decade and to be as close as practicably possible to the years of the Canada Census, in 1851, 1861, 1871, and 1881. The four data-base files contain records of a total of 26,638 doctor-patient encounters. Most of the quantitative statements in this study are based on analysis of these sample years.

In addition, all the daybooks and account books were read. Significant cases involving extraordinary detail, innovation, or controversy were recorded in a fifth data-base file; an attempt was also made to include all deaths, autopsies, inquests, law cases, surgical operations, and consultations in this file, but these figures should be taken as good approximations at best. Another file was constructed to accommodate all long journeys and major financial transactions. A few quantitative statements have been based on these collections.

Any study of Richmond Hill involving use of the Canada Census poses some difficulty, as its Yonge Street situation placed it on the boundary between two districts (Vaughan and Markham townships); moreover, the town lay only slightly south of another boundary defining two more districts (King and Whitchurch townships). Since the village was not incorporated until 1873, the 1881 Census was the first to contain a separate district for the muncipality. All statements involving comparisons with the Census are based on an examination of at least the two districts including or adjacent to the village, that is, the two closest Census districts in Vaughan and Markham. Since Langstaff often went further afield, statements concerning the composition of the population have also included information from the two closest districts in King and Whitchurch. District numbers for specific localities changed from year to year, and the relevant number and microfilm call numbers have been included wherever relevant.

This project did not proceed in as orderly a fashion as the preceding narrative may have implied. When I began in the fall of 1985, the last fourteen years of the daybooks were missing; as a result almost nothing was known of Louisa Palmer Langstaff or of her husband's relationship to the public health movement. To compensate for this loss, I undertook a detailed survey of the two Richmond Hill newspapers, the *York Herald* and the *Liberal*. In the fall of 1988, after three years of searching, James Rolph Langstaff found his grandfather's missing daybooks tucked away in the attic of his house, originally built by James Miles Langstaff in 1849. The nearly complete newspaper survey was subsequently redirected by significant dates indicated in the daybooks; however, the initial newspaper search remained a valuable source for this book.

The real names of patients as written in Langstaff's documents have been used thoughout this work, with the exception of names of patients sent to the Provincial Lunatic Asylum, as the archive of that institution stipulated patient anonymity prior to my examination of the material. I was more than pleased to comply with these rules, recognizing that strict confidentiality has often been included in the terms of manuscript donation or record consultation and that failure to respect the request could jeopardize access for others or dissuade potential donors from making future deposits of case records. I am aware, however, that my decision to use all other names may raise some eyebrows. Even when confidentiality has not been required, some historians have chosen not to use patient names and urge the rest of us to do the same; others have recommended suppressing names of only those patients with 'sensitive' or 'embarrassing' diagnoses; and at least one historian has fabricated names for patients, drawing inspiration from the names of colleagues. For these scholars and perhaps for their anticipated audience, the identification of patients may not have been important. For my work, however, the names were crucial to the research and were the only key to the recognition and understanding of long-term doctor-family relationships. History is difficult enough without make-believe; imposing a double standard of identification, based on late-twentieth century determinations of confidentiality and of what diagnoses might be (or would have been?) 'sensitive' to a mid-nineteenth century person, borders on hubris.

My reasons for using patient names are fourfold. First, not only were the names important parts of the data collected, they were also essential for the interpretation; to exclude them constitutes suppression of a major component of the scholarly apparatus for this work. Second, using the name together with the date provides an additional approach to the daybook source by allowing anyone interested in retracing my steps to 'triangulate' on the manuscript. Third, this form of citation will serve as a preliminary guide for people in the Richmond Hill area, some of whom have already asked me for information about their ancestors. Finally, I believe these personal tales of fear, misery, injury, and death, now all more than one hundred years old, are not shameful – whatever the diagnosis may have been; they are an intrinsic part of the social history of Ontario, which deserves to be told fully.

I am grateful to the Archives of the Royal College of Physicians and to James Rolph Langstaff, the owners of the material, for their permission and their support of this decision, which was informed by the Code of Ethics of the American Association of the History of Medicine, the College of Physicians and Surgeons of Ontario, the example of Barbara Bates, and the generous deliberations and considered opinions of Professor Emeritus Stuart Ryan and Professor Patricia Peppin, both of the Faculty of Law, Queen's University.[1]

Appendix B
Professional Associates of James Miles Langstaff

1 Partners and Medical Students in Langstaff's Practice

Dr J.V. Parker(in?) (partner)	1852
T.C. Scholfield (student)	1852–4
'Kenedy' (student)	1854
Rob Shaw (student)	1859
O'Brien (student)	1861–2
William Comisky (student)	1862–6
Francis 'Rob' Armstrong (student)	1872
William Cross (student)	1875
Ernest Langstaff (student)	1875–85
J. Elliott Langstaff (partner)	1879–81
L. Garibaldi Langstaff (partner)	1884–5
Jerry A. Palmer (partner)	1887–8
Rolph Langstaff (student)	1888–9

2 Women Attendants and 'Nurses' in Langstaff's Practice

Year	Name of Attendant	Type of Care	Patient
1852	Miss Fisher and Miss ____	Obstetrics	Woman
1855	Granny Hall	Paediatrics	Child
1855	Marsh's 'nurse girl' [a patient]	Medicine	Girl
1856	Mrs Motson	Obstetrics	Woman
1858	'The women'	Obstetrics	Woman
1858	Mrs Miller	Obstetrics	Woman
1859	Mrs Hall	Paediatrics	Child
1859	A woman	Obstetrics	Woman
1861	A woman	Obstetrics	Woman
1863	Mrs Newton	Obstetrics	Woman
1863	Mrs Lawson	Medicine	Man

1863	Mrs Doyle	Obstetrics	Woman
1863	Mrs McCague	Paediatrics	Boy
1864	Mrs Johnson	Surgery	Boy
1867	Mrs Webb	Surgery	Woman
1867	'The women'	Obstetrics	Woman
1867	Miss Williamson	Medicine	Man and boy
1869	Mrs Winslow	Paediatrics	Baby
1869	Mrs Holdridge	Medicine	Girl
1870	'R[oman] C[atholic]' woman	Obstetrics	Woman
1870	Mrs Ross	Obstetrics	Woman
1872	Mrs Doner (mother)	Obstetrics	Woman
1873	Mrs Henricks and Mrs B	Obstetrics	Woman
1874	Mrs Gormley	Medicine	Girl
1875	Miss Weldrick	Medicine	Man
1876	Mrs Craig	Surgery	Woman
1879	Mrs Devlin	Obstetrics	Woman
1881	Mrs Jordan 'the nurse'	Medicine	Woman
1883	Mrs Leggett (mother)	Medicine	Woman
1884	Mrs Chapman	Medicine	Man
1885	Mrs Young (mother)	Medicine	Girl
1887	Miss Smith 'the nurse'	Medicine	Girl
1888	One of the girls	Medicine	Man
1888	'Nurse for the baby' [wet nurse?]	Paediatrics	Baby

3 Medical Colleagues, Location, Qualifications, and Dates

Information on education and/or licensing has been found for 101 of these 148 physicians, two dentists, and one pharmacist. The sources include the records of the College of Physicians and Surgeons of Ontario (CPSO), published lists of college graduates held by the archives of the respective institutions, histories of the profession, local histories, and 'business cards' printed in the newspapers.

Of the ninety-three doctors for whom educational information is available, the majority (sixty-three) obtained their training in Ontario and four others studied at McGill University in Montreal. Several of those who began in Canada sought additional training in Britain or the United States. Thus, twenty-eight doctors had at least some British training and nine had American. The majority of those in Langstaff's sphere who studied outside of Canada did so before 1860. Some, especially those in the first decade and fellow graduates of Rolph's school, did not hold a degree. There were eight other doctors who held the Ontario licence, but the CPSO archive contains no information on their education. For the forty-nine doctors without background information, the information provided in the daybooks was insufficient to allow identification of individuals among several possible licensed candidates. Therefore, with only one exception (Dellenbaugh), all the colleagues in Langstaff's daybooks appear to have been 'regular' practitioners.

A few doctors passed the licensing examination of the old Medical Board of Upper Canada. Many who, like James Langstaff, had been in practice for some time, were registered with the General Council of Medical Education and Registration at its creation in 1865. After the Medical Act of 1869, the College held examinations for both matriculation and licensure. Thus, there may be a gap between the date of training and the date of a traceable licence.

'First Date' and 'Last Date' represent the first and last time Langstaff recorded the name in his daybooks. The last date is blank if the name appeared only once. For family teams, such as the Freels, the Hunters, the Lloyds, and the Reids, it is not always possible to determine whether the father or the son was the consultant; dates in these cases are more accurate when combined.

Abbreviations

ae – *ad eundem* (honorary degree)
TSM – Toronto School of Medicine; before 1856 'Rolph's school,' Aikins's after 1856
Toronto – University of Toronto; prior to 1889 either TSM or Trinity
Victoria – Victoria University, Medical Faculty, Toronto
Trinity – University of Trinity College, Toronto
McGill – McGill University, Montreal

Name	Location	Place and Date of Education and/or Licence	First Date	Last Date
Adams	Bradford Simcoe		1853	
Adamson	Markham Village		1875	
Adlington	Eglington [sic]		1867	
Aikins, W.T.	Toronto	TSM, Jefferson U.S. 1850	1868	1881
Alison	Caledon East		1883	
Allen, James	Bradford		1861	
Ardaugh, J.R.	Barrie	Dublin <1843	1863	
Armstrong, F.R.	Stouffville	Toronto 1873, 1874	1873	1884
Barnham			1886	
Beaton, A.	Aurora	Victoria 1864	1876	
Beatty, T.	Lambton	TSM, Victoria 1856	1867	

Name	Location	Place and Date of Education and/or Licence	First Date	Last Date
Beers, James M.			1877	
Bentley, James	Newmarket	Victoria 1856	1856	
Berryman, C.V.	Yorkville	Victoria 1857	1867	
Bethune, N.	Toronto	Edinburgh 1850, 1869	1870	1886
Black, W.S.	Markham Village	Toronto 1871, 1872	1873	1876
Bone	Vaughan		1862	
Bowman, Isaac	Thornhill	Victoria 1861	1862	1863
Brown, George	Richmond Hill	Victoria 1869	1876	1877
Bull, Edward	Weston	Victoria 1855	1854	1865
Burns, James H.	Collingwood, Toronto	Toronto TSM 1867	1874	1884
Cameron	Toronto, Richmond Hill		1864	1887
Campbell	Markham, Toronto		1864	
Clapp	Lochiel?	Toronto 1879, 1879	1884	
Clement, Lewis	Bradford	Victoria 1864, 1868	1871	1885
Closson, L.D.	Scarboro [sic], Woburn	TSM <1851, Jefferson U.S.	1867	
Coburn, W.	Markham Village	Victoria 1864	1868	
Comisky, William	Markham Village	TSM 1867	1867	1876
Corson, John W.	Thornhill	Victoria 1857 ae	1860	1861
Cotter, George		1849?	1853	1854
Coulter, Robert M.	Richmond Hill	Toronto, Victoria	1882	1885
Covey	Stayner		1873	
DeEvelyn, John	Burwick	Victoria 1858, 1869	1861	1870
Delahooke, J.A.	Weston	London 1839	1853	1863
Dellenbaugh, F.	Maple, Buffalo, N.Y.	'Old German doctor'	1869	
Doherty, John	Markham Village	TSM 1847	1859	1875
Duant			1853	
Duncomb, John	Richmond Hill	Edinburgh, Dublin 1847	1852	1868
Durie, W.S.	Thornhill	Edinburgh 1839	1853	1853
Dyre			1852	
Eckhardt, Thomas	Unionville	Toronto 1862, 1874	1873	1880
Edgar			1873	
Emory		1857	1869	1869
Evans, Dr?	Toronto		1874	1879
Farewell, G.W.	Stouffville	McGill	1874	1885
Fife, Joseph		Victoria 1865, 1866	1865	
Forrest, William	Mount Albert	Toronto 1871	1867	1886
Freel, Jr, Sylvester L.	Stouffville	TSM 1866, Victoria 1872	1867	1889
Freel, Sr, James	Markham Village	Ireland, U.S. 1837?	1867	
Fulton, John	Toronto	TSM 1855	1878	

Name	Location	Place and Date of Education and/or Licence	First Date	Last Date
Gapper (the late Dr)			1856	
Geikie, Walter B.	Aurora, Toronto	TSM, Jefferson U.S. <1851	1852	1889
Gordon, H.A.	Vaughan	Glasgow 1859, 1866	1862	
Gould	Victoria, Craigvale		1881	
Graham	Toronto		1885	1885
Grant, D.J.	Woodbridge		1883	
Gunn, R.J.	Whitby	Edinburgh 1842, 1846	1877	
Hackett, Joseph	Newmarket	1851, 1866	1853	1863
Hammil, W.E.	Aurora	Victoria 1880	1884	1884
Hillary, Robert W.	Aurora	Dublin 1866?	1857	1886
Hostetter, John	Richmond Hill	England 1860, 1866	1861	1873
Hunter, Jr, J.W.	Unionville	1876	1876	1886
Hunter, Sr, J.J.	Newmarket	Geneva, NY 1843, 1866	1851	1851
Jackes, G.W.	Unionville	Toronto 1872, 1875	1874	1875
Jameson			1849	
Justice, Charles	Unionville	England 1828, 1875	1857	1865
Kennedy, J.		TSM? 1854, 1866	1856	
Knill, E.B.	Markham Village	Toronto <1884	1884	1889
Langstaff, George A.	Springhill, Thornhill	Toronto 1877	1878	1889
Langstaff, J. Elliott	Richmond Hill	Toronto 1878	1878	1882
Langstaff, L. Garibaldi	Richmond Hill	New York?, U.S. 1884	1884	1885
Langstaff, Lewis	Springhill (King)	Victoria 1858, 1866	1859	1878
Lloyd, Jr, Rolph C.	Stouffville	TSM 1845: Victoria 1868	1867	
Lloyd, Sr, A.C.	Stouffville	Victoria 1864 ae?	1851	1871
Lynd, Adam	Bond Head	Trinity 1875	1887	
Mahaffy, John	Nobleton	1866	1853	1870
McCallum, G.A.	Mount Albert	Victoria 1866	1867	
McCausland	Markham Village		1868	
McConnell, John D.	Thornhill	Toronto 1869	1869	1882
McKinnon, A.		Victoria 1864	1864	1874
McLean, Peter	Woodbridge		1885	1887
McMaster	York Mills		1860	1871
Medill	Alliston		1885	
Mitchell	Wallaceburg		1881	
Mitchell	Unionville		1884	1887
Montgomery, J.W.	Belle Ewart	TSM 1847	1861	1867
Morrison, Thomas D.		1824	1844	
Mortimer			1860	
Morton	Bradford, Painswick (Barrie)		1864	1883
Muter	Thornhill		1864	
Nash, S.L. or John	Newmarket	Victoria 1865	1867	

Name	Location	Place and Date of Education and/or Licence	First Date	Last Date
Nelles, David	Thornhill	1879	1883	1887
Newcomb, Wm	Eglington	Victoria 1864	1867	
Nichols		1879		
Noble(s), C.T.	Sutton	Victoria 1856	1867	
Noble(s), H.	Sharon		1867	
Norman, T.J.	Schomberg	McGill 1887	1887	1889
Orr, Rowland B.	Maple	Toronto 1877	1880	1888
Paget	Thornhill	Edinburgh	1854	1855
Palmer, Jerry A.	Richmond Hill	TSM 1887	1885	1887
Parker(in?), J.V.	Richmond Hill		1852	1852
Peck, N.J. dentist			1863	1868
Philbrick, C.J.	Yorkville	Edinburgh, Dublin, London	1852	1858
Pierson		Victoria 1867	1867	
Pingel, Albert R.	Unionville	1876	1876	1888
Playter, Edward		Toronto 1860, 1866	1871	1880
Primrose, F.S.		Edinburgh 1834	1852	1852
Reeves			1886	1886
Reid, Jr, John N.	Thornhill	TSM, New York U.S. 1854	1853	1882
Reid, Sr, John	Thornhill	Edinburgh, Ireland <1829	1849	1853
Richards	Bradford		1864	
Richards(on), S.R.	York Mills	Victoria 1871	1880	1882
Richardson, J.H.	Toronto	TSM, King's Toronto 1848	1854	1865
Robinson, A. dentist			1876	1883
Robinson, T.H.	Kleinburg	Trinity 1883	1884	1888
Robinson, Wesley	Markham Village	McGill 1874	1873	1889
Rogers, David L.	Newmarket		1867	
Rolph, John	Toronto	London, Cambridge <1832	1859	1870
Ross	Cookstown		1868	
Rowell J.		TSM, New York U.S. 1854	1865	
Rupert, Oliver	Maple	Victoria 1862, 1866	1864	1879
Russell			1878	
Rutherford	Aurora		1878	1887
Ryerson, G.A.S.	Toronto	Trinity, Edinburgh 1876	1878	1886
Sangster, Alex	Stouffville	1884	1887	
Scholfield, T.C.	Bond Head	TSM, Victoria 1855, 1866	1856	1871
Scholfield, William	Lloydtown	Victoria 1858, 1866	1867	
Shaw, J.E.			1884	1884
Small	Toronto		1867	
Smith			1857	
Stevenson, J.D	Kleinburg	Victoria 1857, 1866	1870	1879
Strange, F.W.	Newmarket	England 1866, 1869	1871	1872
Stratford, S.J.		London 1839	1853	
Tabor			1883	
Taylor	Bradford		1878	
Teasdale			1864	

Name	Location	Place and Date of Education and/or Licence	First Date	Last Date
Telfer, Walter	Toronto	Edinburgh 1839	1852	
Thompson, S.G.	Stouffville	Bellevue NY, Edinburgh	1884	1884
Thorburn, J.		Edinburgh 1855, 1866	1864	
Vernon, E.	Thornhill, Newtonbrook	Jefferson U.S. 1851, 1869	1857	1865
Vox	Schomberg		1867	
Widdifield, J.H.	Holland Landing	Victoria 1869, 1870	1872	1878
Williams, Moses H.	Toronto	Victoria 1867	1868	1868
Wilson	Toronto		1882	
Wilson, William J.	Stouffville, Richmond Hill	Toronto 1877	1879	1888
Winstanley, Orlando	Thornhill, Willowdale	London 1844, 1866	1857	1879
Wismer, Henry			1873	
Workman, Joseph		McGill 1834, 1838	1852	
Wright, H.H.	Markham, Toronto	TSM 1839	1850	1887
Zimmerman, Richard	Toronto	Toronto, London 1872	1876	1878

Appendix C
Langstaff's Personal Library and Charities

The study of medical libraries, both personal and institutional, has recently become a separate discipline.[2] A nineteenth-century country doctor might not be expected to have bibliophilic interests, but his books and periodicals were the sources he chose for information and the selection reflected his interests. A study, based on extant volumes, has been made of the library of one of Langstaff's contemporaries, William M. Comfort (1822–99), and Jennifer J. Connor has compared the collections of several physicians, including Langstaff.[3] Unfortunately, Langstaff's own library was almost entirely dispersed at his death; it can be partially reconstructed from a few remainders belonging to the family, items donated to the Academy of Medicine in Toronto, and his account records of purchases and subscriptions.

Langstaff owned at least a few medical books on specific topics, including orthopaedics and breast cancer, and he subscribed to most of the Quebec and Ontario medical journals published during his career. He appears to have made only one contribution to the medical literature himself: a one-paragraph case report in the form of a letter to the editor about a little girl with pneumonia and complete consolidation of the lung.[4] Like Comfort, he also subscribed to the Wood's Library, an 1880s series that offered mainstream medical science in the form of reprints and commissioned works by familiar authors.[5] When the series stopped in 1886, Langstaff purchased Wood's six-volume set on surgery. Even in non-medical matters Langstaff's library bears a striking resemblance to that of Comfort and perhaps that of any educated Ontario gentleman – with agricultural magazines and books on literature, Canadian and British colonial history, and world geography. He read both local newspapers, but his political leanings are reflected in additional subscriptions: the *Globe*, the major liberal paper of Toronto; *Grip*, a satirical weekly; the Montreal *Witness*, a Protestant newspaper given to non-sectarian reporting of international news through a filter of anti-sectarianism, prohibitionism, and liberal principles; and, implying that he read French, *Le semeur canadien*, published by a French-Canadian convert to Protestantism. Ostensibly committed to 'les vrais intérêts des canadiens français,' *Le semeur* was more specifically devoted to attacks on Monseigneur Bourget and 'les catholiques ultramontains.'[6] Langstaff occasionally bought subscriptions to the Montreal *Witness* for other people in his community. A few clippings from these publications are glued to the inside of the daybooks: most concern the ravages of drink; some are on agricultural topics, such as the anatomy of the horse; a few, like the unidentified epigraph to chapter 2 or Tennyson's newly written 'Charge of the Light Brigade,' were literary pieces that appealed.

Donations to charities reflect Langstaff's Protestant (specifically Presbyterian) religion and his concern for temperance. As for the items in his library, the list was compiled from the remaining books and from entries recorded separately in accounts or in the back of his medical daybooks; titles appear as they were written unless the items could be identified with certainty.

Medical Books

Acquired	Title	Author and Date
?	*A treatise on the theory of ulcers*	B. Bell, 1784
?	*Lectures on the theory and practice of physics*	John Bell, W. Stokes, 1845
?	*An outline of the history and cure of fevers*	Robert Jackson, 1798
?	*Observations on fungus haematodes [or soft cancer]*	James Wardrop, 1809
Sept. 1845	*A treatise on dislocations & fractures of the joints*	Astley Cooper, 1832
Dec. 1880	'Medical books'	
March 1882	Woods Library	
April 1883	Woods Library	
June 1885	Woods Library	
Sept. 1887	'6 vols. on surgery' [Woods Library?]	

Other books

Acquired	Title (as written in account)	Probable Author and Date
June 1854	*Imperial Lexicon*	John Ogilvie, 1850
June 1854	*Memoir of Wellington*	W.F. Williams, vol. 1, 1853
Oct. 1858	*England's Battles*	W.F. Williams, vol. 2, 1856

Nov. 1858	*Travels in Africa*	Dr David Livingstone, 1857
April 1860	County map	Tremaine, 1860
July 1861	*Book of Languages*	
Aug. 1861	Map of Canada	
March 1862	Dictionary of dates	J.T. Haydn, 1851
Feb. 1865	*History of Canada*	J. Roy, 1864, or F.-X. Garneau, 1865
Feb. 1866	Maps of British North America	
Oct. 1866	*Great Rebellion*	J.T. Headley, 1863, or H. Greeley, 1865
May 1868	Books for family devotion	
June 1874	Shakespeare, 2 vols	
Oct. 1876	Shakespeare, nos 8 & 9	
Oct. 1876	*Farming Manual*	C.E. Whitcombe, 1874
Jan. 1879	Atlas [of York County?]	Miles and Company, 1878
July 1880	*Leisure Hours*	A.K.H. Boyd, 1863
Dec. 1880	*Loyalists of America*	Egerton Ryerson, 1880
Aug. 1886	*History of the Presbyterian Church*	William Gregg, 1885

Medical Journals

First ordered	Last ordered	Title
Oct. 1860	Sept. 1862	*British American Journal*
April 1877	Aug. 1884	*Canada Lancet*
Dec. 1874	Jan. 1881	*Canada Medical and Surgical Journal*
Nov. 1864	July 1871	*Canada Medical Journal*
May 1877	Jan. 1887	*Canada Medical Record*
Jan. 1876	Jan. 1882	*Canadian Journal of Medical Sciences*
June 1850	June 1887	*Lancet* [discontinuous]
March 1887	Nov. 1887	*Medical Bulletin* (Philadelphia)
March 1859	March 1860	*Medical Chronicle*

Other Periodicals

First ordered	Last ordered	Title
Feb. 1858		*Primitive [Presbyterian?] Missionary*
April 1858		*New York Pulpit*

Sept. 1858	Dec. 1881	*Presbyterian* (Montreal)
Oct. 1858	July 1859	*War in India* (also Indian Mutiny) (instalment book?)
July 1860		*Temperance Advocate* (Montreal)
June 1861		*Eclectic Temperance Journal*
March 1862	Dec. 1862	*Rural Architecture* (instalment book?)
Dec. 1864	Jan. 1868	*Canada Farmer* (Toronto)
Nov. 1871		*Canadian Poultry Chronicle*
Feb. 1872	April 1879	*Farmer's Advocate* (London, Ont.)
Feb. 1872		*Northern Advocate*
Jan. 1875		*New Dominion Monthly* (Montreal)
Jan. 1877		*Poultry Journal*
Jan. 1881	Jan. 1882	*Free Grant Gazette*
Feb. 1861		*Presbyterian Missionary* (London, England)
June 1882	Aug. 1882	*Picturesque Canada* (instalment book, George M. Grant)

Newspapers

First ordered	Last ordered	Title
June 1850		*Colonist* (Toronto)
Jan. 1858	Aug. 1873	*Witness* (Montreal)
March 1858	Oct. 1873	*Globe* (Toronto)
Sept. 1858	July 1862	*Le semeur canadien* (Montreal and Napierville)
Nov. 1870	Oct. 1888	*Economist* (Markham)
June 1878	Jan. 1881	*Canadian Illustrated News* (Montreal)
July 1878		*Liberal* (Richmond Hill)
Sept. 1878	April 1886	*Grip* (Toronto)
Jan. 1881		*Valley Record*

Charities

These are the charities as they appeared in the back of the medical daybooks; some appeared more than once.

Missionary, June 1858
Victoria College subscription, Dec. 1858
Philharmonic Society, Feb. 1859
Sons of Temperance, March 1859

Temperance Society, March 1859
Agricultural Society, July 1861
Bible Society, Dec. 1866
Family Devotion, Jan., Nov. 1868
Lower Canada Mission, Feb. 1877
Bible Society, April 1883
Home Missions, March 1886

Appendix D
Langstaff's Properties

The list excludes many municipal lots in Wallaceburg and Richmond Hill; a = acres.

County	Township	Concession and Lot		Acquired and Sold		Value in 1889 ($)
Kent	Chatham	8	6 (200a)	1865	1873	
Kent	Chatham	13	1 (200a)	1865		1,200
Kent	Chatham	14	3 E ½ (100a)	1865		
Lambton	Dawn	10	19 E ½ (100a)	1856		400
Lambton	Enniskillin	10	31 N ½ (100a)	1856	1865	
Lambton	Enniskillin	11	31 S ½ (100a)	1856	1865	
Muskoka	Draper	7	3	1868		
Muskoka	Draper	8	3	1868		
Muskoka	Draper	6	32	1868		
Muskoka	Draper	8 (&7?)	2	1882		
Muskoka	Stephenson	10	18?			20
Muskoka	McLean	15	?			20
Ontario	Scott	1	16 E ½ (100a)	1880		2,000
Simcoe	Medonte	5	2 W ½	1880		500
Victoria	Somerville	6	18	1881		20
Victoria	Somerville	14	3	1881		23
Victoria	Bexley	5	9	1881		20
York	Toronto	Queen W	446 448	1856		19,626
York	Toronto	Queen W	586 588	1857		12,980
York	Vaughan	2	27 N (80a)	1865		2,600
York	Vaughan	2	28 (10a)	1865		
York	Vaughan	2	30	1863	1874	
York	Whitchurch	1	61 SE (50a)	1887		200
York	Markham	1	60 rear			1,600
York	Markham	1	59 NE	1880	1884?	
York		?		1883		

Appendix E
Therapies in Langstaff's Daybooks

1 Langstaff's Pharmacopoeia: Drugs and preparations for internal and external use

* Mentioned in first decade, but not in last
° Mentioned in last decade, but not in first

acacia (gum arabic)
acetic acid (vinegar)
aconite°
AIO
aloes
alumen
ammonia
ammoniae carbonicum
anis
anodyne
antimony potassium tartrate
  (tartar emetic)
An/z
AO
aqua
argentum nitratum (lunar caustic)
arsenici, liquor (Solution
  F[owler's]*)
asafoetida
aselli (onisci)
astringent

balsamum copaibae
belladonna
benzoin

bismuth (bismuth trisnitras)
bitters
borax
bromide° (potassium bromide°)

calomel (hydargyri chloridum)
calumba
calx
camphor (mistura camphorae)
cantharides (lytta vesicatoria)
carbolic acid°
castor oil (ricini)
catechu, infusion
cathartic
caustic
chicken weed
chloral hydrate°
chloroform°
citric acid
cinchona (kina, peruvian bark,
  quinine)
cinnamon
clyster
cod liver oil
colchicine

collyrium
conium*
cream
creosote
creta
croton oil (ol. tigli) (internal and
    external)

digitalis
Dover's powder* (ipecac and
    opium)
drink, warm

effervescent salts
emetic
enema
enema of raw egg
ergotamine (secale cornutum)
erigeron
ether (or aether)

fer (iron)
ferri carbonas
ferri sulphas
ferri tartarum*
ferrum oxydatum*
flour

gaultheria (wintergreen)
ginger (zingiber)
guaiac*

hellebore* (veratrum viride*)
hyoscyamus

ice
injection (rectal)
iodine (iodi tinctura, Lugol's
    solution*)

ipecac

jalap

laudanum
laxative
liniment
lotion

mentha
magnesium sulphas (S.M.P.)
mistura nigra*
morphine
mustard plaster (sinapism)
myrrh

nitric acid
nitro-hydrochloric acid
    (nitro-muriatic acid)
nux vomica (strychnine)

ointment
olive oil
onion (poultice)
opium

permanganate (gargle)
physic
pills
plaster
plumbi acetas
plumbi enema
potassae bitartras
potassae carbonas
potassae nitras
potassii iodidum
poultice
powders
punch

purgative

quassia, infusion

rhei (rhubarb)

saccharum (sugar)
salicylate of soda°
santonica
salts
sapo
sedative
Sedlitz powders*
scillae (squills)
senegae
senna
shower
soda (sodii carbonas)

spigelia (pink)
stimulant
stramonium
sulphur sublimatum
sulphuric acid

tallow
tartaric acid
terebenthina (turpentine)
tonic

unguentum hydargyri

valerium
vermifuge (worm powder)

zinc sulphate
zinc [oxide] unguent

2 Dietary and Alcohol-Containing Substances

ale
arrowroot
beeftea
beer
brandy (vini gallici)
bread
broth
buttermilk
capria (capers)
chicken broth
cream
egg
gelatine
gin
grapes
gruel
ice cream
lemon

lemon water
light diet
lime
linseed tea
mayweed
milk
milk, boiled
milk punch
milk and water
mutton
oatmeal
oysters
pukeweed
punch
sago
steak
tea
tea, ginger

tea, pumpkin seed
toast
victus

vini (Burgundy, wine)
water, warm and cold
whisky

3 Methods of Bleeding

leeches (hirudo)
cupping (dry and wet)

venesection (phlebotomy,
  bloodletting)

4 Mechanical Methods

atomiser
balneum (bath, fomentation,
  perfusion, wash)
blister (cloche, vesicatoire)
  (see also part 1, cantharides)
electricity (galvanic battery)
elevation (of part of body)
hair, clipped or shaved
heat

hot bricks
hot hop bags
pressure
rest
smoothing iron (as weight and
  for heat)
seton
shower head
snow

Appendix F
Medical Diagnoses in Langstaff's Daybooks

This alphabetical list contains diagnostic terms used by James Miles Langstaff, but not the broader classification of disease he might have used, as there was no indication of it in his record. For some diagnoses more than one term was used.

* Terms that appear in the first decade, but not in the last
° Terms that appear in the last decade, but not in the first

abscess
acne*
ague
amaurosis
anasarca
anaemia
aneurysm
angina
anthrax*
aortic bruit
apoplexy
arthritis
ascites
asthma

bites
bleeding
bloody flux
brain disease, chronic°
brain fever
Bright's disease
bronchitis
bronchocoele*

bruises
bubo*

calculus
cancer
carbuncle*
catarrh
cephalgia
cerebritis°
chickenpox
chlorosis
cholera
cholera morbus
cholera, sporadic
chorea
clap*
colic*
coma
confusion
constipation
convulsions
costive
coxalgia*

croup
cynanche
cystitis

deaf
debility
debility, infantile
delirium
delirium tremens
demiopia
diabetes°
diarrhoea
diphtheria
dropsy
drowsy
drunkenness
dumb
dysentery
dyspnoea
dysuria

earache
ecthyma°
eczema
emaciation
empyema
endocarditis
enlarged gall bladder
enlarged glands
enlarged liver
enlarged spleen
epididymitis
epilepsy
erysipelas
erythema nodosum

fainting
felon
fever
fever, emigrant*

fever, infantile remittent*
fever, intermittent*
fever, puerperal
fever, remittent
fever, rheumatic
fever, scarlet
fits
flatulence*

gangrene
gastritis°
giddy
goitre
gonorrhea
gout

haematemesis
haematuria
haemoptysis
haemorrhage
headache
heart disease
hemicrania
hemiplegia°
hepatitis
hernia
herpes
hiccups
hip disease
hives
humpback
hydatids
hydrocephalus
hydrocoele
hysteralgia
hysteria
hysteritis

idiocy
imperforate anus

indigestion
inflammation
influenza
insanity°
insomnia
intolerance of light

jaundice

lameness
laryngitis°
leucorrhea
liver disease
loss of memory
loss of speech
loss of swallowing
loss of words
lumbago
lunacy
lymphatic

marasmus
mastitis
measles
melaena
meningitis
mental derangement*
mitral bruit
morbus caeruleus
mumps

narcotism
nausea
nephralgia
nervousness

oedema
old age
ophthalmia
orchitis

pain
palpitation
palsy
paraphimosis
paronychia
pericarditis
peritonitis
petechiae
phlebitis
phrenitis
phthisis
piles
pleurisy
pneumonia
pneumothorax
porrigo furfurans*
porrigo scutulata*
pregnancy
prolapsis ani
psoriasis
ptosis
ptyalism
purging
purpura
pustules

quinsy

religious delirium
renal disease
rheumatism, acute
rheumatism, chronic
ringworm
rupture

scabies
scarlatina
scorbutus (scurvy)
shingles
slow to talk

slow to walk
smallpox
sore eyes
sore face
sore throat
spasm
spina bifida
stiff neck
strangury
stroke
stupor
subsultus tendinum
sudden death
suffocation
sunstroke
swelling
sycosis
syphilis

taenia
tenesmus
testicular atrophy

tetanus
tic douloureux*
tuberculosis
tumour
typhoid
typhus

ulcer, skin
ulcer, stomach°
urticaria
uterine rupture
uvula swollen

varicella
vomiting
vomiting of pregnancy°

warts
waterbrash
whooping cough
worms

Notes

Acknowledgments

1 Jacalyn Duffin, 'A Rural Practice in Nineteenth-Century Ontario: The Continuing Medical Education of James Miles Langstaff,' *Canadian Bulletin of Medical History / Bulletin canadien d'histoire de la médecine* 5 (1988): 3–28; '"They Fed Me; Fed My Horse": The Practice of James Miles Langstaff,' *Canadian Family Physician* 36 (1990): 2189–93; 'Keeping Up: Medical Technology in a 19th-Century Rural Practice,' *Annals of the Royal College of Physicians and Surgeons of Canada* 24 (1991): 381–4

Introduction

1 A by no means exhaustive list of works on eighteenth- and nineteenth-century French, English, and North American medicine includes Michel Foucault, *The Birth of the Clinic: An Archeology of Medical Perception*, trans. A.M. Sheridan-Smith (London: Tavistock 1973); John S. Haller, *American Medicine in Transition, 1840–1910* (Chicago: University of Illinois Press 1981); Judith Walzer Leavitt, *Brought to Bed: Childbearing in America, 1750–1950* (New York, Oxford: Oxford University Press 1986); Jacques Léonard, *La France médicale: Médecins et malades au XIX siècle* (Paris: Gallimard 1978); Irvine Loudan, *Medical Care and the General Practitioner, 1750–1850* (Oxford: Oxford University Press, Clarendon Press 1986); Guenter B. Risse, *Hospital Life in Enlightenment Scotland: Care and Teaching at the Royal Infirmary of Edinburgh* (Cambridge: Cambridge University Press 1986); George Rosen and Charles E. Rosenberg, *The Structure of American Medical Practice, 1875–1941* (Philadelphia: University of Pennsylvania Press 1983); Charles E. Rosenberg, *The Care of Strangers: The Rise of America's Hospital System* (New York: Basic Books 1987); Morris Vogel and Charles E. Rosenberg, eds., *The Therapeutic Revolution: Essays in the Social History of American Medicine* (Philadelphia: University of Pennsylvania Press 1979); Paul Starr, *The Social Transformation of American Medicine* (New York: Basic

Books 1982); John Harley Warner, *The Therapeutic Perspective: Medical Practice, Knowledge, and Identity in America, 1820–1885* (Cambridge, Mass. and London, England: Harvard University Press 1986). With respect to Canada, see Jacques Bernier, *La médecine au Québec: Naissance et évolution d'une profession* (Quebec: Presses de l'Université Laval 1989); James T.H. Connor, 'Minority Medicine in Ontario: A Study of Medical Pluralism and Its Decline' (Ph.D. thesis, University of Waterloo, 1989); Wendy Mitchinson, *The Nature of Their Bodies: Women and Their Doctors in Victorian Canada* (Toronto: University of Toronto Press 1991).

2 Most autobiographical accounts pertain to the years after Langstaff's practice. Some have become classics; see, for example, the work of the Americans Arthur E. Hertzler, *The Horse and Buggy Doctor* (New York, London: Harper and Brothers 1938); James Jackson, *A Memoir of James Jackson Jr.*, M.D., *with Extracts from His Letters to His Father; and Medical Cases Collected by Him* (Boston 1835); and Russell M. Jones, ed., *The Parisian Education of an American Surgeon: The Letters of James Mason Warren* (Philadelphia: American Philosophical Society 1978). With respect to Canada, see Abraham Groves, *All in a Day's Work: Leaves from a Doctor's Casebook* (Toronto: Macmillan 1934); Victor Johnston, *Before the Age of Miracles: Memoirs of a Country Doctor* (Toronto, Montreal, Winnipeg, Vancouver: Fitzhenry and Whiteside 1972). Recent Canadian contributions in this genre include Allan Duncan, *Medicine, Madams, and Mounties: Stories of a Yukon Doctor, 1933–47* (np: Raincoast Books 1989); Harold J.G. Geggie, *The Extra Mile: Medicine in Rural Quebec, 1885–1965*, ed. Norma and Stuart Geggie (published privately 1987); Nigel Rusted, *It's Devil Deep Down There* (St John's, Nfld.: Creative Publishers 1987).

3 Charles G. Roland, 'The Diary of a Canadian Country Physician: Jonathan Woolverton (1881–1883),' *Medical History* 14 (1971): 168–180; S.E.D. Shortt, '"Before the Age of Miracles": The Rise, Fall, and Rebirth of General Practice in Canada,' in Charles G. Roland, ed., *Health, Disease and Medicine: Essays in Canadian History* (Toronto: Hannah Institute for the History of Medicine 1984), 123–52; Steven M. Stowe, 'Obstetrics and the Work of Doctoring in the Mid-Nineteenth-Century American South,' *Bulletin of the History of Medicine* 64 (1990): 540–66

4 J.M. Crummey, 'The Daybooks of Robert McLellan: A Comparative Study of a Nova Scotia Family Practice during World War I,' *Canadian Medical Association Journal* 120 (1979): 492–7; Melville C. Watson, 'An

Account of an Obstetrical Practice in Upper Canada,' *Canadian Medical Association Journal* 40 (1939): 181–8

5 Shortt, 'Before the Age of Miracles,' 143n13

6 Evelyn Bernette Ackerman, 'The Activities of a Country Doctor in New York State: Dr. Elias Cornelius of Somers, 1794–1803,' *Historical Reflections / Réflexions historiques* 9 (1982): 181–93; Edna Hindie Lemay, 'Thomas Hérier, a Country Surgeon outside Angoulême at the End of the XVIIIth Century: A Contribution to Social History,' *Journal of Social History* 10 (1976–7): 524–37; Irvine Loudan, 'The Nature of Provincial Medical Practice in Eighteenth-Century England,' *Medical History* 29 (1985): 1–32; Katherine Mandusic McDonell, ed., *The Journals of William A. Lindsay: An Ordinary Nineteenth-Century Physician's Surgical Cases* (Indianapolis: Indiana Historical Society 1989). Medical case studies of individual localities include J. Worth Estes and David M. Goodman, *The Changing Humours of Portsmouth: The Medical Biography of an American Town* (Boston: Francis A. Countaway Library 1986); Hilary Marland, *Medicine in Wakefield and Huddersfield, 1780–1870* (New York, New Rochelle, Melbourne, Sydney: Cambridge University Press 1987); John Norris, 'The Country Doctor in British Columbia: 1887–1975,' *BC Studies* 49 (1981): 15–38.

7 For an analysis of the difference between a physician's daybook account and his personal diary, see Stowe, 'Obstetrics and the Work of Doctoring.'

CHAPTER 1 **The Making of a Doctor**

1 James Miles Langstaff, Langstaff daybook (Daybook), 3 Oct. 1864

2 Daybook, 20 Aug. to 5 Dec., especially 3 Oct., 1864; Archives of Ontario (AO), Journal of Matthew Teefy, MU 2113, folder 16, 1; AO Matthew Teefy scrapbook, MS 120, item 165

3 AO, Minutes of the Municipality of the Township of Vaughan, vol. 2 1853–66, 3 Oct. and 5 Dec. 1864

4 Daybook, 4 Oct. to 5 Dec. 1864

5 James Rolph Langstaff, letter to author

6 Alex D. Bruce and Wesley C. Gohn, eds., *Historical Sketch of Markham Township, 1793–1858* (Markham: *Economist and Sun* 1950), 7–8. See also entries for 25 Sept. and especially 25 Oct. 1793 in Mary Quayle Innis, ed., *Mrs Simcoe's Diary* (Toronto: Macmillan 1965), 108–9.

7 For more on the settlement of Richmond Hill and vicinity, see F.R.

Berchem, *The Yonge Street Story, 1793–1860: An Account from Letters, Diaries, and Newspapers* (Toronto, New York: McGraw-Hill Ryerson 1977); Isabel Champion, *Markham, 1793–1900,* (Markham: Markham District Historical Society 1989); Doris Fitzgerald, *Thornhill, 1793–1863: The History of an Ontario Village* (Thornhill 1964); G. Elmore Reaman, *A History of Vaughan Township* (Toronto: University of Toronto Press 1971); Robert M. Stamp, *Early Days in Richmond Hill: A History of the Community to 1930* (Richmond Hill: Richmond Hill Public Library Board 1991).

8 Craig Heron, 'Abner Miles,' *Dictionary of Canadian Biography* (Toronto: University of Toronto Press 1983) vol. 5, 596–7. The property was lot 36 in the first concession of Markham township, which, at the time of writing, is recognizable as the northeast corner of Yonge Street and Highway 7 (the Langstaff sideroad).

9 Ely Playter's diary is a rich source of early nineteenth-century social history; Edith Firth, *The Town of York, 1793–1815: A Collection of Documents of Early Toronto* (Toronto: University of Toronto Press and the Champlain Society no. 5 1962), 99n, 243–53

10 These properties were on opposite sides of Yonge Street, lots 45 in concession 1 of Markham and Vaughan townships. Possibly speculating on land values, Abner Miles bought or earned the right to further properties in York and the townships of King, Whitchurch, Vaughan, and Markham. Reaman, *History of Vaughan,* 33, 118. On the distribution of Crown Lands, see Leo A. Johnson, 'Land Policy, Population Growth, and Social Structure in the Home District, 1793–1851,' in J.K. Johnson, ed., *Historical Essays on Upper Canada* (Toronto: McClelland and Stewart 1975), 32–57, especially 33–4. Papers of Mrs Eileen Aiken, especially letter from James Miles Langstaff's daughter Mary Lillian McConaghy to Mrs [Homer] Langstaff, 21 Aug. 1904, containing a copy of a letter from 'Mercie,' about early family histroy.

11 A.J. Clark, 'Reverend William Jenkins of Richmond Hill and His Records,' *Ontario History* 27 (1931): 15–76; Patricia Somerville and Catherine Macfarlane, *A History of Vaughan Township Churches* (Maple: Vaughan Township Historical Society 1984), 316, 319

12 James Rolph Langstaff, 'The Langstaffs of Richmond Hill, Thornhill, Langstaff, and King,' 1980, photocopy of typewritten manuscript, gift of James Rolph Langstaff, Richmond Hill, to author ('Langstaff scrapbook'), 233–42.

13 Gerald M. Craig, *Upper Canada: The Formative Years* (Toronto: McClelland and Stewart 1963), 47, 75, 111; S.F. Wise, 'Colonial Atti-

tudes from the Era of the War of 1812 to the Rebellions of 1837,' in S.F. Wise and Robert Craig Brown, eds., *Canada Views the United States: Nineteenth-Century Political Attitudes* (Toronto: Macmillan 1967), 16–43

14 For a discussion of educational issues as they pertain to rural Ontario, see Leo A. Johnson, *History of the County of Ontario, 1615–1875* (Whitby: Corporation of the County of Ontario 1973), 263–80.

15 This was a schoolhouse built by Nicolas Cober and completed in 1815 on lot 34 concession 1, Vaughan, on Yonge Street opposite the Miller homestead. I. Champion, *Markham*, 168

16 'Obituary,' *York Herald*, 15 Aug. 1889. This same report also claims that Langstaff's education was continued in a house slightly north on 'land donated by James Lymburner on lot 41 Concession 1, Vaughan.' No further evidence can be found concerning the existence of this school.

17 I. Champion, *Markham*, 132–3; Reaman, *History of Vaughan*, 286; Stamp, *Early Days in Richmond Hill*, 68–72; Somerville and Macfarlane, *Vaughan Township Churches*, 319

18 Sources on the 1837 Rebellion are legion and the reader should be aware that almost every word in a synopsis can be controversial. For a brief summary, see Colin Read, *The Rebellion of 1837 in Upper Canada* (Ottawa: Canadian Historical Association Booklet no. 46 1988). See also J.C. Dent, *The Story of the Upper Canadian Rebellion*, 2 vols. (Toronto: C. Blackett Robinson 1885); Charles Lindsey, *The Life and Times of William Lyon Mackenzie* (Toronto: P. Randall 1862); Ronald John Stagg, 'The Yonge Street Rebellion of 1837; An Examination of the Social Background and Re-assessment of the Events' (Ph.D. thesis, University of Toronto, 1976).

19 I. Champion, *Markham*, 188

20 Simon Miller's recollections, elicited in an interview with W.L. Smith and published in the Markham newspaper the *Sun*, 14 July 1898, have been widely cited. See, for example, W.L. Smith, *Pioneers of Old Ontario* (Toronto: George N. Morang 1923), 127–32; Reaman, *History of Vaughan*, 231–2; I. Champion, *Markham*, 192; Stamp, *Early Days in Richmond Hill*, 105.

21 Montgomery's recollection was cited in William Canniff, *The Medical Profession in Upper Canada* (reprint of 1894 edition, Toronto: Hannah Institute for the History of Medicine 1980), 520.

22 Simon Miller, cited in Reaman, *History of Vaughan*, 232

23 I. Champion, *Markham*, 99

24 Ibid., 132

25 No date was given for the journey referred to as Langstaff's 'first

school-boy days from home.' 'Obituary,' *York Herald*, 15 Aug. 1889

26 The generally accepted law of 'primogeniture' had been contested as part of the Reform movement. See G.M. Craig 'The American Impact on the Upper Canadian Reform Movement before 1837,' in J.K. Johnson, ed., *Historical Essays*, 324; David Gagan, *Hopeful Travellers: Families and Social Change in Mid-Victorian Peel County, Canada West* (Toronto: Government of Ontario and University of Toronto Press 1981), 51.

27 Jacques Bernier, *La médecine au Québec: Naissance et évolution d'une profession* (Quebec: Presses de l'Université Laval 1989), 37

28 On the history of medical education and professionalization in Ontario, see Canniff, *The Medical Profession in Upper Canada*, 9–38; James T.H. Connor, 'Minority Medicine in Ontario: A Study of Medical Pluralism and Its Decline' (Ph.D. thesis, University of Waterloo, 1989), 189–267; Walter B. Geikie, 'An Historical Sketch of Canadian Medical Education,' *Canada Lancet* 34 (1901): 225–36, 281–7; R.D. Gidney and W.P.J. Millar, 'The Origins of Organized Medicine in Ontario, 1850–1869,' in Charles G. Roland, ed., *Health, Disease, and Medicine: Essays in Canadian History* (Toronto: The Hannah Institute for the History of Medicine 1984), 65–95; Charles M. Godfrey, *Medicine for Ontario: A History* (Belleville: Mika 1979); Ronald Hamowy, *Canadian Medicine: A Study in Restricted Entry* (Vancouver: Fraser Institute 1984), 13–29, 35–45, passim; Elizabeth MacNab, *A Legal History of the Health Professions in Ontario* (Toronto: Queen's Printer 1970).

29 A full biography of John Rolph that combines study of his medical, legal, and political activities is sadly lacking. Various aspects of his life are presented in many sources, including J.M.S. Careless, *The Union of the Canadas: The Growth of Canadian Institutions, 1841–1857* (Toronto: McClelland and Stewart 1967), 172, 181, 186, 218; Gerald M. Craig, 'John Rolph,' *Dictionary of Canadian Biography* (Toronto: University of Toronto Press 1976) vol. 9, 683–90; Jacalyn Duffin, '"In View of the Body of Job Broom": A Glimpse of the Medical Knowledge and Practice of John Rolph,' *Canadian Bulletin of Medical History / Bulletin canadien d'histoire de la médecine* 7 (1990): 9–30; Edith Firth, *The Town of York, 1815–1834: A Further Collection of Documents of Early Toronto* (Toronto: Champlain Society no. 8 1966), 336, 343, 347; Godfrey, *Medicine for Ontario*, 33–44, 56–8, 73–82, passim; Donald Jack, *Rogues, Rebels, and Geniuses: The Story of Canadian Medicine* (Garden City, NY: Doubleday 1981), 69–72; C.B. Sissons, 'John Rolph's Own Account of the "Flag of Truce Incident" in the Rebellion of 1837,' *Canadian Historical Review* 10 (1938): 56–9. It is beyond the scope of this work to resolve the problem

of John Rolph's duplicity in 1837, but those interested in doing so might begin with the portrayal of Rolph as a hero in Dent, *The Story of the Upper Canadian Rebellion*, and contrast it with the view expressed in John King, *The Other Side of the Story, Being Some Reviews of Mr J.C. Dent's First Volume* (Toronto: Murray 1886).

30 Metropolitan Toronto Public Library, Baldwin Room (MTPL), J.H. Richardson, 'Reminiscences of the medical profession in Toronto, 1829–1905,' typewritten manuscript
31 Ibid.
32 Walter Geikie, cited in Godfrey, *Medicine for Ontario*, 56
33 Duffin, 'The Body of Job Broom'
34 MTPL, Richardson, 'Reminiscences'
35 Daybook, back entry, 10 Sept. 1879
36 Lindsey, *Life and Times of William Lyon Mackenzie*, 384
37 The prize was the 1832 revised American edition of Sir Astley Cooper's *Treatise on Dislocations and Fractures of the Joints*, and the bookplate was signed by John Rolph and C[hristopher] Widmer. Property of James Rolph Langstaff, Richmond Hill
38 Connor, 'Minority Medicine,' 207–9; Gidney and Millar, 'Origins of Organized Medicine in Ontario'
39 Anon., 'Toronto School of Medicine,' unsigned, undated, three-page manuscript, property of James Rolph Langstaff, Richmond Hill. The hand is similar if not identical to John Rolph's, and since the document refers to 'seven years' of operation and 'over sixteen' graduates, it was probably written in 1849 or 1850.
40 James Langstaff was named as an occasional student in the 1845–6 session in a list of eighty-two medical students who had studied in the University of King's College from its inception to 1850; *Journals of the Legislative Assembly of Canada*, 1850, vol. 9, part 2, Appendix KK. The author of 'Toronto School of Medicine,' cited above, complains about 'returns before the House,' possibly in reaction to this document.
41 MTPL, Richardson, 'Reminiscences'
42 National Archives of Canada (NAC), MG 24, B24, John Rolph Papers, vol. 2, 143–6, letter from J.H. Richardson to John Rolph, 29 July 1846
43 Langstaff probably did have a letter of some sort. A few years after Rolph had run into difficulties with his own colleagues, his influence abroad was valued by at least one of his former students, who asked for a letter of introduction prior to a trip to England. NAC, John Rolph Papers, vol. 2, 263–6, letter from A.J. Park to John Rolph, 28 March 1858
44 For information pertaining to Guy's Hospital, I am indebted to Andrew

Baster, Assistant Librarian, United Medical and Dental School of Guy's and St Thomas Hospital.

45 H.C. Cameron, *Mr Guy's Hospital, 1726–1948* (London: Longman's 1954), 185–6; Samuel Wilks and G.T. Bettany, *A Biographical History of Guy's Hospital* (London: Ward, Lock, Bowden, and Co. 1982), 461–3

46 Pamela Bright, *Dr Richard Bright, 1789–1858* (London, Sydney, Toronto: Bodley Head 1983), 216

47 James Miles Langstaff, manuscript lecture notes and case records from Guy's Hospital ('Guy's Notes'), property of James Rolph Langstaff, Richmond Hill

48 'Obituary,' *York Herald*, 15 Aug. 1889

49 Cameron, *Mr Guy's Hospital*, 125–41; Wilks and Bettany, *Biographical History*, 245–50

50 Cameron, *Mr Guy's Hospital*, 353–4; Wilks and Bettany, *Biographical History*, 365–71; Maxwell M. Wintrobe, *Blood Pure and Eloquent: A Story of Discovery, of People, and of Ideas* (New York: McGraw-Hill 1980), 666–7

51 Langstaff, 'Guy's Notes,' 285

52 Ibid., 69. No date was given for Syme's visit, but the relationship of this entry to the dated entries suggests it was written during Feb. or March 1848.

53 For the traditional portrayal of Syme, see Fielding H. Garrison, *Introduction to the History of Medicine*, 3rd ed. (Philadelphia: Saunders 1922), 514.

54 'Le lethion' and 'Du lethion,' *La lancette canadienne* 1 (1847): 20, 25; Charles G. Roland, 'Bibliography of the History of Anaesthesia in Canada: Preliminary Checklist,' *Canadian Anaesthetists' Society Journal* 15 (1968): 202–14; James T.H. Connor, '"To Be Rendered Unconscious of Torture": Anaesthesia and Canada' (M.Phil. thesis, University of Waterloo, 1983), 114–15

55 Andrew Baster, letter to author

56 Bernier, *La médecine au Québec*, 161; Russell C. Maulitz, 'Channel Crossing: The Lure of French Pathology for English Medical Students,' *Bulletin of the History of Medicine* 55 (1981): 475–96; John Harley Warner, 'The Selective Transport of Medical Knowledge: Antebellum American Physicians and Parisian Medical Therapeutics,' *Bulletin of the History of Medicine* 59 (1985): 213–31; John Harley Warner, 'Remembering Paris: Memory and the American Disciples of French Medicine in the Nineteenth Century,' *Bulletin of the History of Medicine* 65 (1991): 301–25. For many years, Langstaff subscribed to the French-Canadian newspaper *Le semeur canadien*.

57 'Obituary,' *York Herald*, 15 Aug. 1889
58 MTPL, Richardson, 'Reminiscences'
59 Canniff, *Medical Profession*, 466
60 Toronto School of Medicine, *Annual Announcement*, 1851, from the personal archives of Mrs Wallace Graham, Toronto
61 Toronto Academy of Medicine, Archives, W.T. Aikins Papers, file no. 86, letter from W.T. Aikins to John Rolph, 5 April 1852
62 Recollection of the doctor's brother John Langstaff, Jr, cited in W.L. Smith, *Pioneers of Old Ontario*, 331
63 AO, Estate files, GS 1-959, Cabinet 2, reel 422, no. 191, John Langstaff
64 Miles Langstaff purchased the land in 1830 from John C. Stookes and sold a one-acre portion to Thomas Kinnear, who with his housekeeper, Nancy Montgomery, was murdered by a servant in 1843. Stamp, *Early Days in Richmond Hill*, 117
65 Canada Census 1851, C 11759–60, Vaughan township, District II, 91
66 John Langstaff, Sr, purchased one gallon of whisky from the store of Matthew Teefy on each of the following dates: 31 March 1852, 30 April, 12 May 1853. AO Papers of Matthew Teefy, MU 2953, Ledger 1851, 366, 386

CHAPTER 2 **Professional and Social World of a Nineteenth-Century Doctor**

1 'Obituary,' *York Herald*, 15 Aug. 1889. There is evidence of a mortgage for £217, dated 30 Oct. 1849. I am especially indebted to Janet Fayle, Heritage Advisor to the Town of Richmond Hill, for identifying the records of the real estate transactions of the Langstaff family.
2 Archives of Ontario (AO), Teefy papers, MU 2930, Account book, 86–7, 'Dr John Reid Philadelphia late of Rich'd Hill,' 21 Nov. 1849; MU 2935, Account, 1848–53, 987; MU 2953, 332, 'Dr Reid Thornhill'
3 John Duncomb, also spelled Duncumb, was not related to the more famous medical brothers Drs Charles and Elijah Duncombe, early associates of Rolph and rebel veterans of 1837. William Canniff, *The Medical Profession in Upper Canada* (reprint of 1894 edition, Toronto: Hannah Institute for the History of Medicine 1980), 199; Robert M. Stamp, *Early Days in Richmond Hill: A History of the Community to 1930* (Richmond Hill: Richmond Hill Public Library Board 1991), 165
4 AO, Teefy scrapbook, MS 120, items no. 79, 308, 309
5 In 1840 the physician-to-population ratio was 1: 3,000; by 1871 it had roughly doubled to 1: 1,455; and it continued to increase into the 1890s.

See James T.H. Connor, 'Minority Medicine in Ontario: A Study of Medical Pluralism and its Decline' (Ph.D. thesis, University of Waterloo, 1989), 201–3.

6 James Miles Langstaff's account book (Account book), 1879, 793–4

7 James Miles Langstaff, Langstaff daybook (Daybook), back entry, 10 Sept. 1887

8 Charles M. Godfrey, *Medicine for Ontario: A History* (Belleville: Mika 1979), 73

9 One notable exception is a short diary written in the 1850s by a student who studied with Langstaff's colleagues Drs Freel and Lloyd in nearby Markham. Archives of Toronto Academy of Medicine, Joseph Bascom, 'Diary of a Medical Student.' See also Connor, 'Minority Medicine,' 214–16. Kenneth M. Ludmerer, *Learning to Heal: The Development of American Medical Education* (New York: Basic Books 1985), 16; William G. Rothstein, *American Medical Schools and the Practice of Medicine: A History* (Oxford: Oxford University Press 1987), 33.

10 He gave $10 to his student, Armstrong, 'to get subject,' possibly but not definitely a cadaver, which ultimately cost only $5. Daybook, back entry, 28–9 April 1870

11 It seems that Comisky owed Langstaff 'about $1,000' as of January 1867; part of his chores had included shopping for pharmaceutical supplies. While Armstrong was a student, Langstaff had allowed him to collect and keep the rents from his Toronto properties; the debt he accumulated between 1869 and 1872 was $1,046.68 without interest, which was charged at a rate of eight per cent. Account book, 1866, 23, 39; Account book, 1869, 8

12 Daybook, 27 March 1878, Dr Armstrong

13 East half lot 16 Concession 1 Scott township, from Dr F.R. Armstrong. Langstaff allowed $1,800 as the value of the farm and assumed a mortgage of $1,200; thus, he accepted $600 to settle the debt of more than $1,000. Daybook, back entry, 1 Sept. 1880

14 On these issues, see Jacques Bernier, *La médecine au Québec: Naissance et évolution d'une profession* (Quebec: Presses de l'Université Laval 1989), 162; Connor, 'Minority Medicine,' 211–13, 418, passim; J.T.H. Connor, '"A Sort of *Felo-de-se*": Eclecticism, Related Medical Sects, and Their Decline in Victorian Ontario,' *Bulletin of the History of Medicine* 65 (1991): 503–27; R.D. Gidney and W.P.J. Millar, 'The Origins of Organized Medicine in Ontario, 1850–1869,' in Charles G. Roland, ed., *Health, Disease, and Medicine: Essays in Canadian History* (Toronto: Hannah Institute for the History of Medicine 1982), 65–95; Godfrey, *Medicine for*

Ontario, 195–7; Ronald Hamowy, *Canadian Medicine: A Study in Restricted Entry* (Vancouver: Fraser Institute 1984), 13–29, 35–45, 53–69, 100–30; Larry McNally, 'The First of Its Kind: The Canadian Medical Association,' *Archivist* 19 (1992): 13–14.

15 College of Physicians and Surgeons of Ontario, Historical Register, James Miles Langstaff; Daybook, 14 March 1866, 13 July 1869; *Globe*, 16 March 1866, 15 July 1869; Daybook, back entry, 29 Aug. 1866, fifty cents to W. Geikie

16 James Miles Langstaff, 'Medical Men in York County November 4, 1867,' inside back cover of Account book, 1867

17 Daybook, 11 Dec. 1855, G. Linfoot child; 28 March 1859, Vale child

18 Daybook, 21 April 1854, Mrs Davis using 'quack plaster'; 7 Sept. 1861, Ben Fox, 'eye ruined by quack'

19 Dellenbaugh's practice seems to have been itinerant: for example, he advertised that he would be in Maple at Noble's Hotel, 'available for consultation on all forms of Lingering Diseases,' in the *York Herald*, 15 Nov. 1861. It is not clear what if any sect he adhered to, although the reference to 'German' invites speculation that he may have been subscribed to the rare 'baunscheidtism' or 'life awakening' techniques mediated by needles on a spring-loaded stalk. Connor, 'Minority Medicine,' 330

20 Daybook, 25 Oct. 1881, 'the nurse Mrs Jordan'; Daybook, 4 May 1887, 'Miss Smith the nurse'; Daybook, 18 Oct. 1888, 'Mrs John Klinck has a nurse for [her] baby'

21 Daybook, 12 Oct. 1859, 8 July 1870

22 Daybook, 10 Nov. 1874, 10 Nov. 1875, 10 Nov. 1876, 9 Nov. 1877. Langstaff sent his physician nephew Elliott to the 1880 dinner. Daybook, back entry, 13 Nov. 1880.

23 *Globe*, 11 Nov. 1874, 11 Nov. 1875, 11 Nov. 1876, 12 Nov. 1877

24 Daybook, back entry, 31 May 1876. In Nov. 1992, Langstaff's grandson, Dr James Rolph Langstaff, found a diploma for a Doctor of Medicine degree issued to 'Jacobus Langstaffe [*sic*]' by the Senate of the University of Victoria College and bearing the same date, 31 May 1876. The connection between Aikens and the Victoria diploma has not yet been explained, although it is possible this diploma was available to all students who had studied with Rolph prior to his association with Victoria.

25 Of thirty-nine consultations done between 1849 and 1851, only two took place in the winter months of Jan. and Dec.; of thirty consultations in 1861, only two were done in Jan. and Dec.

26 Daybook, 21 Dec. 1878, John Snider
27 T. Romano, 'The Medical Profession in Upper Canada, 1820–1870,' paper read at the Kingston Conference on the History of Canadian Science and Technology, Kingston, 1989; Connor, 'Minority Medicine,' 211–13, 372–3
28 Daybook, 4 Nov. 1866, Gibson
29 Daybook, 8 Oct. 1869, Mrs Topham, Sr
30 Daybook, 3 May 1869, William Craig
31 Hostetter was defeated in the East York election for the Ontario legislature by the Reform candidate H.P. Crosby, who had been nominated by Langstaff's friend Simon Miller, seconded by Langstaff's student F.R. Armstrong. *York Herald*, 17 March 1871; *Globe*, 22 March 1871
32 'Public Notice,' *York Herald*, 9 May 1862. Teefy's own copy of the newpaper was the issue later microfilmed by the Archives of Ontario.
33 Daybook, 3 May 1868, Christian
34 Doris Fitzgerald, *Thornhill, 1793–1863: The History of an Ontario Village* (Thornhill 1964), 110–11; AO Teefy papers, MU 2955, *Acts Relating to Powers, Duties, and Protection of Justices of the Peace* (Quebec 1853), inside back cover, clipping inscribed in Teefy's hand, '[Toronto] *Star*, 19 June 1906.' The obituary claimed that Preston was a 'Methodist,' a point that for an unknown reason the Catholic Teefy chose to underline.
35 Daybook, 5 July 1874, Miss Eckhardt
36 Daybook, 1 Jan. 1878, William Young
37 Daybook, 8 Sept. 1888, Isaac adopted child
38 Daybook, 14 and 19 July 1884, Dr Armstrong death and funeral; 4 Jan. 1863, Dr Isaac Bowman; 19 Oct. 1872, Dr W. Comisky
39 *York Herald*, 16, 23 Feb., 3 Aug. 1882. Isaac Bowman published a similar announcement about his return to practice following illness. Ibid., 17 Oct. 1862
40 Ibid., 28 Sept. 1882; *Liberal*, 29 Sept. 1882; Canniff, *Medical Profession*, 570
41 *York Herald*, 29 July 1880
42 Daybook, 2 Oct. 1875, Gamble; 7–8 Oct. 1879, Mrs Bowman and Thos Cook; 23–5 Feb. 1884, visit to Jerry Palmer, Whitby
43 S.A. Holling, 'Each Family Its Own Doctor,' in S.A. Holling, John Senior, Betty Clarkson, and Donald Smith, *Medicine for Heroes: A Neglected Part of Pioneer Life* (Mississauga: Mississauga South Historical Society 1981), 31–49
44 AO, Ely Playter diary, 7 Jan. and 25 Jan. to 6 Feb. 1851

45 Charles Ambrose Carter and Thomas Melville Bailey, eds., *The Diary of Sophia MacNab*, (Hamilton: Griffin 1968), 25–53

46 Daybook, 27 Aug. 1888, Miss Deborah Leak

47 Daybook, 24 July 1888, Jesse Baker

48 Daybook, 19 May 1867, Mrs Dan Tipp

49 Daybook, 10 Sept. 1859, Jobbitt son

50 Daybook, 13 Oct. 1861, Lambert hired man

51 Daybook, 28 Oct. 1861, Biggerstaff

52 W.D. Cosbie, *A History of Toronto General Hospital, 1819–1965: A Chronicle* (Toronto: Macmillan 1975), 58–61; Jacalyn Duffin, '"In View of the Body of Job Broom": A Glimpse of the Medical Knowledge and Practice of John Rolph,' *Canadian Bulletin of Medical History / Bulletin canadien d'histoire de la médicine* 7 (1990): 9–30

53 A boom in hospital-building began shortly after Langstaff's death. See Connor, 'Minority Medicine,' 230; David Gagan, *'A Necessity among Us': The Owen Sound General and Marine Hospital, 1891–1985* (Toronto: University of Toronto Press 1990), 11–14.

54 For lists of horses, their value, origins, and foaling records, see especially Account book, 1867, 92; Account book, 1885, 118, 339. The mare was lamed in the winter of 1857, and the large clipping 'How to examine a horse' (from an unidentified newspaper) was kept with patient entries for March 1878. Daybook, 15 Jan. 1857, 21 March 1878

55 Daybook, 5 Aug. 1863, 21 Feb. 1870, 25 Jan. 1884

56 Daybook, 7 Feb. 1861

57 Daybook, 24–5 Feb. 1868, 23 Feb. 1869

58 Daybook, 7 Sept. 1885, Henry Burkitt

59 Daybook, 15–19 Jan. 1887, Dr Mitchell

60 Daybook, 27 Feb. 1876

61 Daybook, 3 April 1887, Mrs P. Boynton

62 Daybook, 23 Dec. 1883

63 Daybook, 26 Jan. 1889

64 The vivid description of the practice of Dr James Alexander Smith (b. 1870) of Shelburne, Ontario, was written by his son. Donald Smith, 'Country Doctor,' in S.A. Holling et al., *Medicine for Heroes*, 89–93, especially 89.

65 *York Herald*, 28 July 1876

66 Daybook, 23 July 1876, Powell

67 Daybook, 2 Dec. 1870, visit to Busby's brother

68 Daybook, 6 Jan. 1871, visit to Isaac Shell

69 Daybook, 15 June 1852, 30 Dec. 1853, Redon; 25 Dec. 1853, Bovair
70 Daybook, 25 Nov. 1852, 'At Ryan's'
71 Daybook, 29 Nov. 1852 and 11–18 Jan. 1854, Andrew Miller
72 AO, Teefy papers, MU 2946, Account book, 1856–61, 410
73 AO, Estate Files RG 22 series G2, B10, MS 638 reel 78, Cabinet 7, reel 221, Mary Burkitt, died 12 Feb. 1852. The file also contains a clipping of the announcement of Langstaff's intent to adopt the children from *Mackenzie's Weekly Messenger*, 27 Oct. 1856.
74 James Rolph Langstaff, 'The Langstaffs of Richmond Hill, Thornhill, Langstaff, and King,' 1980, photocopy of typewritten manuscript, gift of James Rolph Langstaff, Richmond Hill, to author ('Langstaff scrapbook'), 189
75 *York Herald*, 10, 17 Nov. and 15 Dec. 1876. One political joke was a 'double entendre' reference to the 'Big Push' not as the more familiar political manoeuvre, but as the jolt Langstaff felt when the train he was travelling in was struck by another from behind. On the political 'Big Push' of the year before, see *York Herald*, 5 Nov. 1875.
76 Perhaps other Canadians, like John Langstaff, Jr, detected a certain 'angst' behind the upbeat 'illusion of inevitable progress.' The Centennial celebrated technological urbanism, but it took place at a time of massive change; the 'eulogistic rhetoric' has been said to hint at a posturing discord in the American psyche. Dennis Clark, 'Philadelphia 1876: Celebration and Illusion,' in Dennis Clark, ed., *Philadelphia, 1776– 2076: A Three Hundred Year View* (Port Washington, NY, London: Kennikat Press 1975), 61–3
77 *Canada Medical and Surgical Journal* 5 (1876–7): 95–6, 160–77. Lister chaired one of the sessions at this conference. J.T.H. Connor, 'Joseph Lister's System of Wound Management and the Canadian Practitioner' (MA thesis, University of Western Ontario, 1980), 94
78 The article 'How and Where to Take a Vacation' appeared in the local press just as Langstaff began his practice of taking regular holidays. *York Herald*, 10 July 1879. It is not known where Langstaff stayed while in the north. Vacationing in the Ontario wilderness did not become a popular form of leisure until the 1890s, although some resorts were developed in the 1870s. See R.I. Wolfe, 'The Changing Patterns of Tourism in Ontario,' in *Profiles of a Province: Studies in the History of Ontario* (Toronto: Ontario Historical Society 1967), 173–7.
79 *Globe*, 26 Sept. 1872; Daybook, 25 Sept. 1872, Hamilton fair; 5 Oct. 1870, 23 Sept. 1874, Provincial Exhibition (Toronto); back entry, 16 Sept. 1873, Guelph Central Fair

80 According to the newspaper, *The Messiah* was sung to the 'largest and [most] fashionable audience' by 'a chorus of 100,' but Langstaff, who attended with Dr Geikie, thought there had been 'about 60 singers.' 'Kennedy' may have sung at the Provincial Exhibition. See *Globe*, 19 Dec. 1865; Daybook, 11 Sept. 1860, Prince of Wales; 18 Dec. 1865, 'Messiah'; 11 Sept. 1873, Barnum's show; back entry, 27 Sept. 1866, Kennedy.

81 S.E.D. Shortt, 'Physicians, Science, and Status: Issues in the Professionalization of Anglo-American Medicine in the Nineteenth Century,' *Medical History* 27 (1983): 51–68; Bernier, *La médecine au Québec*, 162

82 Daybook, back entry, 28 May 1884. Generous advance publicity heralded the event, suitably held in Toronto's 'Horticultural Gardens Pavilion.' See, for example, *Globe*, 28 May 1884. On Beecher and evolution, see Clifford E. Clark, Jr, *Henry Ward Beecher: Spokesman for a Middle-Class America* (Urbana, Chicago, London: University of Illinois Press 1978), 257–70. On Beecher and Canada, see Ramsay Cook, *The Regenerators: Social Criticism in Late Victorian English Canada* (Toronto: University of Toronto Press 1985), 15, 46. Beecher's obituary appeared in the Richmond Hill press, an honour usually reserved for local people and extended to international figures only of great renown, such as royalty and statesmen. *York Herald*, 24 March 1887

83 George Rosen, 'Fees and Fee Bills: Some Economic Aspects of Medical Practice in Nineteenth-Century America,' *Bulletin of the History of Medicine* supplement 6 (1946): 1–93

84 The 1866 poster of the Medical Tariff for North York and South Simcoe, signed by James Langstaff with thirty of his colleagues, was reproduced in Sydell Waxman, 'Emily Stowe: Feminist and Healer,' *Beaver* 72 (April–May 1992): 26–30, especially 29. Langstaff paid fifty cents to Dr Walter Geikie towards the publication of the fee schedule. Daybook, back entry, 29 Aug. 1866.

85 Charles G. Roland and Bohodar Rubashewsky, 'The Economic Status of the Practice of Dr Harmaunus Smith in Wentworth County, Ontario 1826–67', *Canadian Bulletin of Medical History / Bulletin canadien d'histoire de la médecine* 5 (1988): 29–49. See also Marc Lebel, 'Pectoral Syrup and Cupping Glasses: A Doctor's Account Book, 1862–1868,' *Archivist* 19 (1992): 7–8.

86 Jan Coombs, 'Rural Medical Practice in the 1880s: A View from Central Wisconsin,' *Bulletin of the History of Medicine* 64 (1990): 35–62; E. Brooks Holifield, 'The Wealth of Nineteenth-Century American Physicians,'

Bulletin of the History of Medicine 64 (1990): 79–85; Christian-F. Roques, 'The Professional and Economic Data on the Activity of a Country Physician from the South of France in 1869,' paper read at the 32nd International Congress on the History of Medicine, Antwerp, 1990, to be published in *Acta Belgica Historiae Medicinae*, in press

87 S.E.D. Shortt, '"Before the Age of Miracles": the Rise, Fall, and Rebirth of General Practice in Canada, 1890–1940,' in Charles G. Roland, ed., *Health, Disease, and Medicine*, 123–52, especially 135

88 M.C. Urquhart and K.A.H. Buckley, eds., *Historical Statistics of Canada* (Toronto: Macmillan; Cambridge: Cambridge University Press 1965), 93–4. On the monetary conversion from pounds to dollars, which took place at the end of Langstaff's first decade in practice, see A.B. McCullough, 'Currency Conversion in British North America,' *Archivaria* 16 (1983): 83–94. For the purposes of this study, one pound has been considered equivalent to four dollars.

89 There are several records concerning Langstaff's hired help. The most complete is the account of Alfred Quantz, who earned $1.50 daily from March 1877 to Jan. 1879. Account book, 1875, 362–5. Domestic servants appear to have been paid $3.00 and board each month, until after 1885, when the wage was increased to $5.00 or $6.00 a month.

90 Langstaff declared an income of $2,000 yearly in the 1861 Canada Census. c 1089 Vaughan Township, District II, 42 no. 5

91 *Globe* report cited in Godfrey, *Medicine for Ontario*, 203

92 In 1849–50 Langstaff owed Teefy less than £3, whereas his father owed almost £40. In 1854–8 Langstaff's debt, which had risen to more than £50, was discharged by several different means: an amount brought forward from another account, attendance on Teefy's in-laws the Clarkson family, fifteen and a half cords of wood, and cash. Teefy charged the doctor interest at six per cent and listed his debts among those he considered 'good' as opposed to those that were 'bad' or 'doubtful.' AO, Teefy Papers, MU 2930–2954, Accounts and Ledgers, especially MU 2931, 364; MU 2947, separate list of good and bad debts; MU 2953, 95, 114, 234, 279, 614

93 Langstaff's case for medical or other unknown reasons against the Carruthers' estate seems to have consumed more than the usual amount of time. It was settled in the doctor's favour with an award of $100, $10 of which Langstaff gave to his lawyer Charles Durand. Daybook, 25 Sept. 1873 and back entry, same date

94 Daybook, back entry, 13 Jan. 1862. Langstaff gave his student Armstrong $10 to replace $10 he had lost. Daybook, back entry, 28 Sept. 1869

95 *Liberal,* 27 May 1881

96 Account book, 1885, inside cover

97 See, for example, a list of patients seen at the request of his brother, Dr Lewis Langstaff, kept as account in the brother's name. Account book 1869, 141

98 *York Herald,* 17 April 1884

99 J.T.H. Connor, '"Preservatives of Health": Mineral Water Spas of Nineteenth-Century Ontario,' *Ontario History* 75 (1983): 135–52

100 The information concerning property has been assembled from a tangled collection of sources, including the daybooks, ledgers, archival deed records, property tax payments, newspaper advertisements, and the estate file. The addresses of the Toronto properties changed several times while Langstaff owned them.

101 Edward Phelps, 'Foundations of the Canadian Oil Industry, 1850–1866,' in *Profiles of a Province,* 156–65

102 *York Herald,* 13 May 1859

103 AO, Estate Files, GS 1–959, Cabinet 2, reel 422, no. 191, John Langstaff

104 See especially description in Daybook, back entry, 29 Sept. to 1 Oct. 1859; 16 Sept. 1873.

105 AO, Teefy Papers, MU 2952, Letter Book 1850–53, title page. A registered letter to G.W. Houghton was likely a payment made by Langstaff on his second Toronto property (see note 107 below). Ibid., MU 2949, Letter Book 1855–60, 10 Feb. 1859

106 Pasted in Account book, 1869, 246. Calculations of instalments due were kept with directions to Scadding's well-known residence in Trinity Square. Account book, 1862, 194

107 The property was bounded by Queen Street, Muter (now Palmerston Avenue), Lumley (now Euclid Ave), and Golding Street (now Euclid Place). The seller was G.W. Houghton, who died shortly after this purchase; Langstaff continued his payments to Houghton's executor, R.B. Miller.

108 Unable to resist a comparison with Toronto real estate, I discovered that half of one building located on or near the site of one of Langstaff's five Queen Street stores was listed for sale at $850,000 in the summer of 1988.

109 Account book, 1869, 319; *York Herald,* 29 Oct. and 5 Nov. 1875. The exact number of Richmond Hill lots sold is unknown; more Wallaceburg lots were sold later.

110 Canada Census 1871, C 9967, Vaughan Division II, Schedule 1, p. 45, Schedule 3, p. 5, and Schedule 5, p. 45 no. 14

111 Account book, 1867, 58, entry dated 19 March 1874. For the doctor's

1870–79 experiences with 'Fowls,' see especially Account book, 1867, 52–8, 72, 93–100; Account book, 1885, inside cover.

112 Account book, 1866, 156

113 Account book, 1885, 4, 340–1; 'Big Apple,' *York Herald*, 30 Oct. 1879

114 For more on mills in southern Ontario, see Leo A. Johnson, *A History of the County of Ontario* (Whitby: Corporation of the County of Ontario 1973), 137, 212, 327–9; G. Elmore Reaman, *A History of Vaughan Township* (Toronto: University of Toronto Press 1971), 54–8, 62; I. Champion, ed., *Markham, 1793–1900* (Markham: Markham District Historical Society 1989), 115–130.

115 A 'water powered' sawmill, owned by John Langstaff, with an investment of £500, no other employees, and a capacity of '460 ' " ' [*sic*]. The symbol, ' " , likely represents the term 'feet inch,' written in longhand elsewhere in the same census, signifying the mill had the capacity of 460 board feet in twelve hours. Canada Census 1851, c 11759–60, Vaughan township, District ii. For more on the outfitting and operation of Canadian mills, see Graeme Wynn, *Timber Colony: A Historical Geography of Early Nineteenth-Century New Brunswick* (Toronto: University of Toronto Press 1981), 111 and passim.

116 The history of this mill has been difficult to trace. From the census of 1861 and of 1871, it apparently passed first to the politician Amos Wright and then to Asa Wilson. Langstaff may have held a mortgage on the mill when it was purchased by Wright. See also Langstaff's notes on the 1854 purchase of an 'Estate ... of Brother John Langstaff,' described as having a 'race,' 'floom' [*sic*], and 'dam.' Account book, 1852, 346. See also 1855 and 1856 accounts with John Langstaff concerning 'rent of mill at £100 a year' and a mortgage. Account book, 1847–9 (unpaginated), 27, 29. At the same time, a similar arrangement was made between brothers in neighbouring Ontario county; see W.H. Graham, *Greenbank: Country Matters in 19th Century Ontario* (Peterborough, Ont. and Lewiston, NY: Broadview Press 1988), 56).

117 See especially the bill submitted by John Dancy for 'Travling Expences' incurred on trip 'from Arora' to 'Orilia,' including the cost of 'touls' and staying a 'knight at Fosters' [*sic*]. Langstaff advanced money to Mrs John Dancy during her husband's absence. Account book, 1866, 41

118 See especially Account book, 1867, 217.

119 Daybook, back entry, 11 March 1875

120 Account book, 1869, 326, Francis Kempt

121 Daybook, back entries, 20 Dec. 1875, Sam Mager; 16 July 1879, James

Lawrence; 16 March 1880, Sam Mager. The factory was sold to 'Messrs Daniels and Major,' although Langstaff's tenant Mager seems to have continued working there. *York Herald*, 7 Aug. 1879

122 Statement made 4 Aug. 1885 concerning lot 2, concession 5, Medonte township, Simcoe; Account book, 1885, 160

123 A systematic examination of the estate files of Ontario doctors would lend some comparative meaning to this seemingly large figure. In the course of this study I saw the estate files of a few deceased physicians at the Archives of Ontario. None came close to the value of Langstaff's estate. For example: Dr Lewis Langstaff (died 1878), value $9,095; Dr Lang (died 1880), value $2,800; Dr John N. Reid (died 1882) value $4,900 (of which $2,000 were book debts); Dr James Ross (died 1892), value $39,900. Non-medical comparisons are offered by two estates: that of the Richmond Hill baker, George Soules (died 1880), whose assets, valued at $8,651, were nearly half in the form of 'book debts'; and that of politician-editor-statesman George Brown (died 1880), valued at over $160,000. AO Estate Files, GS1-985, no. 3335, Cabinet 2, reel 448, Dr Lewis Langstaff; GS1-986, no. 3344, Cabinet 2, reel 449, Dr Lang; GS1-991, no. 4677, Cabinet 2, reel 454, Dr John N. Reid; GS1-1028, Cabinet 2, reel 491, no. 9041, Dr James Ross; GS1-986, no. 3597, Cabinet 2, reel 451, George Soules; MS 583, reel 10, vol. 20, 458–9, Cabinet 4, reel 420, George Brown

124 Michael Bliss, *Northern Enterprise: Five Centuries of Canadian Business* (Toronto: McClelland and Stewart 1987), 266, 269

125 Members promised to buy a certain number of shares; in the interval, funds were lent to members, and when all shares were paid up, the society terminated. Ibid., 269

126 AO, Lauder family papers, MS-567, reel 1, letters from Matthew Teefy to John Lauder 21 Nov. 1862, 4 Dec. 1863, 2 Jan. 1864

127 Daybook, back entry, 18 June 1880. In the many entries concerning OILIC a few other board members were partially identified: 'Walton,' 'Fitch,' 'Duggan,' and 'Gormley.'

128 Bliss, *Northern Enterprise*, 265–7

129 Ibid., 279. It would be interesting to discover to what extent Langstaff's diversification to milling and real estate in the 1850s and to industrial shares in the 1880s was typical of Ontario agricultural and professional 'gentlemen' and if it was related in any way to his political leanings. For a discussion of portfolio diversification and its relation to political interests among mid-nineteenth-century British landowners, see Cheryl Schonhardt-Bailey, 'Specific Factors, Capital Markets, Portfolio Diversi-

fication, and Free Trade: Domestic Determinants of the Repeal of the Corn Laws,' *World Politics* 43 (1991): 545–69.

130 In 1885, when Langstaff wrote his will, he anticipated the value of his stocks would be $10,000, but at his death in 1889 they were worth $6,320. In 1886 he claimed to have increased his holdings to 5,000 shares from the original 30. The value of shares seems to have fluctuated. One entry placed it at $50 per share. Daybook, back entry, 7 Jan. 1884. A document printed by Matthew Teefy's stockbrocker listed the 1892 Toronto Stock Exchange figures for OILIC shares as between $108 and $117. AO, Teefy papers, MU 2955, document printed by Pellat and Pellat

131 Daybook, 5 Sept. 1888, Mrs John Fry

CHAPTER 3 **Medical Knowledge in Diagnosis:
Physical Signs at the Bedside**

1 John Harley Warner, *The Therapeutic Perspective: Medical Practice, Knowledge, and Identity in America, 1820–1885* (Cambridge Mass., London England: Harvard University Press 1986), 7. In contrast, reflecting a not unjustified but somewhat positivistic attitude to present diagnostic categories and implying that doctors were unable to make accurate diagnoses earlier, Shorter considers 'the period between 1880 and 1950 ... as "modern"' because of 'the doctors' ability correctly to diagnose disease: not to *cure* it, but to recognize what it was the patient had.' Edward Shorter, *Bedside Manners: The Troubled History of Doctors and Patients* (Harmondsworth, England: Viking Penguin 1986), 75. On the history of diseases and the early nineteenth-century changes in ways of thinking about them, see J.T.H. Connor, 'Medical Technology in Victorian Canada,' *Canadian Bulletin of Medical History / Bulletin canadien d'histoire de la médecine* 3 (1986): 97–123; Michel Foucault, *The Birth of the Clinic: An Archeology of Medical Perception*, trans. A.M. Sheridan-Smith (London: Tavistock 1973); Lester S. King, *Medical Thinking: An Historical Preface* (Princeton, NJ: Princeton University Press 1982); Stanley Joel Reiser, *Medicine and the Reign of Technology* (Cambridge and New York: Cambridge University Press 1978), 23–66; Charles E. Rosenberg, 'Introduction: Framing Disease: Illness, Society, and History,' in Charles E. Rosenberg and Janet Golden, eds., *Framing Disease: Studies in Cultural History* (New Brunswick, NJ: Rutgers University Press 1992), xiii–xvi.

2 National Archives of Canada (NAC), MG 24 B 24, John Rolph, 'Medical Notes,' vol. 3, 92

3 James Miles Langstaff, Langstaff daybook (Daybook), 9 Aug. 1866, Mrs Nicholls, Sr; 19 Feb. 1879, Joseph Espey

4 Daybook, 3 March 1886, Shank child

5 Daybook, 3 Dec. 1861, Fierheller's son Lewis

6 Daybook, 12 July 1873, Johnson son

7 Daybook, 29 March 1880, C. Chamberlain little girl

8 Daybook, 16 Dec. 1865, John Legg

9 Daybook, 11 June 1863, Jo Latter child

10 Daybook, 25 Feb. 1885, Mrs Holmes

11 Daybook, 3 Dec. 1867, Mrs Henry Miller, Jr; 29 Aug. 1881, W.D. Miller

12 Daybook, 19 Feb., 22 Dec. 1853, Mrs Moore

13 Daybook, 22 Dec. 1853, Mrs Wm Birch. Langstaff had already used the words 'erythema nodosum' earlier whether or not he witnessed the rash, while attending a post-partum patient with cough. Daybook, 11 Oct. 1852, Grady

14 Daybook, 31 May 1862, Mrs Phillips. This patient may have suffered from ecthyma gangrenosum, the skin lesions of a widespread infection due to the Pseudomonas organism.

15 Daybook, 7 Nov. 1864, Kinnie; 6 Feb. 1865, Dunn little boy; 25 Sept. 1864, Teefy little girl

16 Daybook, 5–6 Dec. 1853, Morley's son

17 Daybook, 27 May 1886, Mrs John Brown and Dr Bethune

18 Daybook, 8, 24 Dec. 1869, 6 Nov., 20 Dec. 1870, Thos Boynton

19 Daybook, 4 June 1873, Catherine Linn

20 Daybook, 26 Feb. 1885, D.S. Raeman

21 Daybook, 3–4 April 1888, H. Payne

22 Daybook, 26 May 1887, Mrs Wm Vanderburgh

23 Daybook, 17 Sept. 1887, T. Hicks

24 The last sign seems not to have figured in the record prior to 1865.

25 Daybook, 21 Sept. 1872, Mrs Robbs

26 Daybook, 12 March 1884, Miss Pierce

27 Daybook, 16–18 Jan. 1854, M. Teefy

28 Daybook, back entry, 25 May 1865. Bird, who acquired a flexible stethoscope in 1843, is said to have been the first doctor at Guy's to use the instrument. Audrey B. Davis, *Medicine and Its Technology* (Westport, Conn.: Greenwood 1981), 103–4

29 Daybook, 26 May 1865, G.P. Dickson

30 Daybook, 31 Dec. 1864, Clara Teefy. See also Daybook, 18 Sept. 1885, 'a great cavity in top of left lung,' anon.

31 Daybook, 1 July 1869, Mrs Jo Wilmot

32 Daybook, 18 May 1875, H. Hurst
33 Daybook, 10–11 May 1865, Deverick and Dr Reid. See also 18 Nov. 1866, Chris Henrick and Dr Eckhardt.
34 James Langstaff, 'Complete Consolidation of One Lung,' *Canada Lancet* 12 (1880): 198. I am grateful to Jim Connor for drawing this special item to my attention.
35 Urinary 'albumin' was mentioned in the 1850s, but 'heat coagulation' was specifically recorded first in 1864. Daybook, 4 Dec. 1864, Mrs John Gray. See also Reiser, *Reign of Technology*, 127.
36 Daybook, 4–5 May 1887, Miss Wilcocks and 'Miss Smith the nurse'
37 Daybook, 21 Oct. 1865, Miss Bennett; 22 Nov. 1881, 26 July 1882, Mrs widow Reid; 12 Nov. 1886, Hennesey
38 Daybook, 26 March 1861, Major Button
39 Langstaff's first record of specific gravity came in a consultation with Dr Ardah of Barrie, but it was one year later that he used a 'urinometer' in his own practice. Daybook, 1 Dec. 1863, Reverend Samuel Johnson; 5 Dec. 1864, Mrs John Gray
40 Reiser, *Reign of Technology*, 135
41 University of Toronto, Trinity College Archives, Trinity Medical College, 'Announcement, 1855–56'; J. Bernier, *La médecine au Québec: Naissance et évolution d'une profession* (Quebec: Presses de l'Université Laval 1989), 135–6
42 See, for example, 'Blood-stains Detected by Microspectroscope' and J. Baker Edwards 'Microscopic Examination of Flesh,' *Canada Medical Journal* 3 (1866–7): 139–40 and 5 (1868–9): 481–4 respectively.
43 *York Herald*, 8 Feb. 1861; *Markham Economist*, 2 Sept. 1875; John Harley Warner, '"Exploring the Inner Labyrinths of Creation": Popular Microscopy in Nineteenth-century America,' *Journal of the History of Medicine and Allied Sciences* 37 (1982): 7–33
44 Daybook, back entry, 21 Nov. 1879; back entry, 14 Aug. 1889, 'Inventory'
45 Daybook, 7 Feb. 1888, Henry Jennings
46 Daybook, 13 Feb. 1872, Leonard Klinck
47 Daybook, 31 March 1885, Edward Grice
48 Daybook, 9 July 1888, Mrs widow Gid Hislop; 26 March 1886, Lance Nicholls child
49 Daybook, 21–2 Nov. 1861, Davis
50 Daybook, 26 Aug. 1857, Linton child; 25 July 1875, Thomas Wilson
51 Daybook, 23 Oct. 1872, George Hoshel
52 Davis, *Medicine and Its Technology*, 61–2

53 Ibid., 81; Daniel M. Musher, Edward A. Dominguez, and Ariel Bar-Sela, 'Edouard Séguin and the Social Power of Thermometry,' *New England Journal of Medicine* 316 (1987): 115–17.

54 See, for example, 'The Thermometer in Disease,' *Canada Medical Journal* 2(1865–6): 471–5.

55 Daybook, 1 May 1878, Grainger eldest and Dr Rupert

56 Reviewed in *Canada Medical and Surgical Journal* 5 (1877–8): 115–18

57 'Clinical thermometer, to Matthew Teefy,' Daybook, back entry, 10 Jan. 1881

58 Daybook, 18 Jan. 1883, Wm Pogue; 4 July 1884, John Gorman and Dr Gari Langstaff

59 On the impact of insurance companies in the USA, see Davis, *Medicine and Its Technology*, 191; Audrey B. Davis, 'Life Insurance and the Physical Examination: A Chapter in the Rise of American Medical Technology,' *Bulletin of the History of Medicine* 55 (1981): 392–406.

60 Insurance companies in order of appearance in the Daybooks: Hartford, Aetna, Dominion, Atlantic Mutual, Land and Lane, Sun Life, and Mutual.

61 Daybook, 10 May 1871, John Reid Teefy; 23 June 1871, Mr and Mrs Teefy; 8 Aug. 1882, 21 people

62 Daybook, 22 April 1885, Thomas Kirby; 17 June 1881, Charles Chamberlain

63 Daybook, 12 March 1874, Mrs Thos Cook

64 Daybook, 10 Sept. 1859, Jobbitt

65 Daybook, 26 Feb. 1861, Johnathan Shell's son Rob

66 R.T.H. Laennec, *Traité de l'auscultation médiate et des maladies des poumons et du coeur*, 2nd ed., 2 vols. (Paris: Chaudé, 1826), vol. 2, 630

67 Warner, *The Therapeutic Perspective*, 89–91

68 Daybook, 10 Jan. 1853, G. Collard

69 Daybook, 27 June 1882, Thomas Rand boy

70 Daybook, 3 April 1885, Ed Grice and Dr Garibaldi Langstaff

71 Daybook, 10 Aug. 1885, Mrs Coulter

72 Daybook, 28 May 1859, Shell son; 14 Nov. 1884, Maggie Young; 20 Oct. 1861, William Comisky; 13 April 1856, Isaac Watson

73 Daybook, 9 Dec. 1856, Andrew Miller; 18 April 1861, Hugh McLean; 11 Feb. 1866, Conger; 19 Feb. 1867, Thedore Law; 19 May 1864, Newton, Sr; 3 Sept. 1861, Snowdon child

74 Daybook, 14 April 1875, Emily Beynon; 15 Nov. 1873, Mrs Sims; 28 May 1869, Miss Hemmingway at Holdrige home

75 Daybook, 16 June 1880, Mrs Haffey, Sr. John Cheyne (1777–1835)

published the first report of periodic breathing in Dublin in 1818;
William Stokes (1804–78) reaffirmed it in 1846.

76 Daybook, 25 Dec. 1886, Samuel Line. Adolf Kussmaul (1822–1902)
published his observation on the deep breathing of acidosis in 1874.

77 Daybook, 22 May 1854, Mrs H. Stewart. Ludwig G. Courvoisier (1843–
1918) described his sign or 'law' in 1890.

78 Daybook, 30 April 1861, Joseph Mapes, Jr. The sign was described by
Charles McBurney (1845–1913) in 1889.

79 Daybook, 21 Oct. 1876, Sheppard; 31 July 1883, Strebbing. Antonin B.J.
Marfan (1858–1942) published a description of 'dolichosternomelia' in
1896.

80 Daybook, 18 Feb. 1852, Anon; 7 April 1856, Mrs James Gamble and two
other family members; 30 Aug. 1873, Ansley child and several other
cases in Aug. 1873

81 Daybook, 19 July 1859, Johnathan Shell son

CHAPTER 4 **Medical Knowledge in Therapy:**
Old Stand-bys, Innovations, and Intangibles

1 See for example, J. Worth Estes, 'Drug Use at the Infirmary, the
Example of Dr Andrew Duncan, Sr,' in Guenter Risse, *Hospital Life in
Enlightenment Scotland: Care and Teaching at the Royal Infirmary of
Edinburgh* (Cambridge: Cambridge University Press 1986), 351–84;
Morris J. Vogel and Charles E. Rosenberg, eds., *The Therapeutic Revolu-
tion: Essays in the Social History of American Medicine* (Philadelphia:
University of Pennsylvania 1979); John Harley Warner, *The Therapeutic
Perspective: Medical Practice, Knowledge, and Identity in America, 1820–
1885* (Cambridge, Mass., and London: Harvard University Press 1986);
Chauncey D. Leake, *An Historical Account of Pharmacology to the
Twentieth Century* (Springfield, Ill.: Charles C. Thomas 1975).

2 Edward Shorter, *Bedside Manners: The Troubled History of Doctors and
Patients* (Harmondsworth: Viking Penguin 1986), 26–38, 81–6, 92–102

3 Warner, *Therapeutic Perspective*, 83–161, especially 117–20; John Harley
Warner, 'Power, Conflict, and Identity in Mid-Nineteenth Century
American Medicine: Therapeutic Change at the Commercial Hospital in
Cincinnati,' *Journal of American History* 73 (1987): 934–56

4 For details concerning the history and properties of these remedies,
see Estes, 'Drug use at the infirmary'; Warner, *Therapeutic Perspective*;
Leake, *Historical Account*.

5 Accounts with pharmacists Hallamore and Rob Hall can be found in

James Miles Langstaff's account books (Account book), 1862, 103–5; 1867, 83; 1866–9, 73.

6 James Miles Langstaff, Langstaff daybook (Daybook), 27 Oct. 1861, B. Lyons daughter

7 'Narcotism,' Daybook, 12 July 1852, Stephenson; 24 May 1872, Conger little boy; 1 April 1873, George Stephenson

8 Daybook, 3 April 1868, Mrs Wm Stephenson

9 Daybook, 9 April 1886, Mrs Jo Farmer

10 Daybook, 6 Jan. 1869, Ayerst child

11 Daybook, 16 April 1864, Dedman

12 Jacalyn Duffin and Pierre René, '"Anti-moine; Anti-biotique": The Public Fortunes of the Secret Properties of Antimony Potassium Tartrate (Tartar Emetic),' *Journal of the History of Medicine and Allied Sciences* 46 (1991): 440–56

13 Charles E. Rosenberg, 'The Therapeutic Revolution: Medicine, Meaning, and Social Change in Nineteenth-Century America,' in Vogel and Rosenberg, *Therapeutic Revolution*, 3–25, especially 8

14 John S. Haller, *American Medicine in Transition, 1840–1910* (Urbana, Ill., and London: University of Illinois Press 1981), 77–90

15 Daybook, 12 Dec. 1862, Dr Hostetter; 3 Jan. 1868, Dr Reid; 31 Dec. 1875, Dr McConnell

16 'Evidence against Internal Use of Mercury,' *Canada Medical Journal* 1 (1864–5): 143–4

17 Daybook, 27 Dec. 1888, Mrs Ira Baker; 30 Jan. 1889, Adam Wideman child

18 Samuel Strickland, *Twenty-seven Years in Canada West or The Experience of an Early Settler*, ed. Agnes Strickland (Edmonton: Hurtig 1970), 209–10

19 John S. Haller, 'The Use and Abuse of Tartar Emetic in the Nineteenth-Century Materia Medica,' *Bulletin of the History of Medicine* 49 (1975): 235–57

20 Daybook, 12 Dec. 1872, J.K. Smith child; 28 Feb. 1874, Ab Eyer little boy

21 Daybook, 7 Dec. 1861, Davis; 19 Sept. 1868, Lloyd; 29 Nov. 1875, Elias Nigh son

22 Daybook, 9–10 Nov. 1861, Teefy son Baldwin

23 Guenter B. Risse, 'The Renaissance of Bloodletting: A Chapter in Modern Therapeutics,' *Journal of the History of Medicine and Allied Sciences* 34 (1979): 3–22

24 W.D. Cosbie, *A History of Toronto General Hospital, 1819–1965: A Chronicle* (Toronto: Macmillan 1975), 59–60; Archives of Ontario (AO),

pamphlet, *Report of an Investigation by Trustees of Toronto General Hospital into Certain Charges against the Management of that Institution* (Toronto: Globe Book and Job Publishers 1855), Second Day of Testimony, Dr Wright

25 Daybook, 25 Oct. 1888, Fred Quantz

26 Warner, *Therapeutic Perspective*, 115–16. Some physicians were opposed to bleeding therapy. J.T.H. Connor has suggested that bloodletting was rare in Ontario practice. He intriguingly speculates on the possible influence of physicians trained in Scotland, where bleeding was frowned upon. He used evidence from Langstaff's practice, but without further studies it is difficult to say whether or not use of the modality roughly twice a week on a total of 3.5 to 5 per cent of patients would qualify as 'rare.' J.T.H. Connor, 'Minority Medicine in Ontario: A Study of Medical Pluralism and Its Decline' (Ph.D. thesis, University of Waterloo, 1989), 251

27 Daybook, 18 Aug. 1879, Caldwell; 6 May 1886, Mrs John Brown; William Canniff, *A Manual of the Practice of Surgery* (Philadelphia: Lindsay and Blakiston 1866), 76–80

28 Daybook, 11 June 1883, cupping of several patients; 17 July 1888, Mrs Graham

29 Daybook, 19 June 1858, Peter Hizey; 6 Feb. 1861, Mrs Robert Marsh; 6, 22, 23 Nov. 1863 and 18 March 1864, Mrs Wm Stephenson

30 K. Codell Carter, 'On the Decline of Bloodletting in Nineteenth Century Medicine,' *Journal of Psychoanalytic Anthropology* 5 (1982): 219–34; Barbara Duden, *The Woman Beneath the Skin: A Doctor's Patients in Eighteenth-Century Germany* (Cambridge, Mass.: Harvard University Press 1991), 116–18

31 Daybook, 10 Sept. 1870, Glover male child; 9 July 1875, Jack Robinson little boy

32 Daybook, 3 Dec. 1866, Prentiss little boy

33 Daybook, 2 July 1871, McConaghy boy; 14 Aug. 1873, William Harrison child

34 Daybook, 30 Oct. 1881, Mrs Waterfield

35 Daybook, 12 March 1870, David Welsh

36 Daybook, 2 Aug. 1861, Mrs Geo Atkinson

37 Daybook, 14 Jan. 1872, William Alison; 19 Oct. 1872, Comisky

38 Daybook, 6 May 1868, William Clary

39 Daybook, 23 Sept. 1861, Dr Reid and Mrs Richens; 25 Dec. 1875, Dr Reid and Jewsberry; 6 May 1887, Dr Nelles

40 Daybook, 1 Oct. 1886, Wm Boynton, Sr

41 Daybook, 19 April 1875, John Beynon daughter Emily

42 Daybook, 27 Feb. 1887, John Gormley

43 Daybook, 18–19 Dec. 1861, Mrs widow Atkinson

44 Daybook, 19 Dec. 1887, John Elson child; 9 March 1865, Crawford

45 Daybook, 14 Feb. 1876, Sam Williams; 2 July 1887, Thomas Young

46 Daybook, 17 Aug. 1853, Mrs Lawrence; 25 July 1868, Witherford, Sr; 30 Jan. 1875, Ramsay

47 Daybook, 19 Oct. 1862, Miss E. Davis

48 Daybook, 26 Nov. 1867, Mrs P. Basingtwaite

49 Daybook, 21–3 Oct. 1865, Barna Lyons child

50 Daybook, 21 Oct. 1879, Mrs Arch McCollum

51 AO, Teefy Papers, MU 2946, Account book, 1856–61, np 'C. Durant [sic] gargling oil' 3 June 1857; MU 2950, Invoice book, entries on stocks of gargling oil and liniment. Shorter has suggested that families 'loved' using their own 'hokum' treatments as an alternative to medical consultation and would turn to the doctor out of desperation as a conduit to drugs that 'really worked.' Shorter, Bedside Manners, 62–9. On folk remedies, see also S.A. Holling, 'Each Family Its Own Doctor,' in S.A. Holling, John Senior, Betty Clarkson, and Donald Smith, Medicine for Heroes: A Neglected Part of Pioneer Life (Mississauga, Ont.: Mississauga South Historical Society 1981), 31–49; Guenter Risse, Ronald L. Numbers, and Judith Leavitt, eds., Medicine without Doctors: Home Health Care in American History (New York: Science History Publications 1977).

52 J.K. Aronson, An Account of the Foxglove and its Medical Uses, 1785–1985 (Oxford: Oxford University Press 1985), 2, 317–25

53 Digitalis actually declined in popularity from approximately 1820 to 1900. J. Worth Estes, Hall Jackson and the Purple Foxglove: Medical Practice and Research in Revolutionary America, 1760–1820 (Hanover, NH: University of New England 1979), 228–9

54 Daybook, 20 Feb. 1852, Thompson

55 Daybook, 20 Sept. 1883, Mrs Reach; 9 Jan. 1885, Maggie Young

56 Daybook, 11 April 1875, Nelson Bell and Dr Armstrong

57 Daybook, 3 June 1884, John Wright

58 Jacalyn Duffin, '"In View of the Body of Job Broom": A Glimpse of the Medical Knowledge and Practice of John Rolph,' Canadian Bulletin of Medical History / Bulletin canadien d'histoire de la médecine 7 (1990): 9–30

59 Daybook, 12 March 1851, Mrs Josh Atkinson. See also Daybook, 5 March 1865, Nigh; 27 April 1865, Mrs W.H. Lawrence; 17 Jan. 1869, Mrs Friek; 2 June 1880, Mrs Dr Ed Playter; 14 June 1886, Moses Vanderburgh.

60 Daybook, 14 April 1888, Middleton

61 Daybook, 18 June 1886, Maggie Doner

62 Leake, *Historical Account*, 28, 115

63 John S. Haller, 'Aconite: A Case Study in Doctrinal Conflict and the Meaning of Scientific Medicine,' *Bulletin of the New York Academy of Medicine* 60 (1984): 888–904

64 Warner, *Therapeutic Perspective*, 117, 119, 227

65 Daybook, 27 Dec. 1858, Mrs George Wise

66 Daybook, 27 March 1867, Sidon son; 1 Feb. 1869, Jas Newton, Jr; 18 Feb. 1871, Grainger little boy

67 Daybook, 19, 22 Dec. 1869, H. Jenning daughter; 6 May 1874, Reverend Hunt; 18 April 1880, Mrs Wm Ford

68 Daybook, 21 May 1870, Hitchcook

69 Daybook, 5 May 1872, Mrs Dalton; 16 Oct. 1874, Ed Glover

70 Daybook, 4 April 1873, George Dibb; 20 May 1873, Arch Wright little boy; 13 April 1885, Mrs Jesse Baker

71 Warner, *Therapeutic Perspective*, 117, 119

72 Leake, *Historical Account*, 154

73 Daybook, 6 Jan. 1873, Mrs Henry Walker; 1 March 1874, Mrs Sellars; 1 June 1879, 26 Aug. 1881, Mrs Ben Case. Potassium bromide appeared on Langstaff's pharmacy bill in Jan. 1869. Account book, 1866–9, 73, Hallamore

74 Leake, *Historical Account*, 122; Warner, *Therapeutic Perspective*, 270

75 William Wright, 'Chloral Hydrate,' *Canada Medical Journal* 7 (1870–1): 393–405. See also in the same volume remarks about the drug on pages 20, 21, 23, 40, 79, 186, 230, 337, 388, 487.

76 Cheryl Krasnick Warsh, *Moments of Unreason: The Practice of Canadian Psychiatry and the Homewood Retreat, 1883–1923* (Montreal, Kingston, London, and Buffalo: McGill-Queen's University Press 1989), 145–7

77 Roderick E. McGrew, *Encyclopedia of Medical History* (New York: McGraw-Hill 1985), 257

78 Daybook, 26 March 1878, Elizabeth Cook

79 Daybook, back entries, 24 May 1861, galvanic soles; 8 Oct. 1861, electric machine

80 Carlotta Hacker, *The Indomitable Lady Doctors* (Toronto and Vancouver: Clarke, Irwin 1974), 46–7. An advertisement for Dr Trout's galvanic baths appeared in the *Globe*, 6 Aug. 1875

81 Daybook, 12 Oct. 1861, Edward Jourdan

82 Daybook, back entries, 25 March 1867; 4 April 1868

83 Daybook, 15 Feb. 1875, Mrs Wm Devlin

84 Daybook, 23–4 April 1879, Redditt, Coleman, Shaffer, Doner

85 Daybook, 24 May 1872, Conger little boy; 23 Oct. 1878, Mrs Thomas Frizby

86 Daybook, 29 Dec. 1866, Mrs Harrington; 14 June 1867, Sedman little girl

87 Daybook, 24 March 1861, Mrs T. Martin; 30 Oct. 1886, George Morrison

88 Daybook, 18 Sept. 1874, Mrs John Perkins; 1 Feb. 1869, Mrs Jas Newton, Jr; 19 April 1868, Mrs Davy

89 Daybook, 19 Sept. 1868, L[l]oyd; 29–30 Nov. 1875, Elias Nigh son

90 Daybook, 17 Jan. 1886, Thos Cosgrove child

91 Daybook, 28 May 1882, Mrs Lymburner, Sr

92 Daybook, 22 March 1863, Gilmore; 9 July 1881, Mrs Wilton

93 Daybook, 16 Feb. 1869, D.S. MacDonald child; 24 Sept. 1869, Milan child

94 Daybook, 7 Nov. 1866, Thos Frisby son; 19 May 1864, Newton, Sr

95 Daybook, 24 Dec. 1874, Lewis Peterson

96 Daybook, 2 July 1887, Thomas Young; 22 March 1887, Henricks

97 Daybook, 31 Oct. 1887, Brydon little girl

98 Daybook, 8 June 1859, Gamble

99 Daybook, 10 May 1852, Rush child; 6 Feb. 1887, Lance Nicholls child

100 Daybook, 20 April 1869, Miss Hemmingway

101 Daybook, 13 May 1883, Elsworth L[l]oyd

102 Daybook, 4 Oct. 1863, Hawkins; 9 Jan. 1867, Williams

103 Daybook, 17–18 Oct. 1862, Miss E. Davis. See also Daybook, 10 Feb. 1874, Miss Dibb; 13 Jan. 1883, Mrs Ross; 4 April 1887, Henricks.

104 Daybook, 22 Nov. 1880, Pipher son

105 Daybook, 27 Jan. 1885, Maggie Young

106 Daybook, 4 Aug. 1865, James Hunter, Sr; 27 March 1866, Miss Haven

107 Daybook, 27 May 1879, John Walker

108 Daybook, 5 Dec. 1868, C.E. Lawrence; 8 Sept. 1873, Richard Lewis; 19–20 Feb. 1879, Joseph Espey; 17 July 1880, George Soules; 29 May 1882, John Forrester; 15 July 1883, James L[l]oyd

109 Daybook, 30 Jan. 1872, Mrs Colpit

110 Daybook, 15 Nov. 1861, Gaby child and mother; 3 Sept. 1871, Geo Grant little girl and mother; 16 Feb. 1872, Wm Klinck child and family; 15 May 1873, John White and Mrs White; 23 June 1874, Mrs Saunderson; 28, 31 Aug. 1876, Ben Davison and widow

111 Daybook, 6 Aug. 1868, Fennic widow; 26 Aug. 1868, Jesse Baker widow

112 The newspapers of the period were fond of reporting melancholy deaths of mothers and lovers who had pined away for loss of loved ones. Teefy explicitly stated that his widowed mother had died of grief. AO, MU 2113, folder 16, 'The Journal of Matthew Teefy.' Langstaff's

daughter, Mary Lillian McConaghy, attributed the death of her father's widowed sister, Mary Burkitt, to grief. As the death occurred fourteen years before Mary Lillian was born, it seems the doctor himself may have contributed to this family legend. Papers of Mrs Eileen Aiken, letter from 'Lily' [McConaghy] in Richmond Hill to 'Mrs [Homer] Langstaff,' 28 Oct. 1903

CHAPTER 5 **Patients and Their Diseases: Morbidity and Mortality in Children and Adults**

1 Robert P. Hudson, *Disease and Its Control: The Shaping of Modern Thought* (Westport, Conn.: Greenwood, 1983); Charles E. Rosenberg and Janet Golden, eds., *Framing Disease: Studies in Cultural History* (New Brunswick, NJ: Rutgers University Press 1992); Harold Merskey, 'Variable Meanings for the Definition of Disease,' *Journal of Medicine and Philosophy* 11 (1986): 215–32

2 The new classification of the Ontario Provincial Board of Health, with an undated letter from the secretary, Dr P.H. Bryce, enjoining doctors and clerks to respect it, was sent to Richmond Hill village clerk Matthew Teefy and can be found with his papers. Archives of Ontario (AO), Teefy Papers, MU 2955, envelope 'Provincial Board of Health.' In this document, published no earlier than 1883, the category of 'zymotic' diseases, or those caused by fermentation or bacteria, contained a sub-group of 'miasmatic diseases' that incorporated the bacterial and viral infections cholera, diphtheria, erysipelas, scarlet fever, typhoid, and the infantile infections of measles, mumps, chickenpox, and smallpox. Tubercular conditions were not classified as zymotic, but were considered to be 'constitutional' diseases.

3 The concept of 'pathocoenosis' was introduced by Mirko Drazen Grmek to describe the tableau of clinical pathology in a specific place and time. *Les Maladies à l'aube de la civilisation occidentale* (Paris: Payot 1983), 14–17.

4 An alphabetized index to names in the computerized portions of this study will be kept with James M. Langstaff's original daybooks as an aid to those interested in genealogy.

5 In the 1850s there were approximately 40,000 blacks in Ontario, but the welcome they had received in the early part of the century cooled after 1840. James W. St G. Walker, *Racial Discrimination in Canada: The Black Experience* (Ottawa: Canadian Historical Association booklet no. 41 1985), 10–11

6 James Miles Langstaff, Langstaff daybook (Daybook), 8 July 1850, 17 Feb. 1853, Mrs Ben Jenkins deliveries; 20 July 1884, 30 Oct. 1885, Mrs and Mr James Langstaff Jenkins. Matthew Teefy may have named his oldest son, John Read Teefy (b. 1848), for Langstaff's Richmond Hill predecessor; it has been observed that patients in other practices named their children for the doctor or his family. Evelyn Bernette Ackerman, 'The Activities of a Country Doctor in New York State: Dr. Elias Cornelius of Somers, 1794–1803,' *Historical Reflections / Réflexions historiques* 9 (1982): 181–93, especially 191; Steven M. Stowe, 'Obstetrics and the Work of Doctoring in the Mid-Nineteenth-Century American South,' *Bulletin of the History of Medicine* 64 (1990): 561n29

7 A decline in streptococcal virulence has recently been cited as a reason for the decline in childbed fever, in addition to the more obvious reason of the advent of sulphonamides. Irvine Loudan, 'Puerperal fever, the Streptococcus, and the Sulphonamides, 1911–1945,' *British Medical Journal* 295 (1987): 485–90

8 The proportionate rise in paediatric deaths may be an artefact of Langstaff's record-keeping, as he was more diligent about noting births than deaths. However, the 1880s figure may be slightly low, because there was a decline in Langstaff's obstetrical activity.

9 Caution must be exercised when making generalizations on the basis of these figures. The accuracy of the 1851 census is itself suspect. See Queen's University Documents Library, David P. Gagan, 'Enumerators' Instructions for the Census of Canada 1852 and 1861,' *Histoire sociale – Social History* 7 (1974): 355–65. Furthermore, since the census district area was increasingly restricted, especially between 1851 and 1861, some of the changes in attendance may be more apparent than real. Further reasons for caution in trusting either the daybooks or the census rolls for local mortality are the facts that not all people who died according to the census were reported dead by Langstaff, although he did visit them; and conversely, not all deaths that Langstaff reported for a given census year were actually recorded in the census. This last statement is based on a search that included the other districts in both Vaughan and Markham.

10 Neil Sutherland, *Children and English-Canadian Society: Framing the Twentieth-Century Consensus* (Toronto: University of Toronto Press 1976), 6–7. For a discussion of changing perspectives on the death of children, see Edward Shorter, 'Maternal Sentiment and Death in Childbirth: A New Agenda for Psycho-history,' in Paula Branca, ed., *The Medicine Show: Patients, Physicians, and the Perplexities of the Health*

Revolution in Modern Society (New York: Science History Publications 1977), 67–88.

11 Canada Census 1861, C 1088, Markham District III, Schedule of Deaths; Dan Horner seven-month-old male child; Jacob Horner, male infant. In the preceding year, Langstaff attended births in two Horner households. Daybook, 28 May 1860 and 8 Feb. 1860

12 With respect to a history of children, Joy Parr has observed that the biological determination of childhood and family is minimal and that 'inferences drawn from the present about family life in the past are dangerous.' She also cautioned that 'what is easy to find out is not always important to know,' especially since children are rarely in a position to leave their own testimony. Joy Parr, 'Introduction,' in Joy Parr, ed., *Childhood and Family in Canadian History* (Toronto: McClelland and Stewart 1982), 7–16

13 Daybook, 22 Sept. 1853, Hinckson child; 19 May 1853, Cook child

14 Daybook, 16 Dec. 1852, Dickson little girl; 30 April 1861, John Sanderson little girl

15 Daybook, 13 Nov. 1869, Shaver little girl

16 Daybook, 5 Aug. 1868, Edie little girl

17 Daybook, 30 July 1862, John Martin little girl

18 Daybook, 18 April 1865, Linton little boy

19 Daybook, 1 Feb. 1877, John Bowman

20 Daybook, 18 Feb. 1853, Stark child

21 Daybook, 6 Aug. 1862, Dan Raymond child

22 Daybook, 18 Oct., 7 Nov. 1862, Simms little girl

23 Daybook, 21 July 1876, Laird child; 26 June 1882, Knight little boy; 17 July 1886, Charles Reed

24 Daybook, 22 March 1874, Wm Ford family

25 Daybook, 24 Feb. 1859, John Atkinson little girl

26 Daybook, 25 Oct. 1861, D. Remore little boy; 2 March 1863, Gilmore

27 Daybook, 13 Dec. 1864, Neil Kennedy child; 11–15 March 1871, Button grandchild Elliott

28 Daybook, 4 Nov. 1880, Bricknell child

29 Daybook, 22–3 Feb. 1860, Rod McLeod child

30 Daybook, 3 April 1866, Henry Brown little girl

31 Daybook, 29 April 1888, Geo Raeman son

32 Daybook, 31 March to 5 April 1887, John Henricks's Barbara

33 Daybook, 12–16 April 1887, John Henricks's Caroline

34 Daybook, 22 March 1874, Wm Ford children

35 Daybook, 1–4 May 1879, Bell son

36 Daybook, 22 May 1858, Burgess child

37 Daybook, 6 Feb. 1887, Lance Nicholls child. The 'terrified' mother died in Feb. 1889, following childbirth complicated by diarrhoea.

38 Arthur Hertzler, *The Horse and Buggy Doctor* (New York and London: Harper and Brothers 1938), 1

39 Sutherland, *Children and English-Canadian Society*, 42–55

40 Daybook, 11 Nov. 1871, Richard Macy little boy; 8 Jan. 1852, Awyer son; 6 April 1853, Miss Bovair; 24 Jan. 1872, H. Walker son

41 Daybook, 18 April 1873, George Grant little girl

42 Daybook, 27 Nov. 1871, Wm Linfoot little girl

43 Daybook, 13 Nov. to 12 Dec. 1871, John Trudgeon family

44 Daybook, 26 July to 24 Aug. 1882, Duncan Emsley little girl and her mother

45 Daybook, 9 July to 14 Aug. 1882, William Calvert little girl and her mother

46 Daybook, 18 Oct. 1856 to 3 Jan. 1857, 16 Jan. 1862, Teefy family

47 Daybook, 25 March to 3 May 1873, 6–12 June 1874, Charlie Langstaff

48 Daybook, 29 Nov. to 31 Dec. 1856, 28 May 1859 to 26 Feb. 1861, Jonathan Shell family

49 Daybook, 8 Nov. to 19 Dec. 1861, Baldwin Teefy

50 Daybook, 9 April 1874, Mrs John Burr autopsy

51 Daybook, 13 July 1870, Sicily child; 2 Jan. 1879, Mann child; 7 May 1885, Ellis daughter

52 Daybook, 24 Nov. 1862, P. Rupert, Jr, child

53 Daybook, 15 Feb. 1866, H.A. Bernard little boy

54 Daybook, 29 June 1869, Rob Marsh son; 22 Feb. 1879, Elson son

55 Daybook, 12 June 1865, Baldwin Teefy

56 Daybook, 5, 14 Aug. 1851, Thos Bone; 9 June 1852, Tompson's servant girl; 2–22 Nov. 1852, Anon children; 2 Aug. 1861, Mrs Reverend Nattress

57 Daybook, 11 Aug. 1874, Dolmage; 4 May 1872, James McNair child; 29 March 1880, Chamberlain little girl

58 Daybook, 2 March 1866, Hogg family

59 Daybook, 26 May 1868, Fennic child

60 Daybook, 29 Nov. 1864, Isaac Phillips little boy

61 Sutherland, *Children and English-Canadian Society*, 55–7; Bettina Bradbury, 'The Fragmented Family: Family Strategies in the Face of Death, Illness, and Poverty, Montreal, 1860–1885,' in Joy Parr, *Childhood and Family*, 109–28

62 Daybook, 12–21 Aug. 1868, Henry Miller, Jr, child. Isabella's death on

13 Aug. was not mentioned in the daybook; see James Rolph Langstaff, 'Langstaff scrapbook,' 99.

63 Daybook, 28 Aug. 1871, 1 Sept. 1872, T. Kelly children

64 Daybook, 12 Sept. 1864, Ledgerwood daughter; 28 Jan. 1868, Jarret Wylie little girl; 8 Feb. 1870, Tullah child

65 Daybook, 29 Aug. to 3 Oct. 1870, James Duntan little boy and family

66 Daybook, 22 April to 10 July 1887, Sarah Heise

67 Daybook, 26 May to 2 June 1862, Mrs Brett, Sr

68 Daybook, 21–30 Sept. 1865, Mrs Henry Miller, Sr, Dr Rowel, Dr Tempest

69 Daybook, 16–7 Feb. 1868, 24–9 Aug. 1868, Miss Eleanor Miller

70 Daybook, 30 Aug. to 7 Sept. 1868, Mrs Henry Miller, Jr

71 Daybook, 27 Oct. 1858, Joseph Johnson

72 William Osler, *Principles and Practice of Medicine*, 4th ed. (New York: Appleton 1901), 109

73 Daybook, 13 March 1877, Mr Horsley; 17 March 1877, Mrs Horsley

74 Daybook, 18 Oct. 1860, Mrs widow Wilmot

75 James Langstaff, 'Complete Consolidation of One Lung,' *Canada Lancet* 12 (1880): 198. For an explanation of the content of this article see chapter 3

76 Daybook, 17–27 Feb. 1880, 17–20 April 1880, Peter Finney eldest daughter

77 Daybook, 28 Sept. 1857 and 25 Feb. 1862, Mrs Amos Wright

78 Daybook, 19 July 1880, George Soules; 31 May 1885, Reverend Dick

79 Canada Census 1861, C 1088, Markham District II

80 Daybook, 2–13 July 1862, John Langstaff, Sr

81 Daybook, 2 Feb. to 18 May 1865 Langstaff, Sr, and Langstaff family

82 AO, Estate file, GS 1–959, Cabinet 2, reel 422, no. 191, John Langstaff, Sr

83 Daybook, 3, 8 April 1882, Mrs Isaac Crosby. The sign of a distant heartbeat was heard by attendants of René Laennec, the inventor of the stethoscope, shortly before his death. His description of the sign as it occurred in his own condition constituted a 'P.S.' on the final page in his treatise. René T.H. Laennec, *Traité de l'auscultation médiate ou des maladies des poumons et du coeur*, 2 vols. (Paris: Chaudé 1826), vol. 2, 768–9

84 A yearbook published in 1889 listed phthisis as the fourth most common cause of death, but this was after atrophy and debility (combined), diarrhoea, and lung disease. Since tuberculosis can produce the symptoms of all the diseases that preceded it, especially atrophy and debility, it may actually have been the most common cause of death. *The Statistical Yearbook of Canada for 1889* (Ottawa:

Brown Chamberlin, Queen's Printer 1890), 96–7. In a list of the common causes of death in Ontario between 1871 and 1882, 'phthisis' was always first; see Charles M. Godfrey, *Medicine for Ontario: A History* (Belleville: Mika 1979), 254. It was also prominent as a cause of death in cemetery records; see Risa Barkin and Ian Gentles, 'Death in Victorian Toronto, 1850–1899,' *Urban History Review / Revue d'histoire urbaine* 19 (1990): 14–29.

85 Daybook, 26 March 1864, Langton; 14 July 1874, James Duncan; 23 July 1883, Mrs Armstrong; 29 May 1886, John Baker daughter

86 Daybook, 20 Jan. 1867, George Walls

87 The received view about tuberculosis mortality is that Canadian women died more frequently than men until 1922. See Wendy Mitchinson, *The Nature of Their Bodies: Women and Their Doctors in Victorian Canada* (Toronto: University of Toronto Press 1991), 55–6; George Jasper Wherret, *The Miracle of the Empty Beds: A History of Tuberculosis in Canada* (Toronto: University of Toronto Press 1977), 250. Statistics on ninteenth-century tuberculosis mortality as derived from the Canada Census and related yearbooks are notoriously imprecise, since pththisis was confused with many other diseases. Reliable age and sex statistics on nineteenth-century tuberculosis are said to be those of England and Wales, but there is some evidence that female mortality was lower in other European countries; furthermore, it is not known if extrapolation of these figures to North America is justified. Pierre C.A. Louis, *Researches on Phthisis: Anatomical, Pathological, and Therapeutical*, 2nd ed., trans. Walter H. Walshe (London: New Sydenham Society 1844), 377–8, 479–81; Sheila Ryan Johansson, 'Sex and Death in Victorian England: An Examination of Age- and Sex-Specific Death Rates, 1840–1910,' in Martha Vicinus, ed., *A Widening Sphere: Changing Roles of Victorian Women* (Bloomington and London: Indiana University Press 1977), 163–81; Edward Shorter, *A History of Women's Bodies* (New York: Basic Books 1982), 231–3, 233n, 363n19

88 Daybook, 1 Oct. 1868, Don Mackenzie

89 The spelling error occurred only once. Daybook, 1 Nov. 1855, Duncan McKinnon

90 Daybook, 2, 5 Jan. 1861 and 31 Dec. 1864, Clara Teefy

91 Daybook, 4 Nov. 1866, Gibson

92 Daybook, 31 Oct. 1870, Skeel

93 Daybook, 20 May 1868, Miss Matilda Harrington

94 Daybook, 7 July 1875, John Bennett; 20 July 1877, Isaac Munshaw

95 Daybook, 23 Jan. 1869, Mrs Sandvidge, Sr

96 Daybook, 18 March to 21 May 1854, Bloomfield boy; 20, 26 Jan. 1870,

David Welsh; 24 July 1872, Thos Bone son

97 Daybook, 6 June 1863, Hotson

98 Daybook, 13 June 1875 to 28 Dec. 1881, Ansley

99 Daybook, 14 Dec. 1872 to 15 May 1873, John White at Ridgeway

100 Daybook, 12 Sept. 1856 to 26 Jan. 1885, especially 21 June, 29 July, 4–6 Oct. 1884, Frank Boynton and family

101 Daybook, 14 Nov. 1884 to 7 July 1885, Maggie Young

102 Geoffrey Bilson, *A Darkened House: Cholera in Nineteenth-Century Canada* (Toronto: University of Toronto Press 1980); Geoffrey Bilson, 'Canadian Doctors and the Cholera,' in S.E.D. Shortt, ed., *Medicine in Canadian Society: Historical Perspectives* (Montreal: McGill-Queen's University Press 1981), 115–36; Charles E. Rosenberg, *The Cholera Years: The United States in 1832, 1849, and 1866* (Chicago and London: University of Chicago Press 1962)

103 Daybook, 25 July 1875, Thomas Wilson; 9 Oct. 1878, Mrs Kemp

104 Daybook, 24 Aug. 1852, Mitchel

105 Daybook, 29 Oct. 1865, Rob Hall child; 13 Feb. 1886, James M. Langstaff

106 Daybook, 28 Sept. 1863, Hawkins; 29 Sept. 1872, Dalton daughter; 11 Sept. 1876, Arch Wright daughter. Ontario mortality rates for typhoid from 1880 to 1900 appear in Godfrey, *Medicine for Ontario*, 253.

107 Daybook, 28 Sept. to 16 Nov. 1863, Hawkins

108 Daybook, 14–26 April 1882, Mrs David Benson; see also 24 March to 12 April 1875, Mrs Jacob Atkinson; 21 June 1879, Mrs Mary Ann Langstaff. Also see chapter 8.

109 Marianna O'Gallagher, *Grosse Ile: Gateway to Canada* (Ste Foy, Que.: Carraig Books 1984)

110 Daybook, 6 Oct. 1863, R. Raymond little girl; 6 Oct. 1864, Mrs Isaac Bellerby

111 Daybook, 13 Feb. 1857, Wm Clink

112 Anna Brownell Jameson, *Winter Studies and Summer Rambles in Canada*, Clara Thomas, ed. (Toronto: McClelland and Stewart 1965), 28–9, 126–7. See also, H.H. Langton, ed., *A Gentlewoman in Upper Canada: The Journals of Anne Langton* (Toronto, Vancouver: Clarke Irwin 1964), 192–4.

113 Charles G. Roland '"Sunk under the Taxation of Nature": Malaria in Upper Canada,' in Charles G. Roland, ed., *Health, Disease, and Medicine. Essays on Canadian History* (Toronto: Hannah Institute for the History of Medicine 1984), 154–70

114 Daybook, 4 Oct. 1879, Joseph Redman; 29 May 1883, Jas Newton, Jr

115 Daybook, 5 Sept. 1888, Jas Pearson

116 Daybook, 6 June 1863, Hotson

117 Daybook, 15 Nov. 1862, Mrs Jobbitt

118 Daybook, 30 Jan. 1864, Mrs John Bruce

119 Daybook, 14 April 1888, Middleton

120 Daybook, 17 Nov. 1852, Carlisle; 12 April 1853, Fred; 16 Dec. 1853, Lund's guest an English gentleman; 11 Jan. 1854, Nicols; 21 Feb. 1861, Paige; 18 July 1873, Kendrick; 29 Aug. 1881, Miller; 20 Nov. 1888, Anon. A woman had a swollen gland called a 'bubo,' but this did not necessarily mean the lesion was syphilitic. Daybook, 13 Aug. 1853, Mrs Obrien. On venereal disease in late nineteenth-century Canada, see Jay Cassel, *The Secret Plague: Venereal Disease in Canada, 1838–1939* (Toronto: University of Toronto Press 1987), 91–100.

121 'North Ontario Medical Association,' *Canada Lancet* 7 (1874–5): 220–1

122 Jacalyn Duffin, 'The Great Canadian Peritonitis Debate, 1844–47,' *Histoire sociale – Social History* 19 (1986): 407–24

123 Daybook, 2 July 1856, Mrs I. Stokes; 12 Aug. 1865, Miss Elliott

124 Daybook, 15 May 1876, James Miles Langstaff

125 Daybook, 13 July 1867, Geo Atkinson son

126 Daybook, 13 June 1876, Sicily little girl

127 Abraham Groves claimed to have performed the first appendicectomy in Canada in May 1883, but he did not announce his accomplishment until much later. Abraham Groves, *All in a Day's Work: Leaves from a Doctor's Casebook* (Toronto: Macmillan 1934), 20–1; William B. Spaulding, 'Abraham Groves (1847–1935): A Pioneer Surgeon, Sufficient unto Himself,' *Canadian Bulletin of Medical History / Bulletin canadien d'histoire de la médecine* 8 (1991): 249–62

128 Daybook, 19 Feb. 1861, John Woods little girl; 4 April 1885, Mrs Holmes; 12 Nov. 1886, James Henessey

129 John Bell, 'Case of Leukocythaemia – History and Autopsy' and William Osler, 'Remarks on the Histology of the Above Case,' *Canada Medical and Surgical Journal* 4 (1875–76): 435–9 and 439–47, respectively

130 Robert P. Hudson, 'The Biography of Disease: Lessons from Chlorosis,' *Bulletin of the History of Medicine* 51 (1977): 448–63; Karl Figlio, 'Chlorosis and Chronic Disease in Nineteenth-Century Britain: The Social Construction of Somatic Illness in a Capitalist Society,' *Social History* 3 (1978): 167–97

131 Daybook, 17 Oct. 1876, Hosler

132 Daybook, 10 Feb. 1887, Mrs Henry Hopper

133 Daybook, 29 July, 17–25 Dec. 1876, Thos Cook esq

134 Daybook, 4 Aug. 1868, Fennic; 5 Oct. 1880, Fahey, Sr

135 Daybook, 21 May 1878, Miss Francy
136 Daybook, 26 Nov. 1870, Mrs Wideman. See also 21 April 1854,
    Mrs Davis.
137 Daybook, 16 March, 23 Sept. 1867, Mrs Edmund Warren, Sr; 20 June
    1884, Miss Creesor
138 Daybook, 7 Feb. 1879, Dr Hunter's anonymous patient
139 Daybook, 27 Jan. to 8 Feb. 1868, Dr Lewis Langstaff
140 Daybook, 11, 28 Oct., 17 Nov. 1878, Dr Lewis Langstaff; he died
    27 Nov. 1878.
141 Daybook, 4 July 1875, R.J. Hopper
142 Daybook, 24 March 1869, Miss Campbell
143 Daybook, 3 June 1865, Remore, Sr
144 Undated letter from 'Mom' (wife of Homer Langstaff) to 'Dear all,'
    property of her daughter, Mrs Eileen Aiken, Prescott. Homer's wife
    never met James Langstaff; her husband, who, she claimed, had
    'inherited' Bright's disease, was only eighteen months old at his father's
    death. Daybook, 30–1 March, 25 April, 1 May 1889, James Langstaff

CHAPTER 6: **Lunatics, Dreamers, and Drunks**

1 With respect to Canada, especially Ontario, see Thomas E. Brown,
  'Foucault Plus Twenty: On Writing the History of Canadian Psychiatry
  in the 1980s,' *Canadian Bulletin of Medical History / Bulletin canadien
  d'histoire de la médecine* 2 (1985): 23–50; Thomas E. Brown, '"Living with
  God's Afflicted": A History of the Provincial Lunatic Asylum at
  Toronto, 1830–1911' (Ph.D. thesis, Queen's University 1980); Cyril
  Greenland, 'Services for the Mentally Retarded in Ontario, 1870–1930,'
  Ontario History 54 (1962): 267–74; Henry M. Hurd, ed., *The Institutional
  Care of the Insane in the United States and Canada*, 4 vols. (Baltimore:
  Johns Hopkins University Press 1917), vol. 1, 427; vol. 4, 120–202;
  Cheryl L. Krasnick, '"In Charge of the Loons": A Portrait of the London
  Ontario Asylum for the Insane in the Nineteenth Century,' *Ontario
  History* 74 (1982): 138–84; Wendy Mitchinson, 'The Toronto and
  Gladesville Asylums: Humane Alternatives for the Insane in Canada
  and Australia,' *Bulletin of the History of Medicine* 63 (1989): 52–72; S.E.D.
  Shortt, *Victorian Lunacy: Richard M. Bucke and the Practice of Late
  Nineteenth-Century Psychiatry* (Cambridge: Cambridge University Press
  1986); Harvey G. Simmons, *From Asylum to Welfare* (Downsview, Ont.:
  National Institute on Mental Retardation 1982); Cheryl Krasnick Warsh,
  Moments of Unreason: The Practice of Canadian Psychiatry and the

Homewood Retreat, 1883–1923 (Montreal, Kingston, London, and Buffalo: McGill–Queen's University Press 1989).

2 Charles E. Rosenberg, 'Body and Mind in Nineteenth-Century Medicine: Some Clinical Origins of the Neurosis Construct,' *Bulletin of the History of Medicine* 63 (1989): 185–97; Shorter observed that doctors tended to dislike seeing patients with psychosomatic problems because they were difficult to cure; as a result they sometimes resorted to extreme therapies. Edward Shorter, *From Paralysis to Fatigue: A History of Psychosomatic Illness in the Modern Era* (New York: Free Press; Toronto: Maxwell Macmillan 1992), 125–7

3 Mitchinson, 'Toronto and Gladesville Asylums,' 57; Brown, 'Living with God's Afflicted,' 52

4 James Miles Langstaff, Langstaff daybook (Daybook), 4 Nov. 1887, anonymous male at Finches Corners

5 Krasnick Warsh, *Moments of Unreason*, 7–8; Shortt, *Victorian Lunacy*, 38; Brown, 'Living with God's Afflicted,' 181

6 Daybook, 9, 20 Sept. 1859, a young woman; 9, 18 Sept. 1859, a man; 14 Nov. 1863, a man; 25 Nov. 1863, a man; 2 April 1878, a woman; 6 Jan. 1880, a man; 25 Dec. 1881, a man; 12 April 1883, a man; 22, 28 June 1888, a woman. In compliance with the rules of confidentiality applying to Toronto Asylum Medical Records held by Archives of Ontario (AO), names have not been used.

7 Daybook, 9 Sept. 1859, a young woman

8 Simmons, *Asylum to Welfare*, 6

9 Archives of Ontario (AO), Provincial Lunatic Asylum, Admission / Discharge Warrants and Histories, RG 10 Series 20-B-1, registration nos. 2183, 2967, 5246, 5413, 5611. These items were traced by Carolyn E. Gray through the asylum's General Register, RG 10 Series 20-B-3.

10 Brown, 'Living with God's Afflicted,' 187–8, 193, 196–7

11 AO, Provincial Lunatic Asylum, Admission / Discharge Warrants and Histories, RG 10 Series 20-B-1, registration no. 5413

12 Ibid., no. 5611

13 Ibid., no. 2967

14 Daybook, 4 Nov. 1887, anonymous male at Finches Corners

15 Brown, 'Living with God's Afflicted,' 168

16 Daybook, 25 May 1852, Mrs Anon.; 20 Dec. 1852, Miss Hopper; 1 Nov. 1853, Miss Lyon; 7 March 1854, Miss Milburn; 25 July 1856, Miss Tindall; 1 Dec. 1865, Miss Foggan; 14 Aug. 1867, Smith daughter; 5–17 Nov. 1869, Miss Tran; 1 April 1872, Mrs D.S. Raeman, Miss Tran; 8 April 1873, Miss Cochead [?]; 7 Feb. 1883, Julius Seager. According

to Shorter, 'fits' were an earlier version of motor hysteria that were replaced by 'paralysis' in the nineteenth century; males were increasingly seen to have this diagnosis after the acceptance of a theory of reflex irritation that was not dependent on the presence of female reproductive organs. Shorter, *From Paralysis to Fatigue*, 96–108, 117. For more on the history of hysteria, see Harold Merskey, 'Hysteria: The History of an Idea,' *Canadian Journal of Psychiatry* 28 (1983): 428–33.

17 Daybook, 14 Aug. 1867, Smith daughter
18 Daybook, 5–17 Nov. 1869, Miss Tran
19 Daybook, 10 March 1885, Lyman Crosby; 7 July 1886, George Cober daughter
20 Daybook, 1 Nov. 1868, Mrs Bell. In addition, however, there were two others with similar problems: a woman with 'hysteria' after a delivery; a woman who had been hit in the head when she was young and was said to have 'mental derangement' after the birth of a child, and whom Langstaff continued to visit for three months. Daybook, 18 Dec. 1853, Mrs Morley; 1 April 1872, Mrs D.S. Raeman
21 Daybook, 5 Jan. 1870, Mrs Welman
22 Daybook, 27 April 1860, Ash son. In 1877 R.M. Bucke of London, Ontario, instituted aggressive treatments for 'masturbatory insanity.' Shortt, *Victorian Lunacy*, 145–6
23 Daybook, 11 May 1854, Wm Marsh child; 3 April 1868, Matthewson child; 16 July 1874, John Dancy child; 30 Jan. 1889, Adam Wideman child
24 Daybook, 5 Aug., 13 Sept., 16 Oct., 1868, 9 June 1870, 31 Dec. 1875, Catie (or Kate) Edie and Mrs Edie
25 Daybook, 22 June 1888, David Mortson
26 Daybook, 27 Aug., 17 Oct. 1863, Wilson's daughter Mrs Anderson
27 Daybook, 28–9 May 1867, Mrs John Hislop. See also Daybook, 21 March, 5 Aug., 3 Sept. 1861, 10 Oct. 1869, 3 Feb. 1870, 15 March 1874, Mrs John Hislop and son.
28 Daybook, 16 Aug. 1880, Miss Ada Hunter
29 Daybook, 28 June 1873, Jacob Pingle at Albert Quantz home
30 Daybook, 27 June 1861, Shell son
31 Daybook, 27 Sept. 1881, William Weldrick
32 Daybook, 24 July 1867, Mr Alison
33 On the history of suicide and the methodological problems of its study, see Michael MacDonald, 'The Medicalization of Suicide in England, 1500–1870,' in Charles E. Rosenberg and Janet Golden, eds., *Framing Disease: Studies in Cultural History* (New Brunswick, NJ: Rutgers Univer-

sity Press 1992), 85–103; Michael MacDonald, 'Madness, Suicide, and the Computer,' in Roy Porter and Andrew Wear, eds., *Problems and Methods in the History of Medicine* (London: Croom Helm 1987), 207-29.

34 Daybook, 5 Jan. to 19 March 1870, Mrs Welman. The same woman may have attempted suicide a decade earlier with the morphine Langstaff had given her for vomiting and diarrhoea. At that time he wrote that she had 'threatened coma from too much Med[ication].' 2–14 Sept. 1859, Mrs Welman

35 *York Herald*, 15 March 1870

36 Daybook, 16–17 Sept. 1872, Brain, Sr [also John Breen, Sr]; *York Herald*, 16 Sept. 1872

37 Daybook, 8 Oct. 1861, Gardner

38 Daybook, 24 April 1879, Fairchilds

39 Daybook, 14 May 1888, Mrs widow Bowman

40 Daybook, 21 Aug. 1876, Thomas Robinson; *York Herald*, 25 Aug. 1876

41 Daybook, 1 June 1859, Shell son; 30 May 1860, Mrs widow Smith; 25 Dec. 1861, Miss Edith Arnold; 12 Aug. 1861, Wm Ellis child; 19 July 1879, Mrs Ben Jenkins; 1 Jan. 1884, Ellis eleven-year-old girl

42 Daybook, 21 Aug. 1865, Thomas Wilson

43 Daybook, 23 Dec. 1866, Mrs Gilmore; her children had died in the spring of 1863.

44 Daybook, 17 Oct. 1871, McGeachy

45 Lancelot Law Whyte, *The Unconscious before Freud* (London: Tavistock Social Science Paperbacks 1960), 134

46 Daybook, 19–20 Nov. 1866, Chris Henricks

47 Daybook, 28–30 Nov. 1886, Skeele

48 Daybook, 14–18 Oct. 1873, Rob Robinson

49 Daybook, 20–3 May 1874, Emma Enoui; 1 May 1879, Bell eight-year-old boy; 13 May 1883, Lloyd Elsworth

50 W.L. Smith, *The Pioneers of Old Ontario* (Toronto: George N. Morang 1923), 295–300

51 Edith Firth, *The Town of York, 1815–1834: A Further Collection of Documents of Early Toronto* (Toronto: University of Toronto Press and the Champlain Society Ontario Series vol. 8 1966), 342, 347; M.A. Garland and J.J. Talman, 'Pioneer Drinking Habits and the Rise of the Temperance Agitation in Upper Canada prior to 1840,' *Ontario History* 27 (1931): 341–64; James M. Clemens, 'Taste Not; Touch Not; Handle Not: A Study of the Social Assumptions of the Temperance Literature and Temperance Supporters in Canada West, 1839 to 1859,' *Ontario History* 64 (1972): 142–60

52 Cheryl Krasnick, '"Because There Is Pain:" Alcoholism, Temperance, and the Victorian Physician,' *Canadian Bulletin of Medical History / Bulletin canadien d'histoire de la médecine* 2 (1985): 1–19; Cheryl Krasnick Warsh, *Moments of Unreason: The Practice of Canadian Psychiatry and the Homewood Retreat* (Montreal, Kingston, London and Buffalo: McGill-Queen's University Press 1989), 144–54; Graeme Decarie, '"Something Old, Something New"; Aspects of Prohibitionism in Ontario in the 1890s,' in Donald Swainson, ed., *Oliver Mowat's Ontario* (Toronto: Macmillan 1972), 154–71

53 Langstaff Account books, 1847 and 1862, inside covers

54 The figure may be falsely low for two reasons: first, the few barrels that were listed without their capacity were estimated to be the smallest size; second, to facilitate the search, special attention was paid to the invoices of two suppliers, D. MacDonnell and R.D. Macpherson, and there may have been whisky purchases from other merchants. AO, Teefy Papers, MU 2950, Invoice book, 1852–54 and MU 2951, Invoice book, 1855

55 AO, Teefy Papers, MU 2955, *Acts Relating to the Powers, Duties, and Protection of Justices of the Peace* (Quebec 1853), inside cover, clipping from *Whitby Chronicle*, 20 June 1878; Teefy was appointed a magistrate in 1853 and 'never had a decision [reversed] by a higher court.' AO, MU 2113, folder 16, 'Journal of Matthew Teefy,' 1

56 AO, MS 120, Teefy Scrapbook, item 233, 'Magistrates Court, Wed. 20 July 1859'; Daybook, 17 July 1859; back entry, 19 July 1850, 15 shillings to Rob Marsh (the magistrate)

57 Daybook, 15–16 April 1861, Constable

58 Daybook, 24 July 1867, 12–13 Sept. 1869, 14 Feb. 1871, 14 Jan. 1872, Wm Alison

59 Daybook, 4 Jan. 1873, 9 Aug. 1873, Ned Lackey

60 Daybook, 4 Jan. 1863, Dr I. Bowman; 9 April 1874, Dr Wm Comisky; 14 July 1884, Dr F.R. Armstrong; 31 Dec. 1886, Walker, Thornhill hotelkeeper

61 Daybook, 27 Oct. 1858, Jos Johnson

62 Daybook, 5 Sept. 1863, Mrs H. Lever

63 Daybook, 17–31 Oct. 1871, McGeachy

64 Daybook, 3 June 1868, McGravy

65 Daybook, 16 March 1859, Peter Phillips little girl; 7 Aug. 1874, Mrs Wm Frizby

66 Daybook, 27–8 Sept. 1861, Priest's daughter

67 Daybook, 6 May 1860, Mrs David Eyer, Jr

68 Isabel Champion, ed., *Markham, 1793–1900* (Markham, Ont.: Markham District Historical Society 1989), 297

69 The temperance vow had been co-signed by Thomas R[olph] Graham, son of James Graham and a former student of John Rolph. See Langstaff's account book, 1847; William Canniff, *The Medical Profession in Upper Canada, 1783–1850* (reprint of 1894 edition, Toronto: Hannah Institute for the History of Medicine 1980), 392–3.

70 *York Herald* 4, 11 Jan., 22 March, and 5 April 1877

71 Daybook, 6 Jan. 1871, Isaac Shell

72 Daybook, 5 Dec. 1864, 20 Feb. 1865; AO, Minutes of the Municipality of the Township of Vaughan, meetings of 5 Dec. 1864, 20 Feb., and 10 March 1865

73 *York Herald*, 10 Jan. 1878. The authors of an anonymous broadside sent to Richmond Hill may have thought Thornhill's problems stemmed from a different kind of dissolution: 'Morals Good or Bad?' they asked, as they revealed that every other Friday evening 'young men and girls (I beg pardon I meant to say Ladies) do congregate promiscuously in secret conclave in the dark hours of the night.' Readers were invited to 'pause and consider what may be the result.' AO, MS 120, Teefy scrapbook, item 56, 'Thornhill 1860'

74 *York Herald*, 20 Jan. 1871

75 Ibid., 9 June, 24 Nov. 1876

76 Ibid. 7 June 1861 and 8 Sept. 1871; Daybook, back entry, 9 June 1861; 11 Sept. 1871. On medical reaction to 'Ten Nights in a Bar-Room,' see Barbara Leslie Epstein, *The Politics of Domesticity: Women, Evangelism, and Temperance in Nineteenth-Century America* (Middletown, Conn.: Wesleyan University Press 1981), 8–12.

77 On *Grip* and Bengough, see Carl Spadoni, 'Grip and the Bengoughs as Publishers and Printers,' *Papers of the Bibliographical Society of Canada* 27 (1988): 12–37; Ramsay Cook, *The Regenerators. Social Criticism in Late Victorian English Canada* (Toronto, Buffalo, London: University of Toronto Press 1985), 123–51. A discussion of Bengough's Richmond Hill 'chalk talk' on 10 March 1887 appeared in the *Liberal*, 17 March 1887.

78 Daybook, 'D.I.K. Rine' daybook, 9 Jan. 1878; *York Herald*, 24 Jan. 1878; A.J. Birrell, 'D.I.K. Rine and the Gospel Temperance Movement in Canada,' *Canadian Historical Review* 58 (1977): 23–42

79 Daybook, 'Three sermons Gough,' 11 April 1886; *Liberal*, 15 April 1886

80 Daybook, 8 Sept. 1860, 'Toronto to see prince but it rained'; 11 Sept. 1860, 'saw Prince of Wales'

81 *Globe*, 10, 12 Sept. 1860
82 *Quarterly Journal of Inebriety* 1 (1876): 25. Twenty-two volumes of this journal are in the Osler Library, Montreal.
83 Daybook, 10 Nov. 1874, 10 Nov. 1876, 9 Nov. 1877; *Globe*, 11 Nov. 1874, 11 Nov. 1876, 12 Nov. 1877
84 Decarie, '"Something old, Something New,"' 163; Cook, *The Regenerators*, 38–40; Arnold Haultain, *Goldwin Smith, His Life and Opinions* (Toronto: McClelland and Goodchild nd.), 282–3
85 Krasnick, 'Because There Is Pain'
86 Daybook, 2 March 1885. Perhaps the Reverend D.I. MacDonnell was a relative of the family that had been Teefy's importer thirty years before; see note 54 above.
87 *York Herald*, 5 March 1885

CHAPTER 7   **Accidents, Injuries, and Operations: Langstaff's Practice of Surgery**

1 John Duffy, *The Healers: A History of American Medicine* (Urbana, Ill.: University of Illinois Press 1976), 247–59; Paul Starr, *The Social Transformation of American Medicine* (New York: Basic Books 1982), 156–7; Charles E. Rosenberg, *The Care of Strangers: The Rise of America's Hospital System* (New York: Basic Books 1987), 188; Wendy Mitchinson, *The Nature of Their Bodies: Women and Their Doctors in Victorian Canada* (Toronto: University of Toronto Press 1991), 253; Martin Pernick, *A Calculus of Suffering: Pain, Professionalism, and Anesthesia in Nineteenth-Century America* (New York: Columbia University Press 1985)
2 Katherine Mandusic McDonell, *The Journals of William A. Lindsay: An Ordinary Nineteenth-Century Physician's Surgical Cases* (Indianapolis: Indiana Historical Society 1989); Edna Hindie Lemay, 'Thomas Hérier, a Country Surgeon outside Angoulême at the End of the xviiith Century,' *Journal of Social History* 10 (1976–7): 524–37
3 J.T.H. Connor, 'To be Rendered Unconscious of Torture; Anaesthesia and Canada. 1847–1920' (M.Phil. thesis, University of Waterloo, 1983); W. Kirk Colbeck, 'First Record of an Anaesthetic in Ontario,' *Canadian Medical Association Journal* 32 (1935): 84–5; Akitomo Matsuki, 'Chronology of the Very Early History of Inhalation Anaesthesia in Canada,' *Canadian Anaesthetists' Society Journal* 21 (1974): 92–5; Akitomo Matsuki and Elemér K. Zsigmond, 'Bibliography of the History of Surgical Anaesthesia in Canada,' *Canadian Anaesthetists' Society Journal* 21 (1974): 427–30; Akitomo Matsuki and Elemér K. Zsigmond, 'The First Fatal Case of Chloroform Anaesthesia in Canada,' *Canadian Anaesthetists'*

Society Journal 20 (1973): 395–7; Charles G. Roland, 'The First Death from Chloroform at the Toronto General Hospital,' *Canadian Anaesthetists' Society Journal* 11 (1964): 437–9; Charles G. Roland, 'Bibliography of the History of Anaesthesia in Canada,' *Canadian Anaesthetist's Society Journal* 15 (1968): 202–14; David J. Steward, 'The Early History of Anaesthesia in Canada: The Introduction of Ether to Upper Canada, 1947,' *Canadian Anaesthetists' Society Journal* 24 (1977): 153–61

4 James Miles Langstaff, Langstaff daybook (Daybook), 8 July to 28 Aug. 1850, especially 24 July, Mr Craik

5 Daybook, 14 Aug. 1851, Mahlon Phillips; 17 Sept. 1851, Anon; 16 March 1853, Mrs John Cook; 27 May 1853, Fishburn; 3 July 1853, Mrs Maguire

6 Daybook, 13 May 1857, Hamilton boy

7 Daybook, 17–25 Sept. 1859, Arnup little girl

8 *Globe*, 17 Feb. 1858; Matsuki and Zsigmond, 'First Fatal Case'

9 Daybook, 8 Dec. 1872, Mrs Wm Harding

10 Daybook, 30 Oct. 1861, Garden's child

11 Daybook, 2 Aug. 1869, Dr Emroy's son, Fennic's son, J.R. Arnold

12 Daybook, 1 Aug. 1879, the Misses Bowman; 14 Jan. 1870, John Cook

13 Daybook, 7 Nov. 1864, Joel Kinnie; 19 July 1881, Paul Shell second son

14 Daybook, 30 Sept. 1866, Ritter, Sr

15 Daybook, 3 May 1868, Christian

16 Charles Ambrose Carter and Thomas Melville Bailey, eds., *The Diary of Sophia MacNab* (Hamilton: W.L. Griffin 1968), 27, 30, 33

17 Daybook, 21 May 1868, Thos Boynton four-year-old boy

18 Daybook, 25 Jan. 1871, Mrs Ginn

19 Daybook, 15 Jan. 1869, Mrs Ledgerwood; see also Daybook, 24 Aug. 1877, Mrs Reverend Jo Eakins.

20 Daybook, 17 Oct. 1885, Nellie Langstaff

21 *York Herald*, 22 Sept. 1881; *Toronto Telegram*, 21 Sept. 1881

22 Daybook, 18 April 1864, Rob Vanhorn

23 Daybook, 11 July 1879, Leach

24 Daybook, 26 Sept. 1884, John Forrester's son Thomas

25 Daybook, 15 Jan. 1868, George Atkinson; 12 May 1869, William Johnson

26 Daybook, 23 Nov. 1859, Lawson's child

27 Daybook, 8 Dec. 1876, Grainger son

28 Daybook, 6 Nov. 1871, Pointon; 22 April 1866, Duntan two boys; 2 May 1880, Miss Inspector McLellan; *York Herald*, 5 June 1879, 6 May 1880

29 Daybook, 14 June 1877, 'Holland little girl'; 'Mary Bennett,' *York Herald*, 21 June 1877

30 Daybook, 19 July 1868, Slayter; 3 Aug. 1868, Peter Boynton. A woman

in Toronto lost both her legs when she tried to step off a moving train. *York Herald*, 13 Nov. 1879

31 Daybook, 10 June 1873, Joseph Gray; 2 July 1868, John Brown
32 *Liberal*, 8 May 1884
33 *Economist* (Markham), 19 Jan. 1871
34 *York Herald*, 7 Sept. 1866
35 On the rise in threshing machinery, see Richard Pomfret, 'The Mechanization of Reaping in Nineteenth-century Ontario: A Case Study of the Pace and Causes of the Diffusion of Embodied Technical Change,' in Douglas McCalla, ed., *Perspectives on Canadian Economic History* (Toronto: Copp Clark Pitman 1987), 81–95; Graeme R. Quick and Wesley F. Buchele, *The Grain Harvesters* (St Joseph, Mich.: American Society of Agricultural Engineers 1978), 53–62, 103–12; J. Sanford Rikoon, *Threshing in the Midwest, 1820–1940: A Study of Traditional Culture and Technological Change* (Bloomington and Indianapolis: Indiana University Press 1988), 27–38; Alan Skeoh, 'The Ontario Agricultural Implement Industry, 1850–1891,' in T.A.Crowley, ed., *Third Annual Agricultural History of Ontario Seminar Proceedings* (Guelph, Ont.: University of Guelph 1978), 4–21, especially 12.
36 A new steam threshing machine in the area of Richmond Hill received the attention of the *York Herald* on 14 Aug. 1879.
37 Daybook, 11 Aug. 1877, Wm Elliott
38 Daybook, 12–17 Nov. 1878, Michael Obrien, Jr
39 Daybook, 11 Sept. 1884, Thomas Cosgrove
40 *York Herald*, 7 Aug. 1879; *Globe*, 16 Dec. 1873, 21 Jan. 1874
41 Daybook, 27 May to 1 July 1860, James Magill
42 Daybook, 7 Jan. 1880, Mrs Blebbs shot by George Ernest; *York Herald*, 8 Jan. 1880
43 Daybook, 20 Nov. 1872, Fred Martin and Landimore; 24 May 1878, Rob Trench
44 Daybook, 10 Dec. 1858, B. Stephenson
45 Daybook, 7 June 1866, 'pauper Vaughan [township]'
46 Daybook, 28 Dec. 1884, Mrs James Lever; see also Daybook, 9 Aug. 1882, Mrs Jesse Baker
47 Daybook, 4 July 1861, Holladay, Sr
48 Daybook, 11 March 1863, Dan Horner, Jr little boy
49 Daybook, 19 Jan. 1871, Hugh Bennett
50 Daybook, 30 Nov. to 19 Dec. 1868, Charles E. Lawrence
51 Daybook, 9–10 May 1867, Teefy son; 30 Oct. 1885, James L. Jenkins
52 Daybook, 11 June 1869, Mrs Savage

53 Daybook, 28 Dec. 1862, Miss Glass; 21 Sept. 1868, James Munshaw

54 Daybook, 29 Aug. 1862, Welham

55 Daybook, 23 Jan. 1868, Vantassel

56 Daybook, 10 July 1850 to 24 Aug. 1851, Mr Bruce

57 Daybook, 5 Nov. 1853, Gregory's son

58 J.T.H. Connor, 'Joseph Lister's System of Wound Management and the Canadian Practitioner' (M.A. thesis, University of Western Ontario, 1980)

59 See especially the article that appeared in late 1867, William Canniff, 'Some Remarks upon Carbolic Acid as a Remedial Agent in the Treatment of Wounds,' *Canada Medical Journal* 4 (1867–8): 307–11. In the same volume of this journal, carbolic was also discussed on pages 185, 188, 225, 388, 495.

60 Daybook, 28 Aug., 1 Sept. 1868, John Wilson

61 Daybook, 10 Jan. 1869, Welman child

62 Daybook, 25 July 1870, Wm Page child

63 Daybook, 14 Oct. to 27 Dec. 1870, Geo Patterson son

64 J.T.H. Connor, 'Joseph Lister's System,' 19, passim

65 Daybook, 18 Aug. 1870, Mrs Andrew Macbeth; 27 Aug. 1871, Geo Grant little girl

66 Daybook, 15 April 1881, Mrs Jo Gaby; 31 Jan. 1888, Mrs Francis

67 Daybook, 7 Oct. 1883, Mrs Wood

68 Daybook, 3 June 1884, John Wright

69 Daybook, 25 Oct. 1881, Mrs Johnstone; 7 Oct. 1883, Mrs Woods

70 Daybook, 9 Dec. 1873, Brown son; *Economist* (Markham), 11 Dec. 1873

71 Langstaff's account book, 1869–70, 355–7, essay in pencil. If this letter was published, the printed version has not been found.

72 James Miles Langstaff, manuscript lecture notes and case records from Guy's Hospital ('Guy's Notes'), property of James Rolph Langstaff, Richmond Hill, Feb 1848, 69. Joseph Lister himself had published an almost identical case, 21 Sept. 1867, cited in Logan Clendening, *A Source Book of Medical History* (New York: Dover 1960), 619.

73 'The Least Sacrifice of Parts as a Principle of Surgical Practice,' *Canada Lancet* 7 (1875): 238–9

74 Daybook, 21–6 Aug. 1874, H. Wice son

75 Lint, splints, and rollers were mentioned in fracture dressings prior to 'pasteboard and starch,' which were recorded by 1861. Daybook, 26 Oct. 1861, Rob Stephenson

76 Isabelle M.Z. Elliott and James Rawlings Elliott, *A Short History of Surgical Dressings* (London: Pharmaceutical Press 1964), 95

77 Daybook, 25 Aug. 1874, Watson Leak little boy

78 Daybook, 6 Jan. 1883, Mrs Wm Russell, Sr
79 Daybook, 18 Aug. 1857, Duncan Wilkie's negro
80 Daybook, 17 Oct. 1885, Wm Cook Deputy Reeve of Vaughan
81 Daybook, 12 July 1880, Wm Russell
82 Daybook, 12 Nov. 1873, Legget, Jr
83 Daybook, 20 Dec. 1887, Dr Palmer's writing
84 Daybook, 18 Nov. 1858, Watkins, Ambler's ostler
85 Daybook, 1 Feb. 1870, Simms child
86 Daybook, 15 June 1863, Manly and Dr Hostetter
87 Daybook, 23 Sept., 26 Oct., 30 Dec. 1861, 31 Jan., 17 Feb. 1862,
    Rob Stephenson
88 Daybook, 24 Nov. 1876 to 19 Jan. 1877, William Russell
89 Daybook, 26 Feb. 1870, P. Dancy; 28 Oct. 1885, Latimer son
90 Daybook, 17 Aug. 1880, Booth little boy
91 Daybook, 11 May, 27 Sept. 1877, John Craig, Jr
92 Daybook, 27 July 1868, 28 Dec. 1869 to 9 April, 7 June, 4 July 1870,
    25 March to 12 May 1871, David Hart and Mrs Hart
93 Daybook, 16 May 1867, Mrs Webb at operation on Mrs Dews; 17 Nov.
    1876, Mrs Craig at operation on Mrs Morrison
94 Daybook, 29 July 1876, William Falconbridge
95 Daybook, 18–19 Nov. 1858, Watkins, Ambler's ostler
96 Daybook, 17–25 Sept. 1859, Arnup little girl
97 Daybook, 20 May 1882, David Hopper and 'Dr from Maple'
98 Daybook, 19 Dec. 1860 to 3 Jan. 1861, Jo Gaby
99 Daybook, 5 July 1863 to 18 Oct. 1865, Walker
100 Daybook, 31 Oct. 1881, McConnell, Sr
101 Daybook, 26 March 1871, Fox; 13 Sept. 1881, Rutherford
102 Langstaff first used this term in his daybook, on 8 June 1863.
103 Pernick, *Calculus of Suffering*, 216. It has been suggested that elective
    surgery did not appear in Ontario until the 1890s, but if other doctors
    were like Langstaff, perhaps there had been an earlier boom that was
    already on the wane by that date. Connor, 'Minority Medicine,' 251
104 Daybook, 1887–9, back entry, 'Inventory 14 Aug. 1889'
105 Daybook, 20 June 1867, William Glenn son
106 Daybook, 28 March 1881, Elson, Sr
107 Daybook, 27 Nov. 1861, Davis
108 Daybook, 15 Feb. 1881, Mrs Eakins and Dr Aikins
109 'Vitalized air' was a term for nitrous oxide or 'laughing gas.' Daybook,
    24 July 1873, Dr Robinson to draw teeth for Mrs Gregg; 24 Sept. 1873,
    Wm Harrison (twelve teeth); 24 Sept. 1875, Anon (four teeth); 24 Aug.

1876, Rob Lymburner; 24 Aug. 1883, Dennison (six teeth); *Liberal*, 25 Sept. 1884.

110 For example, on a single day he helped Peck draw eleven teeth from Mrs Walker, sixteen from Mr Patterson, and one from Mrs Patterson. Daybook, 27 Feb. 1864

111 Daybook, back entry, 22 March 1862; 2 May 1863; 26 April 1867; 25 July 1887

112 Daybook, 9 July 1863 to 1 Nov. 1873, Clara Teefy; 13 June 1863, Teefy little girl; 15 June 1873, Miss Teefy, Armand Teefy

113 Daybook, 28 Aug. 1868, John Wilson

114 Daybook, 23 May 1857, James Playter child; 2 July 1868, John Brown

115 Daybook, 17 Dec. 1852, Miller of Whitchurch arm; 25 May 1860, Neil Wilkey leg; 2 July 1868, John Brown arm; 17 Aug. 1875, George Sisco arm; 29 Oct. 1875, Miss Dunn leg

116 Daybook, 6 March to 14 May 1872, Gid Hislop

117 Daybook, 15 Feb.1865, James Shaw child

118 Daybook, 27 Oct. 1874 to 9 March 1877, especially 29 Oct. 1875, Miss Dunn

119 Daybook, 23 May 1850, Miss Pollock; 22 Sept. 1851, Mrs Hiltz

120 Robley Dunglison, *A Dictionary of Medical Science* (Philadelphia: Blanchard and Lea 1855), 82

121 Daybook, 2 May 1864, George Dibbs; 26 Sept. 1882, Obrien

122 Daybook, 19 May 1856, Miss Sellars; 21 June to 31 July 1882, Mrs Isaac Snider. The local newspaper reported that a woman in the United States had had this procedure done nearly 200 times over eight years in order to remove 4,969 pounds of water. *York Herald*, 6 Feb. 1879

123 Daybook, 13 June 1876, Sicily little girl

124 Daybook, 27 July 1869, Miss [daughter of] widow Hiltz; 27 June 1882, Rand boy

125 Daybook, 17–24, 26 May 1853, Thos Shaw child and Mrs Thos Shaw

126 Daybook, back entry, 1 Oct. 1870, Mrs Brydon

127 George Buchanan, 'On Tracheotomy in Diphtheria,' *Canada Medical Journal* 1 (1864–5): 434–8

128 Daybook, 12 March 1866, Miss Wm Lawson

129 Daybook, back entry, 14 March 1866

130 Daybook, 15 Feb. 1872, Wm Klinck's son Leonard

131 Daybook, 22 Jan. 1873, John Baker little girl

132 Daybook, 7 Nov. 1877, Wm Dancy and Dr Anderson

133 Daybook, 29 April 1888, Geo Raeman child

134 Daybook, 30 July, 2, 7, 8 Nov. 1861, Teefy child

135 Warner demonstrated a decline in the use of most drastic remedies and related it to a call for physiological therapeutics based on experimental science. Pernick, however, has shown that the advent of anaesthesia altered the equation for medication prior to operative intervention, by making it more likely for a patient to expect and receive pain relief. It would be interesting to learn if other non-specialist practitioners like Langstaff gradually developed an avoidance of older *surgical* procedures, such as lancing gums in teething children or puncturing swollen legs, and if this could be related to a new dilemma: all surgical cases should receive anaesthetic, but anaesthetic was powerful medication. See John Harley Warner, *The Therapeutic Perspective: Medical Practice, Knowledge, and Identity in America, 1820–1885* (Cambridge, Mass. and London, England: Harvard University Press 1986), 12, 17, 35, 258; Pernick, *Calculus of Suffering*, 211–12

136 Daybook, 8, 28 July 1850, Mr Craik

137 Daybook, 8 May 1852, Lyons

138 Daybook, 18 Feb. 1863, Simon Miller assisted; 10 Aug. 1859, 19 Nov. 1873, Rob Law administered anaesthetic for two mastectomies.

139 Daybook, 24 Aug. 1876, Mrs Newberry, Sr

140 Daybook, 13 May 1857, Hamilton boy

141 Daybook, 17–31 Jan. 1867, anonymous boy at Barnard's

142 Daybook, 14 Nov. 1864, John Armour little boy

143 Daybook, 5 May 1864 to 14 May 1888, Jas Bowman daughter and family

144 Daybook, 26 Oct. 1866, Obrien child

145 Daybook, 23 May, 29 Oct, 6 Nov. 1861, Chris Hoover child

146 Daybook, 30 Oct. 1861, Garden child; 29 Oct., Chris Hoover child

147 Daybook, 16, 22 Sept. 1879, Miss Busby

148 Daybook, 8 July 1864, 28 Feb. 1866, Mrs Hunt; 2 March 1868, 20 July 1869, Mrs Ayerst

149 Daybook, 15 Oct. 1864, 20 Oct. 1866, 16 May 1867, 19 Feb. 1868, Mrs Dew. Langstaff appears to have been particularly interested in this patient's type of cancer, since he owned Wardrop's essay on the topic (see Appendix c).

150 Daybook, 21 April, 1854, Mrs Davis

151 Daybook, 22 Sept. 1861, Mrs George Nicholls

152 Daybook, 10–30 Aug. 1859, Mrs Fred Vanhorn

153 Daybook, 16 May 1867, Mrs Dew

154 Daybook, 20 July 1869, Mrs Ayerst

155 Daybook, 19 Nov. 1873, Mrs Polly Klinck

156 Daybook, 2 March 1868, 20 July 1869, Mrs Ayerst
157 Daybook, 13 Dec. 1877, Mrs John Martin. See also Daybook, 24 Aug. 1876, Mrs Newberry.
158 Daybook, 26 Nov. 1870, Mrs Wideman
159 Daybook, 11, 17 April, 3 Sept. 1878, Mrs Dalton
160 Daybook, 25 Nov. 1862, 5 July 1863, Mrs John Mackenzie
161 Daybook, 23 Sept. 1869, Mrs Francis Walker
162 Daybook, 16 Oct. 1875, Anon patient and Dr Geikie; also Daybook, 12 Feb. 1881, Mrs David Eakins and Dr Aikins Toronto
163 Daybook, 8 May 1869, Mrs Enoui
164 Daybook, 14 June 1861, Mrs John Cook; 31 July 1865, Fitzmaurice; 19 June 1880, Mrs Wm Gohn; 30 July 1881, Henry Langstaff
165 Daybook, 11 May 1875, Mrs John Loyd [sic]
166 Daybook, 18 Feb., 18, 23 March 1878, William Spofford
167 Daybook, 17 Nov. 1876, Mrs Morrison
168 Daybook, 22 Sept. 1873, John Barker
169 Daybook, 25 July 1884, John Hislop
170 Daybook, 25 Oct. 1850, Thomas Shaw little girl
171 Daybook, 21 Feb. 1859 to 28 July 1883, Nick Lynot(t)
172 Daybook, 9 May 1862, Miss Duntan; 3 June 1880, Mrs James Watson; 21 June 1882 to 14 Feb. 1884, Mrs Isaac Snider
173 Daybook, 14 Sept. 1886, Richard Jordan. See also Daybook, 17 Dec. 1861, Martin Hoover, Sr.
174 Daybook, 15 June 1862, Mrs Pollack, Sr; 28 Aug. 1876, Ben Davison
175 Daybook, 8 Nov. 1881, Henry Hopper
176 Daybook, 15 Sept. 1883, Blakely

CHAPTER 8 **Birthing and Its Problems in Langstaff's Practice of Obstetrics**

1 William Ray Arney, *Power and the Profession of Obstetrics* (Chicago and London: University of Chicago Press 1982), 1–17; Margaret DeLacy, 'Puerperal Fever in Eighteenth-Century Britain,' *Bulletin of the History of Medicine* 63 (1989): 521–56; Judith Walzer Leavitt, *Brought to Bed: Childbearing in America, 1750–1950* (New York, Oxford: Oxford University Press 1986), 6–7, 36–63; Wendy Mitchinson, *The Nature of Their Bodies: Women and Their Doctors in Victorian Canada* (Toronto: University of Toronto Press 1991), 3–14; Edward Shorter, 'Review of Mitchinson, *Nature of Their Bodies,*' *Bulletin of the History of Medicine* 66 (1992): 158–9;

Steven M. Stowe, 'Obstetrics and the Work of Doctoring in the Mid-Nineteenth-Century American South,' *Bulletin of the History of Medicine* 64 (1990): 540–66, especially 564–6

2 See, for example, Edward Shorter, *A History of Women's Bodies* (New York: Basic Books 1982); Harold Speert, *Obstetrics and Gynecology in America: A History* (Chicago: American College of Obstetricians and Gynecologists 1980), 131–5.

3 See, for example, Mary Daly, *Gyn/Ecology: The Metaethics of Radical Feminism* (Boston: Beacon 1978); Ann Oakley, *The Captured Womb: A History of the Medical Care of Pregnant Women* (Oxford: Basil Blackwell 1986).

4 Leavitt, *Brought to Bed*, 155–6; Mitchinson, *Nature of Their Bodies*, 175–80; Martin Pernick, *A Calculus of Suffering: Pain, Professionalism, and Anesthesia in Nineteenth-Century America* (New York: Columbia University Press 1985), 50–6, 185–7; Mary Poovey, '"Scenes of an Indelicate Character": The Medical "Treatment" of Victorian Women,' in Catherine Gallagher and Thomas Laqueur, eds., *The Making of the Modern Body* (Berkeley, Los Angeles, London: University of California Press 1987), 137–68

5 Twins are born once in every 90 births; triplets once in every 8,100.

6 The 'immediate area' was confined to the census districts of Markham and Vaughan containing the town of Richmond Hill, that is, Vaughan District II in all four decades, Markham District I in 1851 and 1881, Markham District III in 1861, Markham District II in 1871, and the town of Richmond Hill in 1881. These figures have not been corrected for changing borders and population of census district, which were relatively stable except for Markham's smaller District III in 1861. This one discrepancy in district size might tend to make the figure for 1861 slightly high. Nevertheless, these percentages are not estimates, but are based on the absolute numbers of Langstaff's known attendance at births listed in the census.

7 Leavitt, *Brought to Bed*, 12

8 The census may not be entirely accurate on the subject of births. Searching for all Langstaff's births among those listed in all the census districts, not simply the closest districts, for each of the four townships near Richmond Hill (King, Whitchurch, Vaughan, and Markham) might result in a potentially useful 'correction factor' for demographic studies.

9 James Miles Langstaff, Langstaff daybook (Daybook), 10–11 Sept. 1879, Mrs Gilbert Mathieson

10 Audrey Saunders Miller, ed., *The Journals of Mary O'Brien, 1828–1838*

(Toronto: Macmillan 1968), 157, 197, 232, 253–4, 279. Mary O'Brien may not be representative of other colonial women, since both her brother and her brother-in-law were physicians. Contrast the use two different historians have made of her writings: the former claims they show how women desired a doctor's assistance; citing different passages, the latter claims they illustrate how women did not need or want medical help. James T.H. Connor, 'Minority Medicine in Ontario: A Study of Medical Pluralism and Its Decline' (Ph.D. thesis, University of Waterloo, 1989), 138; Mitchinson, *Nature of Their Bodies*, 152, 170

11 Archives of Ontario (AO), MU 2113, Journal of Matthew Teefy, 1, dates of birth of Teefy children: 2 March 1847, 21 Aug. 1848, 2 Jan. 1850, 22 Aug. 1851, 7 Feb. 1853, 29 Dec. 1853, 25 Jan. 1859, 11 June 1860, 14 May 1862; Daybooks, 25 Jan. 1859, 11 June 1860, 14 May 1862, Mrs Teefy

12 The obstetrical notes of Hugh MacKay of Woodstock and Toronto's Burnside Lying-In Hospital are analysed in Connor, 'Minority Medicine,' 153–7. See also Mitchinson, *Nature of Their Bodies*, especially 206–22; Stowe, 'Obstetrics and the Work of Doctoring'; Melville C. Watson, 'An Account of an Obstetrical Practice in Upper Canada,' *Canadian Medical Association Journal* 40 (1939): 181–8. A comparative study of three early nineteenth-century New England practitioners has been made by Dr Paul Berman, 'The Practice of Obstetrics in Rural New England, 1800–1860,' unpublished paper read at the Annual Meeting of the American Association for the History of Medicine, Louisville, KY, May 1993.

13 Daybook, 26 Oct. 1867, Mrs widow Pollock; 22 Nov. 1861, Mrs Jo Williams. See also 24 July 1869, Mrs Thomas Russell; 26 Aug. 1881, Mrs Ben Case

14 Daybook, 24 July 1867, Mrs Thomas Kelly; 25 July 1867, Mrs Frank Cook

15 Daybook, 1 April 1861, Mrs Wm Boynton; 2 April 1861, Mrs Dolmage; 5 April 1861, Miss Steinhof

16 Daybook, 18 Aug. 1861, Mrs Phillips; 21 March 1862, Mrs Bond

17 Daybook, 2 Aug. 1876, Mrs John Young; 12 April 1889, Mrs John Nigh; 31 Dec. 1879, Mrs Stong

18 Daybook, 17 March 1888, Mrs Wilkinson

19 Daybook, 25 Feb. 1850, Mrs Peter Rupert

20 Daybook, 9–16 Nov. 1864, Mrs Jeremiah Nelson

21 Daybook, 21 Dec. 1864, Mrs John Brillinger

22 Daybook, 24 Jan. 1889, Mrs Wm Cosgrove; 6 Feb. 1889, Mrs Lance Nicholls

23 Daybook, 21 Oct. 1873, Mrs Hess. The summons to a birth has been

cited as a significant aspect of physician's stories about obstetrical work. Stowe, 'Obstetrics and the Work of Doctoring'

24 Leavitt, *Brought to Bed*, 101
25 Daybook, 9 Aug. 1873, Mrs Pingle
26 Daybook, 10 Feb. 1868, 1 Dec. 1870, Mrs Francis Button, Jr
27 Daybook, 23, 25 April 1879, Mrs Rob Lymburner
28 Connor, 'Minority Medicine,' 128–87; C. Lesley Biggs, 'The Case of the Missing Midwives: A History of Midwifery in Ontario, from 1795–1900,' *Ontario History* 75 (1983): 21–35; Hélène Laforce, *Histoire de la sage-femme dans la région de Québec* (Quebec: Institut québécois de recherche sur la culture 1985); Jacques Bernier, *La médecine au Québec: Naissance et évolution d'une profession* (Quebec: Presses de l'Université Laval 1989), 99–100; Mitchinson, *Nature of Their Bodies*, 162–9
29 Daybook, 18 May 1867, Mrs Rob Law
30 Daybook, 16 Sept. 1858, Mrs Arch Campbell
31 Leavitt, *Brought to Bed*, 87. See also Laurel Thatcher Ulrich, *A Midwife's Tale: The Life of Martha Ballard Based on Her Diary, 1785–1812* (New York: Knopf 1990), 257–61.
32 Daybook, 10–11 Sept. 1879, Mrs Gilbert Mathieson
33 Daybook, 25 Aug. 1873, Mrs Cross; 31 May 1879, Mrs Jacob Graham
34 Daybook, 16 May 1858, Mrs J. Storm; 14 Sept. 1859, Mrs Gardner
35 Daybook, 22 Dec. 1858, Mrs Gorman
36 Daybook, 30 Nov. 1861, Mrs Bone
37 Daybook, 4 March 1870, Mrs Cook
38 Daybook, 1 Oct. 1879, Mrs Tindall
39 Daybook, 2 Sept. 1884, Mrs Sam Mager
40 Daybook, 19 April 1879, Mrs Young
41 Daybook, 19 April 1883, Mrs Sam Mager
42 Langstaff administered an unnamed medication, perhaps a sedative, to one of these children. Daybook, 17–20 Oct. 1858, Sweetapple; 31 Oct. to 7 Nov. 1885, Mrs John Thompson
43 Daybook, 15 Feb. 1865, 22 May 1867, Mrs James Shaw
44 Daybook, 13 Feb. 1868, Mrs Henry Wice; 19 Aug. 1868, Mrs George Grant; 12, 27 March 1869, Mrs Clary
45 Daybook, 7 Oct. 1866, Mrs Jo Hall; 24 July 1880, Mrs Ben Lyons
46 Daybook, 25 Oct. 1881, Mrs Johnstone
47 This frequency of anencephaly of 2/1,000 births is well within the wide range of 0.3 to 7/1,000 in the contemporary United States. Medical Task Force on Anencephaly, 'The Infant with Anencephaly,' *New England Journal of Medicine* 322 (1990): 669–74

48 Daybook, 18 Aug. 1861, Mrs Phillips; the first anencephalic infant was born 19 May 1858 to Mrs Rob Marsh.
49 Daybook, 21 Nov. 1865, 27 Jan. 1867, Mrs Dresser
50 Daybook, 11 Dec. 1876, 5 Jan. 1877, Mrs Fred Gaby
51 The biblical reference is 2 Kings 4:34; Henning Poulsen, 'Forward,' in J.D. Herholdt and C.G. Rafn, *An Attempt at an Historical Survey of Life-Saving Measures for Drowning Persons* (reprint of 1796 edition, Copenhagen: Aarhuus Stiftsbogtrykkerie 1960), i–xi
52 Daybook, 21 April 1860, Mrs John Wood
53 Daybook, 27 May 1853, Mrs Young
54 Daybook, 1 May 1864, Mrs Wm Sliney
55 Daybook, 13 April 1869, Mrs Thomas Frizby
56 Daybook, 20 Nov. 1883, Mrs Hart; 3 Feb. 1869, Mrs Wm Boyd; 8 April 1866, Mrs Henry Wice
57 Daybook, 14 Nov. 1864, Mrs John Simms
58 Daybook, 12 May 1876, Mrs John Horner. Another child 'breathed for about an hour' before it died and the liver filled two-thirds of the abdomen. This mother had at least one other miscarriage. Daybook, 7 Aug. 1874 and 19–20 March 1886, Mrs Wm Frizby
59 Daybook, 13 Nov. 1852, Mrs Cook; 20 Jan. 1863, Mrs Kirkland; 31 July 1878, Mrs Tran; 14 Nov. 1881, Mrs Jos Stephenson
60 Daybook, 9 March 1852, Mrs Ellis; 28 Nov. 1864, Mrs Paget; 17 June 1873, Mrs Brown
61 Mitchinson, *Nature of Their Bodies*, 216
62 Jo Oppenheimer, 'Childbirth in Ontario: The Transition from Home to Hospital in the Early Twentieth Century,' *Ontario History* 75 (1983): 36–60
63 Daybook, 18 April 1850, Mrs Jas Stewart
64 Mitchinson, *Nature of Their Bodies*, 210–15
65 Daybook, 20 Oct. 1856, Mrs Frank Cook; 9 March 1859, Mrs Jacob Baker
66 Daybook, 25 Dec. 1859, Mrs Wm Anon. On birthing postures, see Mitchinson, *Nature of Their Bodies*, 198.
67 Daybook, 7 Dec. 1859, Mrs H. Wise
68 Daybook, 27 Dec. 1859, Mrs Jacob Atkinson
69 Daybook, 26 Oct. 1863, forceps bought at I. Bowman's sale; 2 Nov. 1865, Mrs R. Vailes
70 Daybook, 24 July 1868, Mrs Michael Wallace; 11 Oct. 1869, Mrs Dr Rupert; 27 Jan. 1882, Mrs John Saunderson
71 Daybook, 27 April 1866, Mrs Frank Wylie; 25 July 1867, Mrs Frank Cook

72 Watson, 'An Obstetrical Practice'; Connor, 'Minority Medicine,' 157–8; Mitchinson, *Nature of Their Bodies*, 212–14

73 Daybook, 16 Dec. 1867, Mrs Yetman; 31 Jan. 1883, Mrs Milton Fierheller

74 Daybook, 5 Jan. 1867, Mrs Hitchcock; 18 June 1880, Mrs H. Brillinger

75 Daybook, 10 July 1887, Mrs Latimer

76 Daybook, 31 July 1878, Mrs James Tran; 30 Oct. 1879, Mrs Henry Heise

77 Daybook, 2 Feb. 1868, Mrs Heacock, Dr Mahafay; 25 March 1884, Miss John Saunderson, Dr Hammil

78 Daybook, 1 Oct. 1872, Mrs Ford; 8 Aug. 1868, Mrs Friek; 14 Nov. 1881, Mrs Josh Stephenson

79 Daybook, 31 July 1878, Mrs James Tran

80 Daybook, 25 March 1872, Mrs Thomas Hopper

81 Mitchinson asked the provocative question: 'If forceps could cause problems, why did some practitioners persist, as critics claimed they did, in using them to the point of abuse?' *Nature of Their Bodies*, 215. The difficulty in answering this question stems from the slippery definition of the pejorative term 'abuse,' which sometimes seems to be defined simply as frequent use of a procedure with little consideration of intent.

82 Daybook, 20–1 June 1881, Mrs John Denison

83 Daybook, 27 Jan. 1882, Mrs John Saunderson; 29 Nov. 1868, Mrs John Henricks

84 On this aspect of nineteenth-century practice, see especially Richard W. Wertz and Dorothy C. Wertz, *Lying-In: A History of Childbirth in America* (London, New York: Free Press, Collier, Macmillan 1977), 77–108.

85 Daybook, 18 Feb. 1863, Mrs Whealon

86 Watson, 'An Obstetrical Practice,' 185; John Burns, *The Principles of Midwifery*, 7th ed. (London: Longman, Rees, Orme, Brown, and Green 1828), 442–6; Charles D. Meigs, *Woman and Her Diseases and Remedies – A Series of Letters to His Class*, 3rd ed. (Philadelphia: Blanchard and Lea 1854), 340–1; Fleetwood Churchill, *Theory and Practice of Midwifery*, 5th ed. (London: Henry Renshaw; Dublin: Fannin 1866), 418

87 Jacques Bernier, *La médecine au Québec: Naissance et évolution d'une profession* (Quebec: Presses de l'Université Laval 1989), 124, 127n51–2, 139, 143n80

88 Daybook, 14 July 1860, Mrs Ludford; 8 Dec. 1883, Mrs Jo Rumble

89 Daybook, 31 Oct. 1859, 3 March 1865, Mrs Wm Bridg(e)man; 6 July 1869, 13 Jan. 1871, Mrs Theodore Reid; 18 March 1873, Mrs Wm Bell

90 Daybook, 6 Feb. 1861, Mrs Rob Marsh; 23 Feb. 1875, Mrs Milton Fierheller; 30 June 1868, F. Helmky, Sr

91 Daybook, 28 Oct. 1862, Mrs Jacob Rupert; 19 Nov. 1864, Mrs Jonah Leak

92 Daybook, 21 Jan. 1870, Mrs Raeman

93 Daybook, 7 June 1865, Mrs John Drury

94 Daybook, 12 Sept. 1873, Mrs Webster

95 Mitchinson, *Nature of Their Bodies*, 206–7

96 Daybook, 20 June 1881, Mrs John Denison

97 Daybook, 18 Jan. 1852, Mrs Farrah

98 Daybook, 11 June 1879, Mrs George Shell

99 Daybook, 11 Nov. 1871, Mrs Ed Saunderson

100 Daybook, 25 April 1860, Mrs D. Eyer, Jr

101 Daybook, 22 July 1863, Mrs Forge

102 John Stearns, cited in Herbert Thoms, *Classical Contributions to Obstetrics and Gynecology* (Springfield: Charles C. Thomas 1935), 24

103 Bernier, *La médicine au Quebec*, 123

104 Daybook, 21 Dec. 1862, Mrs Jos Prentiss

105 Daybook, 11 April 1863, Mrs John Nigh; 30 Sept. 1863, Mrs Arch Campbell; 9 Jan. 1864, Mrs John Legg; 16 July 1864, Mrs T. Reid; 1 March 1866, Mrs George Shaffer

106 Daybook, 30 Oct. 1864, Mrs John Cook; 13 April 1869, Mrs Ben Bennett; 24 July 1869, Mrs Thomas Russell; 17 Jan. 1870, Mrs Fullarton; 30 Oct. 1879, Mrs Henry Heise

107 Daybook, 17 Feb. 1872, Mrs Wakefield; 19 March 1889, Mrs Spaulding

108 Daybook, 27 March 1872, Mrs D.S. Raeman

109 Daybook, 6 Oct. 1879, Mrs Rob Bowman

110 Daybook, 5 Nov. 1856, Mrs Ed Saunderson; 29 March 1867, Mrs Vantassel; 18 June 1880, Mrs H. Brillinger

111 Daybook, 29 June 1863, Mrs Thomas Martin

112 Daybook, 27 Sept. 1882, Mrs Bolin

113 James R. Langstaff, 'Langstaff scrapbook,' 106. Nevertheless, a transfusion attempt has not yet been found in the daybooks.

114 Daybook, 23 Jan., 1 March 1869, Mrs Wm Teasdale; 5 March 1869, Mrs David Lynott; 14 April 1869, Mrs Chris Heise; 16 March 1869, Mrs Doer; 22 April 1869, Mrs Ben Jenkins; 26 April 1869, Mrs John Snider; 1 July 1869, Mrs John Rumble

115 Daybook, 25 Oct. 1881, Mrs Johnstone

116 Burns, *Principles of Midwifery*, 483; Meigs, *Woman and Her Diseases*, 270–7; T. Gaillard Thomas, *Practical Treatise on the Diseases of Women*

(Philadelphia: Henry C. Lea 1878), 610; 'Acetate of Lead in Uterine Haemorrhage,' *Canada Medical Journal* 2 (1865–6): 336

117 *Canada Medical Journal* 6 (1869–70): 89–90, 295, 406–9; 7 (1870–1): 8–9; 8 (1871–2): 139

118 Daybook, 17 Feb. 1865, Mrs Dr James Langstaff

119 Mitchinson, *Nature of Their Bodies*, 214; Leavitt, *Brought to Bed*, 51–2, 121, 182

120 Akitomo Matsuki and Elemer K. Zsigmond, 'The First Fatal Case of Chloroform Anaesthesia in Canada,' *Canadian Anaesthetists' Society Journal* 20 (1973): 395–7

121 Watson, 'An Obstetrical Practice,' 186

122 Daybook, 17 Aug. 1864, Mrs Ough and Dr Hillary

123 Daybook, 15 March 1885, also 24 July 1874, 4 Oct. 1875, 13 Nov. 1878, Mrs Chas Morrison

124 *Canada Lancet* 7 (1874–5): 220

125 Daybook, 26 Dec. 1879, 3 July 1882, Mrs Sturgeon Stewart; 29 April 1882, Mrs Reverend Pickering; 25 July 1883, 8 Jan. 1885, 8 Aug. 1886, Mrs Dr James Langstaff

126 Leavitt, *Brought to Bed*, 118

127 Daybook, 7 Dec. 1873, Mrs Beynon

128 Daybook, 4 July 1878, Mrs Ashton Pingle

129 Daybook, 15 Feb. 1863, Stephen Burr child

130 Daybook, 4 Sept. 1872, Mrs Sellars

131 Daybook, 6 Nov. 1864 to 17 Dec. 1864, Mrs Wm Stephenson; 1–2 June 1879, Mrs Ben Case

132 Daybook, 1–2 June 1879, 26 Aug. 1881, Mrs Ben Case; 1 March 1874, Mrs Sellars; also 5 May 1868, 24 July 1869, Mrs Thomas Russell; 5 July 1865, use of 'cold' Mrs John Nicholls

133 Daybook, 15 Feb. to 9 May 1872, Miss Susannah Doner

134 Oppenheimer, 'Childbirth in Ontario,' 37

135 Daybook, 1 April 1872, Mrs Sam Horner; 31 Jan. 1884, Mrs McBride

136 Daybook, 13–24 Feb. 1864, Peter Remore, Sr, daughter

137 DeLacy, 'Puerperal Fever'; Mitchinson, *Nature of Their Bodies*, 227–8; Sheila Ryan Johansson, 'Sex and Death in Victorian England,' in Martha Vicinus, ed., *A Widening Sphere: Changing Roles of Victorian Women* (Bloomington and London: Indiana University Press 1977), 163–81, especially 168

138 DeLacy, 'Puerperal Fever'; Irvine Loudan, 'Puerperal Fever, the Streptococcus, and the Sulphonamides, 1911–1945,' *British Medical Journal* 295 (1987): 485–90

139 Daybook, 15 Feb. to 9 March 1872, Miss Susannah Doner; 27 March to 3 April, Mrs Raeman; 24–6 March 1872, Mrs Beynon, and 12 April to 8 May 1872, Mrs Dalton; 3–17 June 1879, Mrs George Shell 'baby has erysipelas'

140 For more on the definition, incidence, and impact of hospital treatment on puerperal fever, see DeLacy, 'Puerperal Fever.'

141 Daybook, 19 June 1856, Mrs Legg, Sr; 2 Feb. 1880, Mrs Mortson; 15 April 1881, Mrs Gaby; 25 Oct. 1881, Mrs Johnstone; 4 Feb. 1888, Mrs Francis

142 Daybook, 27 Oct. to 9 Dec. 1874, Mrs D.S. Raeman

143 Daybook, 13 Aug. to 22 Sept. 1866, Mrs Rob Lymburner

144 Daybook, 29 April 1864, Mrs T. Glass; 4 Aug. 1877, Mrs Wm Burr; 8 Feb. 1880, Mrs Joseph Graham

145 Daybook, 12 April 1859, Mrs Wm Fierheller

146 Daybook, 5 April 1858, Mrs Brown; 8 July 1868, Mrs Thos Boynton

147 Daybook, 2 March 1862, Mrs Jacob Strong

148 Daybook, 19 May 1857, Mrs David Johnston

149 Daybook, 21 Dec. 1864, Mrs John Brillinger

150 Daybook, 24 Feb. 1874, Mrs Dresser; 7 Dec. 1859, Mrs Boynton, Sr

151 Daybook, 1 Nov. 1868, Mrs Bell. See also an example of post-partum 'mental derangement' in Daybook, 18 Dec. 1853, Mrs Morley.

152 Daybook, 1–4 May 1879, Bell boy; 4 April 1882, Mrs J. Crosby

153 Daybook, 28 Jan. to 3 Feb. 1889 Mrs John Lung

154 Daybook, 14 Sept. 1865, 'Martin say Mrs?'; 6 Dec. 1872, 'Lewis Arnold's woman'; 21 April 1872, 17 March 1880, Miss Wice or Mrs Griffin

155 Watson, 'An Obstetrical Practice'

156 Daybook, 26 April 1852, Miss Anon; 8 Nov. 1861, Miss Webster; 12 July 1868, Miss Dufoot; 26 Sept. 1882, Miss Sarah McLean

157 Daybook, 23 Feb. 1874, Miss Porteus

158 See especially *York Herald*, 2 Oct. 1879.

159 Alison Prentice, Paula Bourne, Gail Cuthbert Brandt, Beth Light, Wendy Mitchinson, and Naomi Black, *Canadian Women: A History* (Toronto, Orlando, San Diego, Sydney: Harcourt Brace Jovanovich 1988), 124

160 Daybook, 15 Feb. to 9 March 1872, Susannah Doner

161 Daybook, back entry, 27 Nov. 1872, Wm Devlin

162 Daybook, 25 March 1884, Miss John Saunderson

163 Daybook, 29 Jan. 1889, Miss Frizby

164 Daybook, 29 Dec. 1872, Mrs Nolan; 4 Sept. 1881, Mrs John Kaisley

165 The fertility rate in Canada in 1871 was 189 births in 1,000 population

each year; in 1891, it was 145 in 1,000. Connor, 'Minority Medicine,'
167; Mitchinson, *Nature of Their Bodies*, 127

166 Angus McLaren, *Birth Control in Nineteenth-Century England* (London:
Croom Helm 1978), 67, 125; Angus McLaren and Arlene Tigar
McLaren, *The Bedroom and the State: The Changing Practices and
Politics of Contraception and Abortion in Canada, 1880–1980* (Toronto:
McClelland and Stewart 1986), 18; Mitchinson, *Nature of Their Bodies*,
146

167 Daybook, 3 Feb. 1869, Mrs Wm Boyd

168 Daybook, 18 Oct. 1888, Mrs John Klinck 'has nurse for baby'

169 For a discussion of the prevalence of these problems and the related
legal issues, see Mitchinson, *Nature of Their Bodies*, 134–5; Constance
Backhouse, 'Involuntary Motherhood: Abortion, Birth Control, and the
Law in Nineteenth-Century Canada,' *Windsor Yearbook of Access to
Justice* 3 (1983): 61–130; Constance Backhouse, 'Desperate Women and
Compassionate Courts: Infanticide in Nineteenth-Century Canada,'
University of Toronto Law Journal 34 (1984): 447–78; Constance
Backhouse, *Petticoats and Prejudice: Women and Law in Nineteenth-
Century Ontario* (Toronto: Osgoode Society and Women's Press 1991),
112–66; McLaren, *Birth Control in Nineteenth-Century England*, 123–5;
McLaren and McLaren, *The Bedroom and the State: the Changing Practices
of Contraception and Abortion in Canada, 1880–1980*, 32–51.

170 Daybook, 27 June 1866, Miss Rob Raymond; 30 Aug. 1868, Mrs Henry
Miller, Jr.

171 Clusters of first-trimester abortions appeared in November 1859 and
August 1868. Three stillbirths at the seventh month of gestation
occurred within two days in 1877. Daybook, Nov. 1859, Aug. 1868, 22–3
Dec. 1877

172 Daybook, 1 Feb. 1887, Mrs Payne; 17 June 1888, Mrs Hingston

173 Daybook, 2 March 1860, 16 March 1879, 1 Jan. 1880, Mrs John
McKenzie; 13 June 1869, Mrs Geibner

174 Angus McLaren, 'Birth Control and Abortion in Canada, 1870–1920,'
Canadian Historical Review 59 (1978): 319–40

175 Charles M. Godfrey, *Medicine for Ontario: A History* (Belleville: Mika
1979), 57–9; Backhouse, *Petticoats and Prejudice*, 140–66; Mitchinson,
Nature of Their Bodies, 136–40; Jacalyn Duffin, 'The Death of Sarah
Lovell and the Constrained Feminism of Emily Stowe,' *Canadian
Medical Association Journal* 146 (1992): 881–8

176 M.H. Williams graduated as M.D., Victoria University, 1867, and was
licensed 1 Nov. 1867. Archives College of Physicians and Surgeons of
Ontario, Historical Register

177 Daybook, 29 Jan., 9 March, 22 Aug., 14 Sept. 1866; 9, 31 July, 20 Oct., 13 Nov., 9–16 Dec. 1867; 3, 15 Jan 1868, Sabra Wright. There were three visits in 1865 to 'Miss Wm Wright' for similar problems.

178 Leslie J. Reagan, '"About to Meet Her Maker": Women, Doctors, Dying Declarations, and the State's Investigation of Abortion, Chicago, 1867–1940,' *American Journal of History* 77 (1991): 1240–64

179 Daybook, 12 March 1868, Sabra Wright

180 James Rolph Langstaff family archive, letter from James M. Langstaff to W.T. Aikins, 24 March 1868

181 Daybook, 21 Jan., 20–1 March 1868, 'in Toronto,' John Langstaff and Amos Wright

182 *Globe*, 21, 24, 28, 30 March 1868

183 Daybook, 21, 27–8 March 1868, Sabra Jane Wright

184 Daybook, 20 Nov. to 20 Dec. 1867, Mrs P. Basingtwaite [Besingtwait?]

185 *York Herald*, 3 April 1868

186 Ibid., 1 May

187 *Globe*, 1 Nov. 1883; also *Liberal*, 10 April 1884

188 Peter C. Hoffer and N.E.H. Hull, *Murdering Mothers: Infanticide in England and New England, 1558–1803* (New York and London: New York University Press 1981), 159–160. See also Thomas R. Forbes, 'Coroner's Inquisitions from London Parishes of the Duchy of Lancaster: The Strand, Clapham, Enfield, and Edmonton,' *Journal of the History of Medicine and Allied Sciences* 43 (1988): 191–203.

189 Lionel Rose, *The Massacre of the Innocents: Infanticide in Britain, 1800–1939* (London, Boston and Henley: Routledge and Kegan Paul 1986), 46

190 Prentice et al., *Canadian Women*, 91; Thomas E. Jordan, *Victorian Childhood: Themes and Variations* (Albany, NY: State University of New York Press 1987), 72, 90–2, 268

191 See, for example, *Toronto Leader*, 18 July, 10 Oct. 1874; *York Herald*, 7 July 1877, 21 Feb. 1878; Backhouse, 'Desperate Women'; Mitchinson, *Nature of Their Bodies*, 143.

192 *Globe*, 21 March 1870; see also ibid., 15 April 1858.

193 *Canada Medical and Surgical Journal* 5 (1876–7): 93

194 Daybook, 20 March 1880, Miss Wiles

195 *Globe*, 16, 21 April 1858; Daybook, 18 Nov. 1852, 26 Feb., 14, 20 April 1858. On the Peter Rupert family, see 'Golden Wedding,' *York Herald*, 16 Oct. 1879.

196 Less than a year later Langstaff attended Bredin's 39-year-old wife in her first labour and delivery. Daybook, 8 Oct. 1868, Mrs Reverend Bredin

197 *York Herald*, 1 May 1868
198 Daybook, 25 June, 29 July 1871, Mrs Jacob Williams; *York Herald*, 11 Aug. 1871
199 Daybook, 24 Oct. 1871, 'In Toronto on Mrs Williams case'. The 'no bill' decision was reported without details. *Globe*, 25 Oct. 1871
200 Daybook, 24 Sept. 1857, Lucy Dorithea [*sic*]
201 Daybook, 19 June 1859, Mrs T. Folliott
202 Daybook, 15 Aug. 1863, Mrs Dr James Langstaff
203 Ernest was first mentioned in Daybook, 19 March 1864.
204 On pregnancy and nursing in women's lives, see Leavitt, *Brought to Bed*, 15–20.
205 Thomas, *A Practical Treatise*, 48–9; Mitchinson, *Nature of Their Bodies*, 89–94. See also chapter 5, n108, n130, and chapter 6, n16.
206 Daybook, 2 July 1856, Mrs Isaac Stokes, 'peritonitis ... from exposure to strong wind during menstruation'; 12 April 1875, Mrs Jacob Atkinson; 21, 24 June 1879, Mrs Dr James Langstaff; 25–6 April 1882, Mrs David Benson
207 Daybook, 21, 24 June 1879, Mrs Dr James Langstaff
208 *York Herald*, 26 June 1879
209 Daybook, 21 June 1882

CHAPTER 9 **Therapy through Social Action: Lawyers, Politics, and Public Health**

1 George Rosen, *A History of Public Health* (New York: MD Publications 1958), 294–343; Heather MacDougall, '"Health is Wealth": The Development of Public Health Activity in Toronto' (Ph.D. thesis, University of Toronto, 1982); Heather MacDougall, 'Public Health and the "Sanitary Idea" in Toronto, 1866–1890,' in Wendy Mitchinson and Janice Dickin McGinnis, eds., *Essays in the History of Canadian Medicine* (Toronto: McClelland and Stewart 1988), 62–87; Heather MacDougall, *Activists and Advocates: Toronto's Health Department, 1883–1983* (Toronto: Dundurn Press 1990), 10–15
2 Nancy Tomes, 'The Private Side of Public Health: Sanitary Science, Domestic Hygiene, and the Germ Theory, 1870–1900,' *Bulletin of the History of Medicine* 64 (1990): 509–39, especially 514
3 Jacques Bernier, *La médecine au Québec: Naissance et évolution d'une profession* (Quebec: Presses de l'Université Laval 1989), 134–5
4 The recitation of the 1843 double murder of Thomas Kinnear and his common-law wife, Nancy Montgomery, appears in virtually every

history of the Richmond Hill region, but other murders are not mentioned. Perhaps the demise of a wealthy landowner who was 'living in sin' acquired the powerful status of a 'moral tale,' in contrast to the more forgettable stories of battered wives. For the most recent version, see Robert Stamp, *Early Days in Richmond Hill: A History of the Community to 1930* (Richmond Hill, Ont.: Richmond Hill Public Library Board 1991), 117

5 James Miles Langstaff, Langstaff daybook (Daybook), 23 Jan. 1860, Haton; 16, 21 May 1875, Davy Horner; *York Herald*, 27 Jan. 1860; 28 May 1875

6 Archives of Ontario (AO), MS 120, Teefy scrapbook, items 277, 288. Other women in the region were murdered in a brutal fashion. See 'Old Woman Beaten to Death,' *York Herald*, 10 April 1879.

7 Daybook, 27 Dec. 1855, Mrs Heatherington autopsy for 'Queen The'; 30, 31 Aug. and 1, 3, 12, 30 Sept. 1859, Mrs Moore, autopsy, inquest, Robert Moore; Langstaff's account book 1852, 290; *Globe*, 24 Jan. 1856, 26 Oct. 1859; *York Herald*, 28 Oct., 11 Nov. 1859

8 Editorial, 'Coroners' Inquests and Medical Fees,' *Canada Medical Journal* 5 (1868–9): 567; 'Medical Evidence in Criminal Cases,' *Canada Lancet* 7 (1874): 87–8

9 Daybook, back entry, 24 April 1876, payment for Simms autopsy, done 15 Nov. 1873, and Lawson autopsy, done 11 May 1864

10 Kenneth A. DeVille, *Medical Malpractice in Nineteenth-Century America* (New York and London: New York University Press 1990)

11 James T.H. Connor, 'Minority Medicine in Ontario: A Study of Medical Pluralism and Its Decline' (Ph.D. thesis, University of Waterloo, 1989), 248

12 Jacalyn Duffin, '"In View of the Body of Job Broom:" A Glimpse of the Medical Knowledge and Practice of John Rolph,' *Canadian Bulletin of Medical History / Bulletin canadien d'histoire de la médecine* 7 (1990): 9–30

13 *York Herald*, 23 June 1871. Langstaff had been a witness in Andrew Macbeth's suit against his father's estate just four years before. Daybook, 11–17 April 1867, 20 June 1871, Macbeth

14 'Inquest into the Death of Jno. Bowman,' *York Herald*, 12 June 1879

15 *Economist* (Markham), 15 May 1884. On Armstrong's death, see chapter 2.

16 Daybook, 16, 20 Aug., 4 Sept., 27 Oct. 1856, trips to Toronto 'to get Mrs Burkitt's will recorded'

17 Daybook, 5 March 1867, 'Dr Coburn and Robinson's trial'; 29 Sept. 1884, 'For Dr. Grant against McClure'

18 Daybook, 11, 18 March 1885, six interviews with Aetna Insurance against Mrs McNair; 12 Jan. 1886, Mutual Aid vs Thos Jackson

19 Daybook, back entry, 16 Nov. 1882

20 Daybook, 22 Aug. and 3 Oct. 1883
21 Daybook, 25 Nov. 1856, 'Trial with Smith'
22 Daybook, 27 April 1877
23 *Globe*, 27 April 1877; *York Herald*, 3 May 1877
24 Daybook, 17–18 March, 8 May 1884
25 There were sixty-one votes for Langstaff and fifty-nine for his opponent John Brown. *York Herald*, 8 Jan. 1880
26 The inside cover of the earliest daybook is lined with undated newspaper clippings from the *Toronto Leader* concerning a controversy between Egerton Ryerson and the Reverend J.M. Bruyère. Also Daybook, 8 Feb. 1861, 'Elected [to] grammar school board'; 20–1 March 1873; *York Herald*, 28 March 1873; AO, Teefy scrapbook, item 165. Several earlier comments in the daybooks, including the remarks 'school meeting,' 'with Mr Bleakley,' and 'trustees,' suggest the doctor may also have served on the school board in 1851–3. *Liberal*, 21 Jan. 1886; AO, GS 6412, microfilm, Minutes of the Municipality ot the Township of Vaughan, 18 Jan. 1864 to 10 Dec. 1866; Daybook, 26 Nov. 1851, 31 May, 5 June, 15 Aug. 1853; 14 June 1872, 'with road commissioners'; back entries, 19 Dec. 1872, 22 Dec. 1873, paid as road commissioner.
27 *York Herald*, 3 Oct. 1878; see also ibid., 15 Sept. 1876 and 10 Jan. 1884.
28 Quebec physicians also engaged in politics; see Bernier, *La médecine au Québec*, 54, 57, 133–5.
29 *Globe*, 15 Dec. 1857. This petition appeared on the front page for several issues.
30 Donald Swainson, 'Introduction' and A. Margaret Evans, 'Oliver Mowat: Nineteenth-Century Ontario Liberal,' in Donald Swainson, ed., *Oliver Mowat's Ontario* (Toronto: Macmillan 1972), 1–11 and 34–51 respectively
31 Daybook, 'Tory meeting,' 9 Feb. 1887; *York Herald*, 20 Sept. 1877. Langstaff witnessed the prime minister's visit to a Markham meeting on 27 June 1877. Isabel Champion, ed., *Markham, 1793–1900* (Markham, Ont.: Markham District Historical Society 1989), 196
32 Daybook, 2 June 1866
33 Daybook, 28 Aug. 1858; 3 Jan. 1860; 19 Aug. 1872, vote for McLellan (lost); 15 Dec. 1873, 29 Jan. 1874, vote for Moss (won both times); back entry, 28 Aug. 1880, vote for Ryan (lost). Details concerning the electoral battles can be found in the *Globe*.
34 Daybook, 15 Dec. 1857, nomination for W.P. Howland; 29 Sept. 1860, nomination for Amos Wright with Mrs Wright; 20 Dec. 1867, at Unionville Reform meeting; 14 March 1871, nomination for H.P. Crosby

in East York; 8 Oct. 1878, nomination for Crosby; 2 Dec. 1881, East York nomination; *Globe*, 15–16 Dec. 1857, 2 Dec. 1881

35 Daybook, 15 June 1861, at convention; 26 June, 18 July 1867, at Unionville; at Weston Reform convention for Howland; *Globe*, 17 June 1861, 19 July 1867; *York Herald*, 19 July 1867

36 Daybook, 3 July 1877, Unionville Reform picnic

37 Daybook, 7 Jan. 1873, Toronto Reform banquet. Concerning this 'most brilliant and successful affair' held at Toronto's Music Hall, see *Globe*, 8 Jan. 1873; Daybook, 13 June 1879, at Masonic Hall, Richmond Hill. To celebrate election of three members, 300 persons sat down to 'an excellent spread.' *York Herald*, 19 June 1879

38 Daybook, 2 Feb. 1887, 'with Dr Lynd'

39 Daybook, back entry, 11 Aug. 1869, 25 Sept. 1873, 16 Nov. 1882. Although Drs Rolph, Morrison, and Aikins figure in Durand's memoir, there is no mention of his medical client in Richmond Hill. Charles Durand, *Reminiscences* (Toronto: Hunter, Rose and Company 1897)

40 Daybook, 7 Feb. 1866, 'Toronto to see Blake'; 22 Sept. 1881, at Maple, Blake spoke; 2 Dec. 1881, 'saw Alex McKenzie' at East York nomination. The first visit may actually have been on legal business as Blake did not enter politics until 1867. *York Herald*, 6 Oct. 1881; *Globe*, 2 Dec. 1881

41 Evans, 'Oliver Mowat: Nineteenth-Century Ontario Liberal,' 50

42 Daybook, 9 July 1879, 'Ed Blake spoke for nearly 3 hours'; *Globe*, 10 July 1879

43 Daybook 18 July 1867; *Globe*, 19 July 1867; *York Herald*, 19 July 1867; J.M.S. Careless, *Brown of the Globe*, 2 vols. (Toronto: Macmillan 1959), vol. 1, 246

44 AO, MU 2113, 1858, folder 16, 'The Journal of Matthew Teefy,' 2–3; AO, Teefy papers, MU 2955, folder 'Letters 1857–58,' letter from David Reesor to Matthew Teefy, 16 Jan. 1859. Reesor was the Reeve of Markham township and three years earlier had founded Markham's Reform newspaper, the *Economist*. Champion, *Markham*, 341

45 Daybook, back entry, 22 March 1881; AO, MS 120, Teefy scrapbook, item 109

46 Dennis Guest, *The Emergence of Social Security in Canada* (Vancouver: University of British Columbia Press 1985), 12–14 passim

47 See, for example, letter from 'Scrutator' to *York Herald*, 6 Dec. 1877.

48 *York Herald*, 11, 25 Oct. 1877

49 Daybook, 7 Jan. 1878, 'Law and I put in 24 votes'; *York Herald*, 3, 10 Jan. 1878. Abraham Law had nominated the doctor to council.

50 AO, GS 5956, microfilm, Richmond Hill Minute Book, 21 Jan. 1878 to
    19 Dec. 1878
51 *York Herald*, 8 Aug. 1878
52 Ibid., 21 Feb.
53 Ibid., 1, 8 Nov. 1883; 'A Blaze at the Liberal Office,' *Liberal*, 2 Nov. 1883;
    AO, Richmond Hill Minute Book, 5 Nov. 1883, re *Telegram*, 31 Oct. 1883
54 Daybook, 21 March 1879, 'Ambler's house, Pollack's tavern burned this
    a.m.'; *York Herald*, 27 March 1879
55 *York Herald*, 2 Oct. 1879. The village heard many complaints about
    robberies during that year.
56 Daybook, 24 Oct. 1879; *York Herald*, 23, 30 Oct., 13 Nov. 1879
57 *York Herald*, 26 June 1879. Langstaff may also have been 'Viator,' author
    of a letter on the cost of sprinkling stones. Ibid., 18 Sept.
58 Ibid., 14 March 1878. MacDougall, 'Health is Wealth,' 155–7, 223;
    MacDougall, 'Public Health and the "Sanitary Idea,"' 62–87
59 *York Herald*, 4 Aug. 1887. See ibid., for articles on the following:
    typhoid-like disease of horses, 3 Nov. 1876; a strange disease of cows,
    16 May 1878; typhoid in Newtonbrook, 22 Sept. 1881; prevalence of
    typhoid in Toronto, 29 Sept. 1881; typhoid, 29 Jan. 1885.
60 Tomes, 'Private Side of Public Health'; MacDougall, 'Public Health and
    the "Sanitary Idea"'
61 Daybook, 18 Nov. 1880, to County Council; *Globe*, 19 Nov. 1880. This
    issue had interested the doctor for a long time. Langstaff had clipped
    an unidentified newpaper report dated 15 Feb. 1867 concerning
    institutions for the poor and pasted it to the inside cover of his account
    book, 1862. The association of occupation with age at death was an
    object of interest for the Richmond Hill paper in 1879. Weavers,
    'gentlemen,' and 'paupers' were found to live longest; telegraph
    operators, milliners, and dressmakers, the shortest; while doctors and
    lawyers on average died at the moderate age of fifty-five. 'How We
    Die,' *York Herald*, 3 April 1879. For an exploration of changing attitudes
    concerning the causal relationship of poverty and disease in late
    nineteenth-century Britain, see, John M. Eyler, 'The Sick Poor and the
    State: Arthur Newsholme on Poverty, Disease, and Responsibility,' in
    Charles E. Rosenberg and Janet Golden, eds., *Framing Disease: Studies in
    Cultural History* (New Brunswick, NJ: Rutgers University Press 1992),
    275–96
62 *Economist* (Markham), 12 Feb. 1880
63 Daybook, 14 June 1880, 'addressed assembly of whole'; *Globe*, 17 June
    1880; *York Herald*, 17 June 1880

64 *York Herald*, 30 Aug. 1877. One year after the 'battle' with Langstaff, Jordan was accused of illegally impounding yet another cow. Ibid., 28 July 1881

65 *York Herald*, 24 June, 1, 8 July, 19 Aug., 25 Nov., 2 Dec. 1880; AO, Richmond Hill Minute Book, 22 Nov. 1880

66 Daybook, 18 March, 14 Oct. 1881, 2 Aug., 21 Oct. 1882, 20 Dec. 1883, 21–2 Sept. 1884, 14 Sept. 1886, Richard Jordan family

67 Daybook, 2 Feb. 1880, John Horner

68 MacDougall, 'Health is Wealth,' 230–47, 256; A.A. Riddel, 'Small-pox in Ontario,' *Canadian Journal of Medical Science* 4 (1879): 355–60

69 *Economist* (Markham), 12 Feb. 1880

70 Ibid., 19 Feb., 4, 11, 18 March 1880

71 Daybook, 15 March 1880, Jo Powell

72 Daybook, 15 Feb. 1880, Elliott Langstaff

73 *York Herald*, 19 Feb. 1880. The two diseases were often confused by Ontario doctors. MacDougall, *Activists and Advocates*, 117

74 Daybook, 18 March 1880; *York Herald*, 26 Feb. 1880

75 *Economist* (Markham), 29 Oct. 1885. On the 1885 epidemic in Montreal, see Michael Bliss, *Plague: A Story of Smallpox in Montreal* (Toronto: Harper Collins 1991); Michael Farley, Peter Keating, and Othmar Keel, 'La vaccination à Montréal dans la seconde moitié du 19e siècle: Pratiques, obstacles et résistances,' in Marcel Fournier, Yves Gingras, and Othmar Keel, eds., *Sciences et médecine au Québec: Perspectives sociohistoriques* (Quebec: Institut québécois de recherche sur la culture 1987), 87–128. On reactions in Ontario, see Barbara Craig, 'Smallpox in Ontario: Public and Professional Perceptions of Disease, 1884–1885,' in Charles G. Roland, ed., *Health, Disease, and Medicine: Essays in Canadian History* (Toronto: Hannah Institute for the History of Medicine 1984), 215–49.

76 *York Herald*, 12 Feb. 1880; MacDougall, *Activists and Advocates*, 117

77 *Economist* (Markham), 19 Feb. 1880

78 MacDougall, *Activists and Advocates*, 122–3; Bliss, *Plague*, 157–8, 163–5, 169–70, 207–15, 263–4; William B. Spaulding, 'The Ontario Vaccine Farm, 1885–1916,' *Canadian Bulletin of Medical History* / *Bulletin canadien d'histoire de la médicine* 6 (1989): 45–56; Charles M. Godfrey, *Medicine for Ontario: A History* (Belleville: Mika 1979), 159

79 The Public Health Act of 1884 and a four-page pamphlet summarizing the recommendations, of which compulsory vaccination was item 8, was read by Matthew Teefy at the village council meeting on 7 Nov. 1885 and filed with his papers. AO, Teefy papers, MU 2955, folder 'Board of Health, Circulars, 1883-93'

80 Dr James Edmunds of London, interview for *Globe*, cited in *Economist* (Markham), 22 Oct. 1885. On the dependence of public health on political circumstances and the detrimental effects of an epidemic on the public health movement, see Judith Walzer Leavitt, 'Politics and Public Health: Smallpox in Milwaukee, 1894–1895,' in Susan Reverby and David Rosner, eds., *Health Care in America: Essays in Social History* (Philadelphia: Temple University Press 1979), 84–101.

81 *York Herald*, 22 Dec. 1881

82 MacDougall, *Activists and Advocates*, 18, 23

83 Edward Playter, 'On Relations of the Medical Profession to Public Health,' speech to York Medical Association, 12 Oct. 1875, *York Herald*, 5 and 12 Nov. 1875; MacDougall, *Activists and Advocates*, 18. See also Charles G. Roland and Paul Potter, *An Annotated Bibliography of Canadian Medical Periodicals, 1826–1975* (Toronto: Hannah Institute for the History of Medicine 1979), 32, 56.

84 Simon Szreter, 'The Impact of Social Intervention in the Decline of Mortality,' *Social History of Medicine* 1 (1988): 1–38

85 Daybook, 19 Feb. 1870, Tullah; 22 Jan., 2, 8, 14 Feb. 1886, John Cook family – four were sick and 'Dr Forrest concluded poison came from privy and perhaps waste pipe of sink'; 9 Oct. 1888, Kerlake boy

86 Daybook, Vaughan Council meeting, 20 Sept. 1882; *York Herald*, 28 Sept. 1882

87 AO, Teefy papers, MU 2955, 'Board of Health, Circulars,' questionnaire and responses, 30 May 1883; unanswered questionnaire, 21 Oct. 1884

88 Stamp, *Early Days in Richmond Hill*, 211

89 AO, Richmond Hill Minute Book, 3 Sept. 1883

90 Ibid., 10 Oct.

91 *Liberal*, 11 Sept. 1884

92 Ibid., 4, 11 Aug. 1887. This problem was not unique. In April 1887, only five of the twenty-five slaughterhouses in Toronto met the standards of cleanliness of the health department MacDougall, 'Public Health and the "Sanitary Idea,"' 84

93 *York Herald*, 3 April 1879

94 *Liberal*, 10, 24 Dec. 1885, 7, 21 Jan. 1886

95 Ibid., 21 Jan. 1886

96 Ibid., 7 Jan. The superintendent's letter had appeared in the 31 Dec. 1885 issue, which is now missing from the series microfilmed by the Archives of Ontario. Langstaff's draft reply is in the back of his account book, 1879, together with a manuscript document testifying to the success of a road experiment (probably from 1880).

97 *Liberal*, 28 Jan. 1886
98 *York Herald*, 8 June 1882
99 William Buckingham and George W. Ross, *The Honourable Alexander Mackenzie: His Life and Times* (reprint of 1892 edition, New York: Greenwood 1969), 588–9, 602–3; Dale C. Thomson, *Alexander Mackenzie, Clear Grit* (Toronto: Macmillan 1960), 373–4
100 *Liberal*, 15 Aug. 1889. The prominent doctor may have been Langstaff's old friend H.H. Wright, who is mentioned several times in the Mackenzie biography. Thomson, *Alexander Mackenzie*, 365
101 *Globe*, 10 June 1882
102 Ibid., 12 June
103 Ibid., 7, 9, 10, 12, 14, 16, 17, 19, 20, 21 June 1882
104 Daybook, 6–26 June 1882, Hon A. Mackenzie
105 Thomson, *Alexander Mackenzie*, 374
106 Queen's University Archives, Alexander Mackenzie papers, coll. 2112, box 4, file 2408–44, letter to 'Mary,' 29 Aug. 1882
107 *Economist* (Markham), 12 Oct. 1882
108 *York Herald*, 26 July 1888. See also *Liberal*, 14 July 1887.
109 Buckingham and Ross, *The Honourable Alexander Mackenzie*, 628
110 *York Herald*, 8 June 1882. On the origins of voting rights for Canadian women, see Catherine Cleverdon, *The Woman Suffrage Movement in Canada* (Toronto: University of Toronto Press 1974), 19–24.
111 In 1871 J.W. Palmer was forty-four years old, his spouse, Mary Ann was thirty-nine, and the children were Louisa, age nineteen, Antoinette, eighteen, Amy, thirteen, Adda, eleven, Franklin, ten, Milton eight, and Jeremiah, six. In 1881 another son, Murray, was seven years old. Canada Census 1861, c1058, Whitby, Division IV; Census 1871, c9974, Whitby, District 48, Division I, 32; Census 1881, c13244, District 132, Whitby Town Division II, 59
112 Mount Allison University was the first to grant higher degrees to Canadian women: a B.Sc. to Grace Annie Lockhart in 1875; a B.A. to Harriet Starr Stewart in 1882. Stewart's achievement was the subject of an article in the Richmond Hill papers, just a few weeks before Louisa was hired. *Liberal*, 11 Aug. 1882; see also Alison Prentice, Paula Bourne, Gail Cuthbert Brandt, Beth Light, Wendy Mitchinson, and Naomi Black, *Canadian Women: A History* (Toronto, Orlando, San Diego, Sydney: Harcourt Brace Jovanovitch 1988), 157–62.
113 *York Herald*, 10 Oct. 1878. Unfortunately, the Ontario Ladies' College of Whitby has no record of Louisa's sojourn in its records.
114 *Liberal*, 7 Nov. 1878

115 *York Herald*, 25 Sept. 1879, 29 July 1880
116 Ibid., 10 Aug. 1882
117 Unknown to the Richmond Hill Langstaffs until the spring of 1991, this story was family tradition among the descendants of the Palmer brothers. Mrs Evelyn Bentley, granddaughter of Louisa's brother Milton Palmer, personal communication
118 *York Herald*, 28 Sept., 5 Oct. 1882; *Globe*, 30 Sept. 1882. How Langstaff came to know Rogers is not clear. In 1861 he had lent money to Rogers; when it was returned the doctor used some of it to buy a subscription to the Montreal *Witness* from the clergyman. On two other occasions Langstaff had travelled to Collingwood to tend Rogers in sickness. Daybook, 24–7 April 1867, 30 Sept. to 1 Oct. 1874
119 *Liberal*, 6 Oct. 1882
120 *York Herald*, 5 Oct. 1882. The darker skies of nineteenth-century Ontario made star-gazing accessible to all: Langstaff recorded seeing another large comet in the sky north-by-northeast while out on his rounds one summer night. Daybook, 1 July 1861. The 1882 comet was a large 'sun-grazing' comet of long periodicity, variously called the Great September Comet, Crul's Comet, and 1882 II. It occasioned a scientifico-religious tract published by an anonymous Quebec author who determined that the comet was 'gentille' because it served as a reminder to marvel at how God governs his Creation with *'number, weight, and measure!'* [my translation]. See A.M. *La Grande Comète de 1882* (Quebec: J.N. Duquet 1882). David A. Seargent, *Comets: Vagabonds of Space* (Garden City, NY: Doubleday 1982), 118–19, 127–8
121 Teachers tended to move between families, but according to the 1881 Census, Louisa and another young woman were residents at the home of James M. Davis. Langstaff was summoned to the Davis home at least five times during 1881, but never for a boarder. Census 1881, C-13248, Richmond Hill, District 136a, 6, family 25; Daybook, 28 March to 25 Nov. 1881, J.M. Davis
122 Daybook, 2 Oct. 1875, 'to Brooklyn'; *York Herald*, 30 Aug. 1877
123 Daybook, 24 Aug. 1877, Mrs Eakins at Whitby 'staid [*sic*] at Dr Gunn's and Mrs L at Mrs Chambers where Mrs Eakins was sick.' Mrs Eakins was the daughter of Richmond Hill's Reverend James Dick.
124 *York Herald*, 15 July 1880, 27 Jan., 3 Feb. 1881
125 Cleverdon, *Woman Suffrage Movement in Canada*, 5; Mary Beacock Fryer, *Emily Stowe: Doctor and Suffragist* (Toronto and Oxford: Hannah Institute and Dundurn Press 1990), 104; Wendy Mitchinson, *The Nature of Their Bodies: Women and Their Doctors in Victorian Canada* (Toronto:

University of Toronto Press 1991), 82–7; Beth Light and Joy Parr, eds., *Canadian Women on the Move, 1867–1920* (Toronto: New Hogtown Press and Ontario Institute for Studies in Education 1983), 51, 197–203; Prentice et al., *Canadian Women*, 174–9

126 *York Herald*, 17 July, 25 Dec. 1879
127 Ibid., 3 Feb. 1881
128 The local inspector, Fotheringham, railed against the school board for its negative attitude towards education and for spending too much time on the high school at the expense of the public school. Ibid., 8 June, 17 Aug., 30 Nov. 1882, 11 Jan. 1883
129 On Rolph's first high school entrance exam, in 1882, the newpaper indicated that a passing mark was 280, but he had obtained only 166; his chronically low standings had already appeared repeatedly. The paper printed the erroneous anwers given by the students in the examination as comic material. Ibid., 1 April 1880, 2 June, 14 July, 20 Oct. 1881, 13 July 1882
130 Mrs Carroll Davis, Langstaff's granddaughter, personal communication
131 *York Herald*, 26 July 1883, 16 Aug. 1883
132 Private schools were still quite common for higher education. A.M. Lafferty, the director of Ernest's academy at Guelph, gave up teaching for law and moved to Chatham. His mother-in-law, Mrs Isabella Campbell, had directed a private girls school in Richmond Hill since she was widowed in 1848. Both Langstaff's daughters, Lily and Nelly, and possibly also his niece, Susannah, had taken music and other lessons from Mrs Campbell; she had been a tenant of the doctor. *Liberal*, 19 Nov. 1885, 15 Dec. 1887
133 Ernest was in Guelph from the age of eleven to thirteen. He may have attended the Richmond Hill high school from 1873 to 1875, but he was taken to Upper Canada College in March 1875. He boarded with his widowed aunt, Mrs Lewis Langstaff, while he was at University College. Daybook, front and back entries, especially 15 June 1871, 19 Aug. 1873, 8 March 1875, 14 Nov. 1877, 23 Feb. 1885
134 *York Herald*, 23 May 1882 to 20 Dec. 1883; Census 1881, C-13248, Richmond Hill, 18; Account book, 1879, 598
135 Daybook, back entry, 6 March and 27 June 1883
136 Daybook, back entry, 5, 28 Jan. 1884, 'Ernest in Guelph'; *Liberal*, 8 May 1884; *York Herald*, 11 Oct. 1883, 7 Feb., 8 March, and 7 Aug. 1884
137 *York Herald*, 5 Aug. 1880, 28 June 1883, and 12 Jan. 1888; Daybook, Ernest to Chicago, 8 Aug. 1879; *Liberal*, 1 Oct. 1885
138 *Liberal*, 20 Jan. to Sept. 15 1887, especially 30 June

139 Ibid., 18 Feb. 1886

140 *York Herald*, 20 Dec. 1877

141 Ibid., 22 March 1883

142 This debate had to be postponed; the press took the opportunity to tease an 'esteemed citizen' about how he woke in the night shouting: 'Mr Chairman I have the floor.' The maligned individual claimed this was base slander, 'since he was up all night studying.' Ibid., 29 Nov., 6 Dec. 1877

143 *Economist* (Markham), 4 March 1880

144 *York Herald*, 7 March 1878. The same topic had been debated in Markham eleven years before. *Economist* (Markham), 28 Feb. 1867

145 *York Herald*, 14 March 1878

146 Ibid., 29 March 1883. Earlier the same paper had reported on Henry Ward Beecher's statement on the supremacy of women, at least in biblical times. Ibid., 13 March 1879

147 Daybook, back entry, 20 Nov. 1882, '$128, balance of Mrs L's salary from when she was Miss Palmer'

148 *York Herald*, 24 Aug. 1882 to 5 July 1883, especially 21 Dec. 1882; 27 Oct., 10 Nov. 1887. For an analysis of gender and wages in the two Ontario industrial towns of Paris and Hanover, see Joy Parr, *The Gender of Breadwinners: Women, Men, and Change in Two Industrial Towns, 1880–1950* (Toronto: University of Toronto Press 1990).

149 *York Herald*, 1 Nov. 1883

150 Daybook, scribbling, 22 April 1885, 4–8 Nov. 1888; back entry, undated c. 22 Oct. 1888

151 James Rolph Langstaff, stories told by his father Rolph Langstaff, personal communication

152 Daybook, back entry, 5 Nov. 1879, 'girls clothing in Toronto $21.50'

153 The Board of Health meeting read a letter from Mrs Louisa Langstaff, regarding a 'dangerous nuisance,' following which McNair's tenant, Whitlock, was given a warning. *Liberal*, 18 June 1885

154 *York Herald*, 6 Aug. 1885. While still a widower Langstaff hosted a 'social' that collected $70; perhaps he had invested less in decorations than had the ladies. When the Church of England held a party at his residence, $36 was gathered for a new organ. Ibid., 27 Jan., 7 July 1881

155 Ibid., 27 May 1886

156 *Liberal*, 15 May 1884

157 Barabara Leslie Epstein, *The Politics of Domesticity: Women, Evangelism and Temperance in Nineteenth-Century America* (Middletown, Conn.:

Wesleyan University Press 1981), 115, 121; Light and Parr, *Canadian Women on the Move*, 219–21

158 Wendy Mitchinson, 'The WCTU: "For God, Home, and Native Land": A Study in Nineteenth-Century Feminism,' in Linda Kealy, ed., *A Not Unreasonable Claim: Women and Reform in Canada, 1880s–1920s* (Toronto: Women's Press 1972), 151–67. On Canadian women and missionary societies, see Wendy Mitchinson, 'Canadian Women and Church Missionary Societies in the Nineteenth Century: A Step Towards Independence,' *Atlantis* 2 (1977): 57–77

159 *York Herald*, 15 Oct. 1885

160 Ibid., 1 Nov. 1883

161 Ibid., 20 Oct. 1887

162 Ibid., 8 Jan. 1885

163 *Liberal*, 21 July 1887 [my emphasis]

164 Daybook, 12 June 1888, court day 'Judgement against Alva, $30'

165 Edwin was released on bail to await trial, but no further mention of this case has been found. *Liberal*, 28 July 1887

166 According to the daybook the trial took place 23 Sept. 1885, but the troubles dated back to February 1884 and did not end until late November 1886, after another legal dispute between Burkitt and McLean in March 1886. The newspapers are disappointingly silent on the details of this case.

167 *York Herald*, 19 Feb.; *Liberal*, 18 June, 6 Aug., 10 Sept., 15 Oct. 1885

168 AO, GS1-1015, 478, cabinet 2, Estate File of James Miles Langstaff, no. 7529

169 The presumed date of this marriage is 5 Nov. 1888, but no announcement seems to have been made. Lily's first child was born in November 1890; she was included as a member of the McConaghy family in the 1891 Census.

170 Daybook, 16–17, 23–5 Feb. 1884, Jerry Palmer. On the second trip Langstaff wrote that he reached 'Whitby at 4 a.m. having gone from evening of Sunday about 110 miles.'

171 Presumably they visited Langstaff's sister Mercy and his brother Miles; Mercy returned the visit a few months later. *Liberal*, 21 July, 8 Sept. 1887

172 Daybook, 12, 30, 31 March 1889

173 Daybook, 1 May 1889

174 Daybook, 18–19 June 1889, Mrs David Henry Gillim

175 Daybook, 5 Oct. 1888, 'Judge on poultry'

176 Phyllis Grosskurth, daughter of Milton Langstaff, personal communication

177 *Liberal*, 8, 15 Aug. 1889

178 AO, Estate File of James Langstaff, caveat 28 August 1889. Probate was granted 25 October 1889.

179 Langstaff's account book, 1887 to 1889. Some tracing of debts seems to have been done by the nephew, Dr George Langstaff of Thornhill.

180 *Globe*, 29 April 1890. The mill was sold to William Leslie and John Innes for $1,440 on 4 June 1890.

181 Census 1891, T-6380, Richmond Hill, 27, 29

182 *Globe*, 21 April 1892. The second will is missing, but its text was copied into 'Langstaff-and-Langstaff: Petition,' 26 Feb. 1904, papers of Mrs Eileen Aiken.

183 Ibid., 26 Sept.

184 Daybook, 26 June 1893 (95?), 'Langstaff vs Langstaff'; *Globe*, 1 March 1904, 'Langstaff vs Langstaff'; see also note 182 above.

185 Anon., *Major J.M. Langstaff, Barrister at Law: A Memorial*, published by friends and business associates. Photocopied portions are in James R. Langstaff, 'Langstaff scrapbook,' 139–48.

186 AO, 'Journal of Matthew Teefy,' 1; Miss L. Teefy, 'Historical Notes on Yonge Street,' *Papers and Records of the Ontario Historical Society* 5 (1904): 53–60

187 Anon., *Dr Lillian: A Memoir*, the Langstaff Medical Heritage Committee, 1979

Appendices

1 Kenneth Kiple, 'American Association for the History of Medicine Report of the Committee on Ethical Codes,' *Bulletin of the History of Medicine* 65 (1991): 565–70; Barbara Bates, *Bargaining for Life: A Social History of Tuberculosis* (Philadelphia: University of Pennsylvania Press 1992), 5

2 For an introduction to this field, see Jennifer J. Connor, 'Medical Library History: A Survey of the Literature in Great Britain and North America,' *Libraries and Culture* 24 (1989): 459–74; Phillip J. Weimerskirch, 'Libraries of Physicians: A Review of the Literature,' AB *Bookman's Weekly*, 20 April 1987, 1705–7.

3 E.T. Peer, 'A Nineteenth-Century Physician of Upper Canada and His Library,' *Bulletin of the Cleveland Medical Library* 19 (1972): 78–85; Jennifer J. Connor, 'To Advocate, To Diffuse, and To Elevate: The

Culture and Context, of Medical Publishing in Canada, 1630–1920 (Ph.D. thesis, University of Western Ontario, 1992), 239–57

4 James Langstaff, M.D. 'Complete Consolidation of One Lung,' *Canada Lancet* 12 (1 March 1880): 198 (for more on this article, see chapter 3).

5 Philip Teigen, *Wood's Library of Standard Medical Authors, 1879–1886* (Bethesda: National Library of Medicine 1985)

6 André Beaulieu and Jean Hamelin, *La presse québécoise des origines à nos jours*, 8 vols. (Ste Foy: Presses de l'Université Laval 1973), 1: 147–9, 171–3

List of Manuscript
and Printed Sources

James Miles Langstaff Records and Papers

Most documents are the property of the family of Dr James Rolph Langstaff, Richmond Hill. Some items (indicated **) are held by the Archives of the Royal College of Physicians and Surgeons of Canada. The papers can be divided into daybooks, account books, and miscellaneous documents.

Medical Daybooks of James Miles Langstaff

These volumes contain the daily entries concerning visits to patients. A daily register of financial transactions covering the same period can be found at the back of each volume, usually proceeding from back to front. Citation of financial entries from the daybooks as opposed to the account books is indicated in the reference notes by the term 'Daybook, back entry.' The Langstaff daybooks are bound in the following order:

4 May 1849 to 7 February 1852
7 February 1852 to 3 December 1853 **
5 December 1853 to 6 June 1854
– missing –
1 November 1855 to 29 February 1860 **
1 March 1860 to 24 March 1861 **
25 March 1861 to 31 January 1862 **
1 February 1862 to 30 July 1863 **
August 1863 to 18 May 1866 **
19 May 1866 to 22 September 1869
23 September 1869 to 3 February 1872
4 February 1872 to 28 February 1875 **
1 March 1875 to 21 November 1877

22 November 1877 to 14 October 1880
15 October 1880 to 21 June 1882
21 June 1882 to 10 May 1885
13 May 1885 to 31 October 1887
1 November 1887 to 10 December 1889

Account Books of James Miles Langstaff

These documents contain the information concerning patient debts organized by family in a roughly alphabetical order, the doctor's real estate
transactions, some information on his farming and milling activities, draft
letters, and an eclectic variety of other records. From the considerable
overlap between volumes, it appears that Langstaff used more than one
book at a time. The account books cannot be dated as precisely as the
daybooks, but the pages were usually numbered and the information
contained in each seems to conform to the chronology below. In the
reference notes, the account books are cited by the first year and the page
number wherever possible.

1847–52 (includes accounts of John Reid) **
1852–62
1862–6
1866–71
1867–9
1869–70
1871–4
1875–8
1879–84
1885–9
1887-90

Miscellaneous Documents

James Miles Langstaff, Lecture Notes and Case Records, Guy's Hospital,
    1846–8
Letters and other documents, including correspondence with John Rolph
    and W.T. Aikins

Ledger concerning debts owed to estate of James Miles Langstaff, 1889
James Rolph Langstaff, 'The Langstaffs of Richmond Hill, Thornhill,
   Langstaff, and King,' 1980, genealogical scrapbook

Other Manuscript Sources

Archives of Ontario (AO), Estate Files, MS 583, reel 10, vol. 20, pp. 458–9,
   Cabinet 4, reel 420, George Brown
AO, Estate Files, RG 22, series G2 B10, MS 638, reel 75, Cabinet 7, reel 221,
   Mary Burkitt
AO, Estate Files, GS1-959, Cabinet 2, reel 422, no. 191, John Langstaff, Sr
AO, Estate Files, GS1-985, Cabinet 2, reel 448, no. 3335, Dr Lewis Langstaff
AO, Estate Files, GS1-986, Cabinet 2, reel 449, no. 3344, Dr Lang
AO, Estate Files, GS1-986, Cabinet 2, reel 451, no. 3597, George Soules
AO, Estate Files, GS1-991, Cabinet 2, reel 454, no. 4677, Dr John N. Reid
AO, Estate Files, GS1-1015, Cabinet 2, reel 478, no. 7529, Dr James Langstaff
AO, Estate Files, GS1-1028, Cabinet 2, reel 491, no. 9041, Dr James Ross
AO, Ely Playter Diary
AO and the Greenland-Griffith Archive, Provincial Lunatic Asylum, Toronto,
   General Register and Admission Warrants; Case Histories
AO, GS 5956, Richmond Hill Minute Book
AO, GS 6412, Minutes of the Municipality of the Township of Vaughan
AO, Matthew Teefy papers, MU 2929–55, invoices, daybooks, account books,
   and postal records
AO, Journal of Matthew Teefy, MU 2113
AO, Matthew Teefy scrapbook, reel MS 120
AO, Lauder family papers, letters from Matthew Teefy, MS 567, reel 1
Archives of Trinity College, University of Toronto, Trinity Medical College
   Announcement, 1855–6
Canada Census 1851, Vaughan, Markham, King, Whitchurch
Canada Census 1861, Vaughan, Markham, King, Whitchurch, Whitby
Canada Census 1871, Vaughan, Markham, King, Whitchurch, Whitby
Canada Census 1881, Vaughan, Markham, King, Whitchurch, Whitby,
   Richmond Hill
Canada Census 1891, Vaughan, Markham, King, Whitchurch, Whitby,
   Richmond Hill
College of Physicians and Surgeons of Ontario, Historical Register
Queen's University Archives, Alexander Mackenzie papers

Queen's University Documents Library, David P. Gagan, 'Enumerators'
   instructions for the Census of Canada, 1852 and 1861,' *Histoire sociale /
   Social History* 7 (1974): 355–65
Mrs Eileen Aiken, Prescott, Ontario, passport, papers, and photographs of
   Louisa Palmer Langstaff and her descendants
Metropolitan Toronto Public Library, Baldwin Room, J.H. Richardson,
   'Reminiscences of the medical profession in Toronto, 1829–1905'
National Archives of Canada, John Rolph papers, MG 24 B24, vols. 1, 2, and 3
Toronto Academy of Medicine, W.T. Aikins Papers
Toronto Academy of Medicine, Joseph Bascom diary

Newspapers

Economist (Markham)
Globe (Toronto)
Liberal (Richmond Hill)
Le semeur canadien
Mackenzie's Weekly Messenger
Toronto Leader
Toronto Telegram
Upper Canada Gazette
Whitby Chronicle
York Herald (Richmond Hill)

Medical Journals

Boston Medical and Surgical Journal
British American Journal
Canada Lancet
Canada Medical and Surgical Journal
Canada Medical Journal
Canada Medical Record
Canadian Journal of Medical Science
Canadian Medical Association Journal
Lancet
Medical Chronicle
New England Journal of Medicine
Quarterly Journal of Inebriety
Upper Canada Medical Journal

Select Bibliography

Ackerman, Evelyn Bernette, 'The Activities of a Country Doctor in New
York State: Dr Elias Cornelius of Somers, 1794–1803,' *Historical Reflections
/ Réflexions historiques* 9 (1982): 181–93
Backhouse, Constance, 'Involuntary Motherhood: Abortion, Birth Control,
and the Law in Nineteenth-Century Canada,' *Windsor Yearbook of Access to
Justice* 3 (1983): 61–130
– 'Desperate Women and Compassionate Courts: Infanticide in Nineteenth-
Century Canada,' *University of Toronto Law Journal* 34 (1984): 447–78
– *Petticoats and Prejudice: Women and Law in Nineteenth-Century Ontario*
(Toronto: Osgoode Society and Women's Press 1991)
Barkin, Risa, and Ian Gentles, 'Death in Victorian Toronto, 1850–1899,'
Urban History Review / Revue d'histoire urbaine 19 (1990): 14–29
Bernier, Jacques, *La médecine au Québec: Naissance et évolution d'une profession*
(Quebec: Presses de l'Université Laval 1989)
Bilson, Geoffrey, *A Darkened House: Cholera in Nineteenth-Century Canada*
(Toronto: University of Toronto Press 1980)
Bliss, Michael, *Northern Enterprise: Five Centuries of Canadian Business*
(Toronto: McClelland and Stewart 1987)
– *Plague: A Story of Smallpox in Montreal* (Toronto: Harper Collins 1991)
Brown, Thomas E., '"Living with God's Afflicted": A History of the
Provincial Lunatic Asylum at Toronto, 1830–1911' (Ph.D. thesis, Queen's
University, 1980)
– 'Foucault Plus Twenty: On Writing the History of Canadian Psychiatry in
the 1980s,' *Canadian Bulletin of Medical History / Bulletin canadien de
l'histoire de la médecine* 2 (1985): 23–50
Buckingham, William, and George W. Ross, *The Honourable Alexander
Mackenzie, His Life and Times [1892]* (New York: Greenwood 1969)
Cameron, H.C., *Mr. Guy's. Hospital, 1726–1948* (London: Longman's 1954)
Canniff, William, *The Medical Profession in Upper Canada, 1783–1850* (reprint of
1894 edition, Toronto: Hannah Institute for the History of Medicine 1980)

Carter, Charles Ambrose, and Thomas Melville Bailey, eds., *The Diary of Sophia MacNab* (Hamilton: W.L. Griffin 1968)

Carter, K. Codell, 'On the Decline of Bloodletting in Nineteenth Century Medicine,' *Journal of Psychoanalytic Anthropology* 5 (1982): 219–34

Cassel, Jay, *The Secret Plague: Venereal Disease in Canada 1838–1939* (Toronto, Buffalo, London: University of Toronto Press 1987)

Champion, Isabel, ed., *Markham, 1793–1900* (Markham, Ont.: Markham District Historical Society 1989)

Champion, Mary B., ed., *Markham Remembered* (Markham, Ont.: Markham District Historical Society 1988)

Clemens, James M., 'Taste Not; Touch Not; Handle Not: A Study of the Social Assumptions of the Temperance Literature and Temperance Supporters in Canada West, 1839–1859,' *Ontario History* 64 (1972): 142–60

Cleverdon, Catherine, *The Woman Suffrage Movement in Canada* (Toronto: University of Toronto Press 1974)

Connor, J[ames].T.H., 'Joseph Lister's System of Wound Management and the Canadian Practitioner' (M.A. thesis, University of Western Ontario, 1980)

– '"To Be Rendered Unconscious of Torture": Anaesthesia and Canada,' 1847–1920, (M. Phil. thesis, University of Waterloo, 1983)

– 'Minority Medicine in Ontario: A Study of Medical Pluralism and Its Decline' (Ph.D. thesis, University of Waterloo, 1989)

– '"A Sort of Felo-De-Se": Eclecticism, Related Medical Sects, and Their Decline in Victorian Ontario,' *Bulletin of the History of Medicine* 65 (1991): 503–27

Connor, Jennifer J., 'Medical Library History: A Survey of the Literature in Great Britain and North America,' *Libraries and Culture* 24 (1989): 459–74

– 'To Advocate, To Diffuse, and To Elevate: The Cuture and Context of Medical Publishing in Canada, 1630–1920' (Ph.D. thesis, University of Western Ontario, 1992)

Cook, Ramsay, *The Regenerators: Social Criticism in Late Victorian English Canada* (Toronto, Buffalo, London: University of Toronto Press 1985)

Coombs, Jan, 'Rural Medical Practice in the 1880s: A View from Central Wisconsin,' *Bulletin of the History of Medicine* 64 (1990): 35–62

Cosbie, W.D., *A History of Toronto General Hospital, 1819–1965: A Chronicle* (Toronto: Macmillan 1975)

Craig, Barbara, 'Smallpox in Ontario: Public and Professional Perceptions of Disease, 1884–85,' in Charles G. Roland, ed., *Health, Disease, and Medicine: Essays in Canadian History*, 215–49

Craig, G.M., 'John Rolph,' *Dictionary of Canadian Biography* (Toronto: University of Toronto Press 1976), vol. 9, 683–90

Crummey, J.M., 'The Daybooks of Robert McLellan: A Comparative Study of a Nova Scotia Family Practice during World War I,' *Canadian Medical Association Journal* 120 (1979): 492–7

Davis, Audrey B., 'Life Insurance and the Physical Examination: A Chapter in the Rise of American Medical Technology,' *Bulletin of the History of Medicine* 55 (1981): 392–406

– *Medicine and Its Technology* (Westport, Conn.: Greenwood 1981)

DeLacy, Margaret, 'Puerperal Fever in Eighteenth-Century Britain,' *Bulletin of the History of Medicine* 63 (1989): 521–56

Duffin, Jacalyn, 'The Great Canadian Peritonitis Debate, 1844–47,' *Histoire sociale – Social History* 19 (1986): 407–24

– '"In View of the Body of Job Broom": A Glimpse of the Medical Knowledge and Practice of John Rolph,' *Canadian Bulletin of Medical History / Bulletin canadien d'histoire de la médecine* 7 (1990): 9–30

– 'The Death of Sarah Lovell and the Constrained Feminism of Emily Stowe,' *Canadian Medical Association Journal* 146 (1992): 881–8

Duffy, John, *The Healers: A History of American Medicine* (Urbana, Ill.: University of Illinois Press 1976)

Elliott, Isabelle M., and James Rawlings Elliott, *A Short History of Surgical Dressings* (London: Pharmaceutical Press 1964)

Epstein, Barbara Leslie, *The Politics of Domesticity: Women, Evangelism, and Temperance in Nineteenth-Century America* (Middletown, Conn.: Wesleyan University Press 1981)

Estes, J. Worth, and David M. Goodman, *The Changing Humours of Portsmouth: The Medical Biography of an American Town* (Boston: Francis A. Countaway Library 1986)

Firth, Edith, *The Town of York, 1815–1834: A Further Collection of Documents of Early Toronto* (Toronto: University of Toronto Press and the Champlain Society vol. 8 1966)

Fitzgerald, Doris, *Thornhill, 1973–1863: The History of an Ontario Village* (Thornhill, Ont.: npub 1964)

Foucault, Michel, *The Birth of the Clinic: An Archeology of Medical Perception*, trans. A.M. Sheridan-Smith (London: Tavistock 1973)

Gagan, David, *Hopeful Travellers: Families and Social Change in Mid-Victorian Peel County, Canada West* (Toronto: Government of Ontario and University of Toronto Press 1981)

Geikie, Walter B., 'An Historical Sketch of Canadian Medical Education,' *Canada Lancet* 34 (1901): 225–36; 281–7

Gidney, R.D., and W.P.J. Millar, 'The Origins of Organized Medicine in Ontario, 1850–1869,' in Charles G. Roland, ed., *Health, Disease, and Medicine: Essays in Canadian History*, 65–95

Godfrey, Charles M., *Medicine for Ontario: A History* (Belleville: Mika 1979)

Graham, W.H., *Greenbank: Country Matters in 19th Century Ontario* (Peterborough, Ontario and Lewiston, NY: Broadview Press 1988)

Groves, Abraham, *All in a Day's Work: Leaves from a Doctor's Casebook* (Toronto: Macmillan 1934)

Guest, Dennis, *The Emergence of Social Security in Canada* (Vancouver: University of British Columbia Press 1985)

Haller, John S., *American Medicine in Transition, 1840–1910* (Urbana, Ill., and London: University of Illinois Press 1981)

Hamowy, Ronald, *Canadian Medicine: A Study in Restricted Entry* (Vancouver: Fraser Institute 1984)

Herholdt, J.D., and C.G. Rafn, *An Attempt at an Historical Survey of Life-Saving Measures for Drowning Persons [1796]* (Copenhagen: Aarhuus Stiftsbogtrykkerie 1960)

Hertzler, Arthur, *The Horse and Buggy Doctor* (New York and London: Harper Brothers 1938)

Hoffer, Peter C., and N.E.H. Hull, *Murdering Mothers: Infanticide in England and New England, 1558–1803* (New York and London: New York University Press 1981)

Holifield, E. Brooks, 'The Wealth of Nineteenth-Century American Physicians,' *Bulletin of the History of Medicine* 64 (1990): 79–85

Holling, S.A., John Senior, Betty Clarkson, and Donald A. Smith, *Medicine for Heroes: A Neglected Part of Pioneer Life* (Mississauga, Ont.: Mississauga South Historical Society 1981)

Hudson, Robert P., *Disease and Its Control: The Shaping of Modern Thought* (Westport Conn.: Greenwood 1983)

Hurd, Henry M., ed., *The Institutional History of the Insane in the United States and Canada*, 4 vols. (Baltimore: Johns Hopkins University Press 1917)

Innis, Mary Quayle, ed., *Mrs Simcoe's Diary* (Toronto: Macmillan 1965)

Jack, Donald, *Rogues, Rebels, and Geniuses: The Story of Canadian Medicine* (Garden City, NY: Doubleday 1981)

Jameson, Anna Brownell, *Winter Studies and Summer Rambles in Canada*, ed. Clara Thomas (Toronto: McClelland and Stewart 1965)

Johansson, Sheila Ryan, 'Sex and Death in Victorian England: An Examination of Age- and Sex-Specific Death Rates, 1840–1910,' in Martha Vicinus, ed., *A Widening Sphere: Changing Roles of Victorian Women* (Bloomington and London: Indiana University Press, 1977), 163–81

Johnson, Leo A., *History of the County of Ontario, 1615–1875* (Whitby: Corporation of the County of Ontario 1973)

Johnston, Victor, *Before the Age of Miracles: Memoirs of a Country Doctor*

(Toronto, Montreal, Winnipeg, Vancouver: Fitzhenry and Whiteside 1972)

King, Lester S., *Medical Thinking: An Historical Preface* (Princeton: Princeton University Press 1982)

Krasnick, Cheryl, '"In Charge of the Loons": A Portrait of the London Ontario Asylum for the Insane in the Nineteenth Century,' *Ontario History* 74 (1982): 134–84

– '"Because There Is Pain": Alcoholism, Temperance, and the Victorian Physician,' *Canadian Bulletin of Medical History / Bulletin canadien d'histoire de la médecine* 2 (1985): 1–19

Krasnick Warsh, Cheryl, *Moments of Unreason: The Practice of Canadian Psychiatry and the Homewood Retreat, 1883–1923* (Montreal, Kingston, London, and Buffalo: McGill-Queen's University Press 1989)

Laennec, R.T.H., *Traité de l'auscultation médiate et des maladies des poumons et du coeur*, 2 vols. (Paris: Chaudé 1826)

Laforce, Hélène, *Histoire de la sage-femme dans la région de Québec* (Quebec: Institut québécois de recherche sur la culture 1985)

Leake, Chauncey D., *An Historical Account of Pharmacology to the Twentieth Century* (Springfield, Ill.: Charles C. Thomas 1975)

Leavitt, Judith Walzer, *Brought to Bed: Childbearing in America, 1750-1950* (New York and Oxford: Oxford University Press 1986)

Lemay, Edna Hindie, 'Thomas Hérier, a Country Surgeon outside Angoulême at the End of the xviiith Century: A Contribution to Social History,' *Journal of Social History* 10 (1976–7): 524–37

Léonard, Jacques, *La France médicale: Médecins et malades au xixe siècle* (Paris: Gallimard 1978)

Light, Beth, and Joy Parr, eds., *Canadian Women on the Move, 1867–1920* (Toronto: New Hogtown Press and Ontario Institute for Studies in Education 1983)

Lindsey, Charles, *The Life and Times of William Lyon Mackenzie* (Toronto: P. Randall 1862)

Loudan, Irvine, *Medical Care and the General Practitioner, 1750–1850* (Oxford: Oxford University Press and Clarendon Press 1986)

– 'Puerperal Fever, the Streptococcus, and the Sulphonamides, 1911–1945,' *British Medical Journal* 295 (1987): 485–90

McDonell, Katherine Mandusic, *The Journals of William A. Lindsay: An Ordinary Nineteenth-Century Physician's Surgical Cases* (Indianapolis: Indiana Historical Society 1989)

MacDougall, Heather, '"Health is Wealth": The Development of Public Health Activity in Toronto' (Ph.D. thesis, University of Toronto, 1982)

– 'Public Health and the "Sanitary Idea" in Toronto,' in Wendy Mitchinson

and Janice P. Dickin McGinnis, eds., *Essays in the History of Canadian Medicine*, (Toronto: McClelland and Stewart 1988), 62–87
- *Activists and Advocates: Toronto's Health Department, 1883–1983* (Toronto: Dundurn Press 1990)
McLaren, Angus, *Birth Control in Nineteenth-Century England* (London: Croom Helm 1978)
- 'Birth Control and Abortion in Canada,' *Canadian Historical Review* 59 (1978): 319–40
McLaren, Angus, and Arlene Tigar McLaren, *The Bedroom and the State: The Changing Practices and Politics of Contraception and Abortion in Canada, 1880–1980* (Toronto: McClelland and Stewart 1986)
MacNab, Elizabeth, *A Legal History of the Health Professions in Ontario* (Toronto: Queen's Printer 1970)
Marland, Hilary, *Medicine in Wakefield and Huddersfield, 1780–1870* (Cambridge, New York, New Rochelle, Melbourne, Sydney: Cambridge University Press 1987)
Matsuki, Akitomo, and Elemér K. Zsigmond, 'The First Fatal Case of Chloroform Anaesthesia in Canada,' *Canadian Anaesthetists' Society Journal* 20 (1973): 395–7
- 'Bibliography of the History of Surgical Anaesthesia in Canada,' *Canadian Anaesthetists' Society Journal* 21 (1974): 427–30
Maulitz, Russell C., 'Channel Crossing: The Lure of French Pathology for English Medical Students,' *Bulletin of the History of Medicine* 55 (1981): 475–96
Miller, Audrey Saunders, ed., *The Journals of Mary O'Brien, 1828–1838* (Toronto: Macmillan 1968)
Mitchinson, Wendy, 'The WCTU: "For God, Home, and Native Land": A Study in Nineteenth-Century Feminism,' in Linda Kealy, ed., *A Not Unreasonable Claim: Women and Social Reform in Canada, 1880s – 1920s* (Toronto's Women Press 1972)
- 'Canadian Women and Church Missionary Societies in the Nineteenth Century: A Step Towards Independence,' *Atlantis* 2 (1977): 57–77
- 'The Toronto and Gladesville Asylums: Humane Alternatives for the Insane in Canada and Australia,' *Bulletin of the History of Medicine* 63 (1989): 52–72
- *The Nature of Their Bodies: Women and Their Doctors in Victorian Canada* (Toronto: University of Toronto Press 1991)
Mitchinson, Wendy, and Janice P. Dickin McGinnis, eds., *Essays in the History of Canadian Medicine* (Toronto: McClelland and Stewart 1988)

Norris, John, 'The Country Doctor in British Columbia: 1887–1975,' BC
   Studies 49 (1981): 15–38
O'Gallagher, Marianna, Grosse Ile: Gateway to Canada (Ste Foy, Que: Carraig
   Books 1984)
Oppenheimer, Jo, 'Childbirth in Ontario: The Transition from Home to
   Hospital in the Early Twentieth Century,' Ontario History 75(1983): 36–60
Parr, Joy, ed., Childhood and Family in Canadian History (Toronto: McClelland
   and Stewart 1982)
Peer, E.T., 'A Nineteenth-Century Physician of Upper Canada and His
   Library,' Bulletin of the Cleveland Medical Library 19 (1972): 78–85
Pernick, Martin S., A Calculus of Suffering: Pain, Professionalism, and Anesthe-
   sia in Nineteenth-Century America (New York: Columbia University Press
   1985)
Prentice, Alison, Paula Bourne, Gail Cuthbert Brandt, Beth Light, Wendy
   Mitchinson, and Naomi Black, Canadian Women: A History (Toronto,
   Orlando, San Diego, Sydney: Harcourt Brace Jovanovitch 1988)
Reaman, G. Elmore, A History of Vaughan Township (Toronto: University of
   Toronto Press 1971)
Reiser, Stanley Joel, Medicine and the Reign of Technology (Cambridge and
   New York: Cambridge University Press 1978)
Risse, Guenter B., 'The Renaissance of Bloodletting: A Chapter in Modern
   Therapeutics,' Journal of the History of Medicine and Allied Sciences 34
   (1979): 3–22
– Hospital Life in Enlightenment Scotland: Care and Teaching at the Royal
   Infirmary of Edinburgh (Cambridge: Cambridge University Press 1986)
Roland, Charles G., 'Bibliography of the History of Anaesthesia in Canada:
   Preliminary Checklist,' Canadian Anaesthetists' Society Journal 15 (1968):
   202–14
– 'The Diary of a Canadian Country Physician: Jonathan Woolverton
   (1881–1883),' Medical History 14 (1971): 168–80
– ed., Health, Disease, and Medicine: Essays in Canadian History (Toronto:
   Hannah Institute for the History of Medicine 1984)
Roland, Charles G., and Paul Potter, An Annotated Bibliography of Canadian
   Medical Periodicals (Toronto: Hannah Institute for the History of Medicine
   1979)
Roland, Charles G., and Bohodar Rubashewsky, 'The Economic Status of
   the Practice of Dr Harmaunus Smith in Wentworth County,' Ontario,
   1826–67,' Canadian Bulletin of Medical History / Bulletin canadien d'histoire de
   la médecine 5 (1988): 29–49

Roques, Christian-F., 'Professional and Economic Data on the Activity of a Country Physician from the South of France in 1869,' 32nd International Congress on the History of Medicine, Antwerp, Belgium, *Acta Belgica Historiae Medicinae*, in press

Rose, Lionel, *The Massacre of the Innocents: Infanticide in Britain, 1800–1939* (London, Boston, and Henley: Routledge and Kegan Paul 1986)

Rosen, George, 'Fees and Fee Bills: Some Economic Aspects of Medical Practice in Nineteenth-Century America,' *Bulletin of the History of Medicine* supplement 6 (1946): 1–93

– *A History of Public Health* (New York: MD Publications 1958)

Rosen, George, and Charles E. Rosenberg, *The Structure of American Medical Practice, 1875–1941* (Philadelphia: University of Pennsylvania Press 1983)

Rosenberg, Charles E., *The Cholera Years: The United States in 1832, 1849, and 1866* (Chicago and London: University of Chicago Press 1962)

– 'The Therapeutic Revolution: Medicine, Meaning, and Social Change in Nineteenth-Century America,' in Morris J. Vogel and Charles E. Rosenberg eds., *The Therapeutic Revolution: Essays in the Social History of American Medicine* (Philadelphia: University of Pennsylvania 1979), 3–25

– *The Care of Strangers: The Rise of America's Hospital System* (New York: Basic Books 1987)

Rosenberg, Charles E., and Janet Golden, eds., *Framing Disease: Studies in Cultural History* (New Brunswick, NJ: Rutgers University Press 1992)

Rusted, Nigel, *It's Devil Deep Down There* (St John's, Nfld.: Creative Publishers 1987)

Shorter, Edward, *A History of Women's Bodies* (New York: Basic Books 1982)

– *Bedside Manners: The Troubled History of Doctors and Patients* (Harmondsworth, England: Viking Penguin 1986)

– *From Paralysis to Fatigue: A History of Psychosomatic Illness in the Modern Era* (New York: Free Press; and Toronto: Maxwell Macmillian 1992)

Shortt, S.E.D., '"Before the Age of Miracles": The Rise, Fall, and Rebirth of General Practice in Canada,' in Charles G. Roland ed., *Health, Disease, and Medicine: Essays in Canadian History* (Toronto: Hannah Institute for the History of Medicine 1984) 123–52

– *Victorian Lunacy: Richard M. Bucke and the Practice of Late Nineteenth-Century Psychiatry* (Cambridge, London, New York, New Rochelle, Melbourne, Sydney: Cambridge University Press 1986)

– ed., *Medicine in Canadian Society: Historical Perspectives* (Montreal: McGill-Queen's University Press 1981)

Smith, W.L., *The Pioneers of Old Ontario* (Toronto: George N. Morang 1923)

Somerville, Patricia, and Catherine Macfarlane, eds., *A History of Vaughan Township Churches* (Maple, Ont.: Vaughan Township Historical Society 1984)

Spaulding, William B., 'The Ontario Vaccine Farm, 1885–1916,' *Canadian Bulletin of Medical History / Bulletin canadien d'histoire de la médecine* 6 (1989): 45–56

– 'Abraham Groves (1847–1935): A Pioneer Surgeon, Sufficient unto Himself,' *Canadian Bulletin of Medical History / Bulletin canadien d'histoire de la médecine* 8 (1991): 249–62

Stamp, Robert, *Early Days in Richmond Hill: A History of the Community to 1930* (Richmond Hill, Ont.: Richmond Hill Public Library Board 1991)

Starr, Paul, *The Social Transformation of American Medicine* (New York: Basic Books 1982)

Stowe, Steven M., 'Obstetrics and the Work of Doctoring in the Mid-Nineteeth-Century American South,' *Bulletin of the History of Medicine* 64 (1990): 540–66

Sutherland, Neil, *Children and English-Canadian Society: Framing The Twentieth-Century Consensus* (Toronto and Buffalo: University of Toronto Press 1976)

Swainson, Donald, ed., *Oliver Mowat's Ontario* (Toronto: Macmillan 1972)

Thomas, T. Gaillard, *Practical Treatise on the Diseases of Women* (Philadelphia: Henry C. Lea 1878)

Thomson, Dale C., *Alexander Mackenzie: Clear Grit* (Toronto: Macmillan 1960)

Tomes, Nancy, 'The Private Side of Public Health: Sanitary Science, Domestic Hygiene, and the Germ Theory, 1870–1900, '*Bulletin of the History of Medicine* 64 (1990): 509–39

Vogel, Morris J., and Charles E. Rosenberg, eds., *The Therapeutic Revolution: Essays in the Social History of American Medicine* (Philadelphia: University of Pennsylvania Press 1979)

Warner, John Harley, *The Therapeutic Perspective: Medical Practice, Knowledge, and Identity in America, 1820–1885* (Cambridge, Mass., and London, England: Harvard University Press 1986)

– 'Power, Conflict, and Identity in Mid-Nineteenth-Century American Medicine: Therapeutic Change at the Commerical Hospital in Cincinnati,' *Journal of American History* 73 (1987): 934–56

Watson, Melville C., 'An Account of an Obstetrical Practice in Upper Canada,' *Canadian Medical Association Journal* 40 (1939): 181–8

Wilks, Samuel, and G.T. Bettany, *A Biographical History of Guy's Hospital* (London: Ward, Lock, Bowden 1892)

Illustration Credits

Archives of the Richmond Hill Public Library: Richmond Hill (no. 206);
  road near Richmond Hill (no. 939073); supper at Harry Rumble's barn
  raising (no. 404); men of Richmond Hill with steam-powered farm
  machinery (no. 939128); Matthew Teefy with his three daughters
Dr James Rolph Langstaff: James Miles Langstaff (frontispiece);
  J.M. Langstaff with his first wife; John Langstaff with his family; Yonge
  Street, Richmond Hill
Mrs Eileen Aiken: Langstaff's second wife; announcement of Langstaff's
  death
Medical Art Photography, Queen's University: instruments; Langstaff's
  daybooks and account book
Isabel Champion, ed., *Markham, 1793–1900* (Markham District Historical
  Society 1989) 73: parents of Langstaff's first wife
Miles and Co., *Illustrated Historical Atlas of York County* (Belleville: Mika
  1972): Langstaff's house
J.C. Dent, *The Story of the Upper Canadian Rebellion* (Toronto: C. Blackett
  Robinson 1885): John Rolph
Robert Stamp, *Early Days in Richmond Hill: A History of the Community to
  1930* (Richmond Hill Public Library Board 1991) 166: Matthew Teefy
J.W. Bengough, *A Caricature History of Canadian Politics* (Toronto: Grip
  Printing and Publishing Company 1974) 83: Liberal politicians portrayed
  as doctors
York Herald, 26 February 1885, Archives of Ontario microfilm: announce-
  ment of Langstaff's credit sale

Index